The Design of a Health Maintenance Organization

Allan Easton

The Praeger Special Studies program—
utilizing the most modern and efficient book
production techniques and a selective
worldwide distribution network—makes
available to the academic, government, and
business communities significant, timely
research in U.S. and international economic, social, and political development.

The Design of a Health Maintenance Organization

A Handbook for Practitioners

PRAEGER SPECIAL STUDIES IN U.S. ECONOMIC, SOCIAL, AND POLITICAL ISSUES

Joanna and Harry Streiter

7/13/77

Praeger Publishers   New York   Washington   London

Library of Congress Cataloging in Publication Data

Main entry under title:

The Design of a health maintenance organization.

  (Praeger special studies in U.S. economic, social,
and political issues)
    Bibliography: p.
    1. Health maintenance organizations—United States.
I. Easton, Allan, 1916-   [DNLM: 1. Health main-
tenance organizations—United States.   W275 AA1 D4]
RA413.5.U5D47   1975   362.1'0973   74-17893
ISBN 0-275-05460-8

PRAEGER PUBLISHERS
111 Fourth Avenue, New York, N.Y. 10003, U.S.A.

Published in the United States of America in 1975
by Praeger Publishers, Inc.

Printed in the United States of America

PREFACE

This study is one of a continuing series resulting from MBA research seminars conducted at the School of Business at Hofstra University. Under this program, students work on subdivisions of a group project under the guidance of a faculty adviser who also serves as the editor of the final report. Each student is completely responsible for his part of the research and on completion of his field and library work, each undertakes the writing of a chapter of a final project report.

The work extended over three semesters, beginning in February of 1971 and ending in June of 1972. During the first part of this interval, each participant engaged in his individual investigation and exploration on the topic he had selected for his chapter. The remaining time was devoted to the assessment of the findings and to report writing. These student reports, in edited form, comprise the main body of this volume.

Because this project was undertaken in a business school and not in a school of medicine, hospital or public administration, the orientation and viewpoints of the student were closer to the business rather than the medical side of the problems involved in the design of health care delivery systems. The student researchers preferred to examine various aspects of one special form of health care delivery system. the Health Maintenance Organization (HMO), from their particular viewpoints as specialists in marketing, personnel, finance, public relations, and others. These preferences account for the business flavor of most of the chapters in this volume.

None of the business-trained, student-authors of these chapters have had any professional training in medicine or its allied fields. This obvious lack presented the editor and several of the authors with a delicate judgmental problem. The problem arose when the business and managerial aspects of their specific sub-topics were found to be inextricably intertwined with medical matters beyond their competence. In a few chapters, cross-disciplinary transgressions of this sort proved to be unavoidable if the materials were to be of any real value and were to be related to the real world of health-care delivery systems. In those cases, the authors consulted competent authorities both by personal interview and through extensive library research. Any errors the medically sophisticated reader may find in material dealing with medical technology and practice cannot be charged to the persons or authorities consulted, but are more properly attributed to misinterpretations, mistranslations and misapplications caused by the very meager medical knowledge possessed by the chapter authors and the editor.

In a multi-authored collection such as this, devoted to a single topic, some overlap and repetition is unavoidable. Certain subjects are touched upon by more than one author. Unnecessary redundancies were ruthlessly blue-penciled by the editor, but others were allowed: (1) if they contributed to the integrity and logical organization of the chapter, (2)

v

to save the reader from the annoyance of too-frequent cross-referencing among chapters, or (3) when the common material was given a different slant in relation to the adjacent subject matter.

We wish to express our gratitude to the many persons who generously aided the student researchers in finding data and much new information; who gave their time and energy in counselling and otherwise smoothing the researchers' paths to obtaining widely scattered evidence and statistical information. Much of the success we have enjoyed in illuminating this exceptionally complex topic is due, in large part, to their unstinting cooperation. Specific acknowledgements are contained in each chapter.

Allan Easton, B.S., Ph. D.
Hempstead, New York

TABLE OF CONTENTS

The Design of a Health Maintenance Organization

INTRODUCTION

Allan Easton

Today's American, concerned about the delivery of health care, is faced with a dual problem. While he is aware that high quality medical treatment is at least potentially available, he may not be able to gain access to it or, once having entered the system, he may not be able to afford the costs. Actually, as many writers on the subject have noted, our system of health care delivery is not a coherent system at all. It is really an un-coordinated collection of physicians, medical groups, hospitals and insurers who present the unsophisticated consumer with a bewildering array of alter-native service and payment plans, all of which are designed to help provide or pay for health care.

In recent years, the growing inadequacies of the ongoing system (or nonsystem) have come under increasing fire. Part of the strain which threatens to further disrupt a deteriorating situation has been the result of medical progress in the control of infectious diseases. This success has increased average life expectancy and consequently has changed the character of our national health problem. Congenital handicaps, mental illnesses and diseases of the aged which require prolonged treatment and a broad range of services have become more prominent, while the changes in the system needed to cope with the altered challenges have developed more slowly than needed.

Even the term "health care" is a misnomer because, with few exceptions treatment is geared toward the correction of existing medical or surgical conditions rather than to the maintenance of good health. The medical profession has long recognized that prevention and health education are extremely important for keeping people healthy, but since most financing mechanisms do not allow for these essential functions, they have been largely ignored or underplayed in the system.

As late as the turn on the century, it was still possible for a physician to possess all of the knowledge available for the treatment of most common ailments. Since the first World War, however, the rapid growth of medical knowledge and the development of medical technology have made it impossible for any one person to master all of the skills needed to provide truly comprehensive care. As a result, many physicians have become specialists in a few restricted areas of medical practice. Such specializa-tion has made higher quality care more feasible, but only at the expense of further fragmentation of the delivery system. And the proportionate increase in the number of specialists has been matched by a decline in the proportion of physicians in general practice, a phenomenon which has reduced the access to high quality medical care for many Americans.

New medical knowledge has led to the development of new equipment which is extremely costly. It is not possible for every physician or every hospital to support all of the equipment needed for the treatment of all diseases.

1

With the proliferation of new medical knowledge, new physician specialties, new technique, and new equipment requirements, it is no longer realistic to ask the unsophisticated consumer to determine his own health needs. In the traditional approach to health care, the consumer usually secures the services of a "family doctor," buys some form of health insurance, and hopes that his choices were good ones. In some cases, where the illness may be complicated, the general practitioner refers the patient to a specialist. But as a rule, he sees his physician only if he feels very sick and typically fails to receive the benefits of preventative medicine.

Finding a fully competent physician can be an ordeal. The patient has no way of evaluating the quality of the care he receives; he has no way of knowing if all of the treatments he received were necessary or effective.

Those fortunate enough to find the correct treatment and those with health insurance, may face further hazards. Many health insurance plans exclude certain treatments, they have deductible and co-insurance clauses all of which may leave the hapless patient with large, unexpected, and unplanned-for out-of-pocket costs.

With the passage of time, more and more Americans are beginning to think of adequate health care as a basic right. And this growing consciousness of the great benefits to be obtained from good health care has been picked up by many political leaders. As a result there are several proposals before the congress of the United States for expanding the scope of the health care available to the average citizen.

"It must be our goal," declared President Richard M. Nixon in his health message to Congress in February 1971, "not merely to finance a more expensive medical system, but to organize a more efficient one. ..We should work to maintain health and not merely to restore it."

The President's chosen instrument for achieving this praiseworthy goal is the increasingly discussed Health Maintenance Organization (H.M.O.). Mr. Nixon's H.M.O. development program includes such details as:

1. H.M.O. planning grants and contracts for public and private H.M.O.'s;

2. H.M.O. operating grants, contracts and loans for public and private H.M.O.'s serving medically underserved areas;

3. H.M.O. grants to medical schools;

4. H.M.O. loan guarantees for ambulatory facilities.

One goal of the Nixon administration is to develop 450 H.M.O.'s in the next few years, 100 of which would serve areas critically short of health care facilities. And in later years, the plans call for between one and two thousand H.M.O's with the potential of enrolling 40 million people.

Even if these very ambitious plans do not materialize, the H.M.O. in some form seems to be upon us. This means that many groups will seek to organize such entities, and if past experience is any guide, some will be very successful and some will fail.

Organizing an H.M.O. is in many ways similar to organizing a business firm. It is necessary to develop an organizational structure; to acquire competent leadership; to obtain proper financing; to staff the entity with competent, dedicated people; to obtain customers (subscribers); to deliver the services contracted for at reasonable cost; to constantly renew the organization's vitality; to replace equipment as it becomes worn out and obsolete; to guarantee that the services delivered are of the proper quality, et cetra.

The purpose of this volume is to bring the specialized skills and knowledge possessed by well-trained business students to the solution of the problems likely to be encountered in the establishment of a new organizational entity for delivering high quality health care to a subscriber population. The task has been divided into several sub-specialties, as a quick reading of the table of contents will reveal.

The student-authors traveled widely and interviewed people engaged in the operation of many kinds of health plans. They have drawn on these interviews and upon many of the publications sponsored by on-going plans. However, in essence, the principal model for the H.M.O. described in this volume is the Kaiser-Permanente plan which is flourishing so vigorously in the Western United States. In order to develop a sharper focus, Nassau and Suffolk Counties of Long Island, New York are used by some authors as a prototype of a geographical region suitable for the establishment of one or more H.M.O.'s. The reader should be able to adapt the materials in these chapters to his own locality with little difficulty.

*   *   *   *   *

The first chapter of this volume contains introductory materials intended to place the H.M.O. development in historical perspective. The remaining chapters deal with specific sub-topics in the Design of a Health Maintenance Organization.

In his comprehensive study entitled, "A Survey of Health Care Financing and Delivery Systems," Walter Schweikert reviews the variegated history of systems for health care delivery and financing in the United States: identifies their advantages and limitations; and reviews the newly expanding role of prepaid group practice arrangements in correcting the short-comings of earlier plans.

Richard Suess, in his chapter, "An Organization Plan for the H.M.O." offers his conception of a basic four-component structure. He discusses the internal functions and suggests how the organization might be altered as the size of the membership grows.

"Reaching the Operational Stage" is the title of a chapter by Robert Brier. Mr. Brier focuses on the money problems a budding H.M.O. will encounter. He identifies some sources of funds that are becoming average to H.M.O. organizers and the many obstacles that must be overcome.

"A Plan for Marketing H.M.O. Services" is the name of a chapter by Alan J. Gartner. He brings together many well-known marketing principles and applies them to the problem of building a subscribership for the H.M.O. His specific recommendations are derived from a factor-analytic study of questionnaire results from a Long Island attitude survey.

In his chapter, "The Manpower Plan," Jack Abeshouse adapts time-tested principles of organizational staffing and personnel procedures to the manpower problems peculiar to a Health Maintenance Organization. Skillful application of this knowledge can assist in the building of a vigorous health care entity.

Harry Maccarone, in his chapter, "Financial Information and Control Procedures" applies knowledge of accounting and managerial controls to the operation of the four-component H.M.O. structure. Use of such procedures can aid the H.M.O. management in keeping a tight rein on financial operations.

A chapter entitled, "The Public Relations Plan" by James A. Kirklin deals with the problem of gaining and nurturing public acceptance of an emerging H.M.O. The new entity has many publics that must be reached with the H.M.O. story.

A final chapter by Jeffrey M. Caro, "The Quality Assurance Plan" concentrates upon the means an H.M.O. can use to guarantee that its high-quality health care potential is realized and maintained. When deviations from standards do occur, the paper shows how the quality control system can point up the need for timely and appropriate corrective action.

In their totality, the eight chapters in this volume comprise a substantial portion of a handbook devoted to the nonmedical aspects of the design of a health maintenance organization.

CHAPTER I

A SURVEY OF HEALTH CARE FINANCING AND DELIVERY SYSTEMS

Walter L. Schweikert

THE EVOLUTION OF HEALTH CARE FINANCING
AND DELIVERY SYSTEMS*

Fraternal or Mutual Aid Plans

The earliest form of protection against the cost of medical care, which dates from the latter half of the 19th century, was the fraternal or mutual aid plan.[1] To avoid "passing the hat" to raise money for friends and co-workers who had been injured or who were ill, many individuals, through their employers, fraternal societies or consumer groups, made regular con- tributions to funds designed to help them budget for medical 'costs. Although these plans were secondary to the overall purposes of the groups, they grad- ually became so important that they overshadowed the primary purposes of the organizations.[2] Many such organizations hired their own physicians to care for their members, but the principal coverage was through indemnity payments.

Union Health and Welfare Funds

The second stage in the evolution of health care plans was the development of union health and welfare funds. The earliest of these was started about 1860, but it was not until the wage freezes of World War II that union funds achieved national prominence.[3] Since wage bargaining was

---

*There are two basic types of organizations financing medical care: (1) those either directly supplying medical services or closely allied with suppliers, and (2) those which are primarily insurers and are independent of the medical profession. Blue Cross, Blue Shield and prepaid group practice plans are examples of the first type; cash indemnity plans run by insurance companies are examples of the second. The distinction is important because it under- lies the divergence in philosophy between the two types.

[1] Edwin J. Faulkner, Health Insurance, (New York, N.Y.: McGraw-Hill Book Co., 1960), p. 20.

[2] Ibid. p. 22.

[3] Ibid.

temporarily halted, fringe benefits became more important in labor negotiations. Although union health programs are usually either fully or partially underwritten by insurance companies, several of the larger unions became self insurers. Most union plans pay specified sums to the insured member for specified illnesses or injuries but some provide direct services to their members. The programs run by the United Mine Workers and the International Ladies' Garment Workers are typical of the direct service plans.

Prepayment Service Plans

During the depression of 1929-1937, vast numbers of people, with experience in mutual aid and union plans, became receptive to prepaying for medical expenses. Organizations known as prepayment service plans were established which made payments directly to the physicians or hospitals providing services rather than to the insured persons. Health plan historians trace the origins of the prepayment service plans to the agreement reached in 1929 between the school teachers of Dallas, Texas and Baylor University Hospital.[4] For the modest sum of $3.00 per semester, the hospital agreed to furnish a limited number of services to any member of the group who needed hospitalization. By the mid-1930's, hospital plans had experienced a phenomenal rate of growth and had achieved national recognition. In 1946, a coordinating body known as the Blue Cross Commission, was established to integrate the activities and policies of a number of these plans and thus the system of Blue Cross Plans were born.[5]

As the hospital service plans grew in popularity, public attention focused on the parallel concept of medical service plans. The best known of these plans is Blue Shield, the so-called "doctors' plan." As in Blue Cross, Blue Shield makes payments directly to the providers of services rather than to subscribers. Both plans operate under special enabling laws which provide relief from state and local taxation and which differentiate them from normal insurance plans.[6]

Government Programs

There are three important types of government programs: (1) state compulsory disability insurance, (2) federal benefits under the Social Security Act, particularly Medicare and Medicaid and (3) federal insurance programs. All of these are financing mechanisms which help large groups of people to defray the high costs of medical care.

State Laws. State compulsory disability insurance laws were first passed in 1942 to cover those who are unable to work because of nonoccupational sickness or accidents.[7] They were designed to provide benefits to those who were ineligible for either unemployment insurance or workmen's compensation. In New York, these benefits are provided under the 1949 Nonoccupational Disability Benefits Law. Under this law, the employer is responsible for

---

[4]Ibid., p. 25.

[5]Ibid., p. 27.

[6]Ibid., p. 29.

[7]Ibid., p. 43.

providing the required benefits and may select either the state fund or a
private plan as the carrier. Benefits, in the form of cash income payments,
are based on the employee's earnings and are financed through payroll deductions and through contributions from the employer. All employers of four or
more persons must provide coverage under this act. Although state compulsory
disability compensation is not health insurance, per se, it does pump funds
into the medical care delivery system.

Social Security. The most important governmental mechanism for
financing the cost of medical care is the Social Security Act, particularly
those sections commonly referred to as Medicare and Medicaid. Both operate
on the insurance principle in that they transfer individual risks to a broad
population base. Both programs make cash indemnity payments which are
directly tied to the cost of the medical services received by the beneficiary.
Almost everyone today agrees that some form of health care coverage was needed
for the aged and the needy who are unable to pay for private insurance.[8]
While much progress has been made, a number of severe deficiencies exist in
the two programs. Many services needed for comprehensive care are not covered,
some legitimate costs are excluded from reimbursement through the use of
deductibles and co-insurance, and medical costs have risen sharply because
there are few controls over utilization rates. Moreover, both programs impede
progress in reorganizing the delivery system. As one author, analyzing
Medicare, wrote:

> It not only accepts the traditional separateness of
> hospital and medical practitioner; it requires the
> separate payment of physician and hospital, and even
> excludes from the hospital payment the cost of the
> physician employed by the hospital. This contradicts
> the congressional declaration of policy not to inter-
> fere in the practice of medicine, or in the manner in
> which medical service is provided, or in the compen-
> sation of any employee, or in the operation of an
> institution. More serious, this imposes restraints
> on the development of organizational patterns that
> could contribute to efficient utilization of man-
> power and dollars, to better organization for the
> delivery of care and to the containment of rising
> costs.[9]

The same criticism also has been made of Medicaid. The limitations
noted above are especially important since they indicate the responsiveness
of the government to the medical and insurance lobbies that are opposed to
reforming the health care delivery system.[10] These programs perpetuate the
prevailing fee-for-service reimbursement method and conflict with the
philosophy of the prepaid group practice plans.

---

[8]I. S. Falk, "Beyond Medicare," American Journal of Public Health, Vol. 59.
(April 1969), p. 608.

[9]Ibid., p. 609. *① Apparently fee - for - service vs. prepaid is a key distinction w/ organizational implications*

[10]Ibid.

Federal Insurance Programs. Federal insurance programs, the third type of governmental plans, include disability provisions of National Service Life insurance, veterans' benefits, and Old Age, Survivors' and Disability Insurance under Social Security and the medical and disability provisions of Workmen's Compensation. Although Workmen's Compensation originally was a federal project, its development was accomplished largely through state laws. As a result, benefits vary from state to state, but all Workmen's Compensation laws provide for weekly income payments and substantial medical payments.[11]

Health Insurance

The most popular form of protection against the financial consequences of illness traditionally has been, and continues to be, health insurance. Private health insurance growth rates, measured in terms of number of persons enrolled, have been spectacular. In 1969, more than 14 times as many persons had some form of health insurance protection than in 1940.[12]

Interest in private health insurance is the result of the financial pressures produced by sickness and disability. This form of protection is a relatively recent development. Notwithstanding the long history of the general insurance industry, it was not until 1903 that the first indemnification clauses covering surgical expenses were added to disability income policies.[13] In 1905, hospital expense benefits were added and in 1910, the first group accident and sickness policy was issued.[14] Hospital and surgical coverage as we know them today were first offered in the 1930's and medical expense coverage in its modern form was introduced in the 1940's.[15]

Prepaid Group Practice

As health insurance grew in popularity, a new form of health care financing mechanism appeared which would eliminate some of the disadvantages of earlier forms of protection. Generally known as prepaid group practice, it combines insurance principles with the delivery of actual health care services. The best known of the prepaid group practice plans are the Kaiser-Permanente Plan which operates on the West Coast, and the Health Insurance

---

[11] Edwin J. Faulkner, op. cit., p. 50.

[12] Source Book of Health Insurance Data, 1970, (New York, N.Y.: Health Insurance Institute, 1970), p. 16.

[13] Franz Goldmann, Voluntary Medical Care Insurance in the United States, (New York, N.Y.: Columbia University Press, 1948), p. 68.

[14] Source Book of Health Insurance Data, 1970, p. 53.

[15] Ibid., p. 54.

Plan of Greater New York. These organizations, and others like them, offer the greatest potential for the provision of truly comprehensive care in the United States.[16]

HEALTH INSURANCE

Background

The most common form of protection against the financial hazards of illness is health insurance. In 1969, more than 61 per cent of those with some form of hospital and surgical protection were covered by insurance companies. The balance were covered by Blue Cross, Blue Shield, medical society plans or independent plans, including prepaid group practice plans.[17]

In contrast with other forms of insurance which are designed to give protection against specific hazards, health insurance seeks to cover a wide range of losses and expenses caused by accident or illness. Benefits ranging from extremely limited to fairly comprehensive are offered under 11 different types of coverage of which the most important are commercial, semi-commercial and group contracts.[18]

Commercial Contracts. Commercial contracts are fairly comprehensive in coverage, having relatively high benefits and ceilings, and are usually offered only to individuals classified as preferred risks. These individuals have few occupational hazards and generally are business, professional or clerical workers. Premium payments under commecial contracts are usually made annually.

Semi-commercial Contracts. Semi-commercial contracts are similar to commercial contracts but offer lower limits and less liberal benefits and are issued to individuals in all insurable occupations. Premiums are generally paid on a quarterly basis.

Group Policies. Group policies, sometimes referred to as "wholesale insurance," involve simultaneous enrollment of a large proportion of the members of a union, employees of a company or members of any other type of organization. After initial enrollment has been completed, new members of the group may be enrolled in the plan after a qualifying period. At the end of 1969, approximately 74 per cent of those with hospital insurance, 82 per cent of those with surgical insurance, 91 per cent of those with regular medical

---

[16]The U. S. Department of Health, Education, and Welfare and the Public Health Service, have been impressed by the accomplishments of prepaid group practice plans and actively encourage their development. Similarly, many unions, impressed by the comprehensiveness of the coverage offered, give their members the option of choosing such plans. See, e.g., D.M. Landay, "Trends in Negotiated Health Plans; Broader Coverage, Higher Quality Care," Monthly Labor Review, (May 1969), p. 7.

[17]Source Book of Health Insurance Data, 1970, pp. 15, 18.

[18]Edwin J. Faulkner, op. cit., p. 64.

insurance and 92 per cent of those with major medical protection were enrolled in group plans.[19] These plans are tailored to meet the needs of the group. Since they are usually offered as part of a "package deal," including life insurance and disability income protection, they seek to eliminate the possibility that only poor risks would enroll while good risks would stay out.[20] Administration of group policies is simple because they are issued to the enrolling organization rather than to the participants of the group. Consequently, the insurer's overhead expenses are lower than they would be under individual enrollment and a larger portion of the premium income can be paid out as benefits. One study comparing expenses under group and individual policies showed that, in 1958, only 48.1 per cent of the premium received in individual policies was returned as benefits as compared to 89.4 per cent for group policies.[21] Lower risks and lower overhead expenses also allow insurers to offer lower premiums under group policies.

In contrast to individual commercial and semi-commercial contracts which are restricted by underwriting rules regarding age, sex, race, occupation, pre-existing conditions and "moral hazard," group policies cover a relatively unrestricted cross-section of the population. They do, however, have a severe eligibility related disadvantage since most such policies are written to cover only employed persons. In recent years, the insurance industry has responded to this criticism through experimental programs which would extend coverage to the temporarily disabled or unemployed and to the retired, but the adequacy of these experiments is questionable.[22]

Other Types. In addition to commercial, semi-commercial and group contracts, health insurance is offered under industrial, travel ticket, newspaper, fraternal, athletic, and special contracts and under credit and overhead expense insurance. Generally, these contracts have limited coverage, low premium rates and short payment periods and are not significant in terms of number of persons covered.[23]

Insurance Theory

Basic Concepts. Insurance is a device for accumulating funds to meet losses through the transfer of individual risks to a large number of persons.[24] It has also been defined as "protection by written contract against the financial hazards (in whole or in part) of the happenings of specified

---

[19]Computed from data in the Source Book of Health Insurance Data, 1970, pp. 17-21. All data on the number of persons covered has been adjusted to eliminate duplication resulting from individuals having the same type of coverage under more than one policy.

[20]Herman M. Somers and Anne R. Somers, Doctors, Patients and Health Insurance, (Washington, D.C.: Brookings Institution, 1961), p. 254.

[21]Ibid., p. 272.

[22]Ibid., p. 274.

[23]Edwin J. Faulkner, op. cit., pp. 64-68.

[24]Oscar N. Serbein, Jr., "The Nature of Prepayment Plans," in Fundamentals of Voluntary Health Care, ed. By George B. DeHuszar, p. 404.

fortuitous events."[25] Implicit in these definitions are the concepts that only large, infrequent, chance losses should be insured. Insurance operates on the law of large numbers. Even though the fortuitous needs of a particular individual cannot be predicted accurately, the needs of a large group can. For this principle to work, there must be a large number of independent chance events.[26]

Contrast With Prepayment. Insurance is sometimes confused with prepayment but there is an important distinction. Insurance is probabilistic in nature while prepayment is a budgeting technique which can accommodate events that are planned by and within the control of the subscribers. Consequently, prepayment plans can cover routine examinations and preventive medicine while pure insurance cannot. The philosophy of insurance can be seen in the following statement by an insurance company executive:

> One must ... question the wisdom of expecting the
> insurance mechanism to pay for preventive service.
> The original purpose of insurance is to protect
> against some unforeseeable event, which, when it
> occurs, can cause substantial financial loss or
> disaster. Health supervision, however, is a fore-
> seeable, relatively minor medical expense that can
> be budgeted as readily as food, shelter and clothing -
> basics for which everyone allows, without question.
> Certainly, if paid out-of-pocket, it will be less
> expensive than to incorporate it as a benefit in an
> insurance plan.[27]

Rate Philosophy. Insurance carriers protect themselves against catastrophe and moral turpitude by setting limits on both the total amount of benefits and on the size of medical and hospital fees. Fees may be paid either on a "reasonable and customary" basis with some review or control mechanism, or as fixed amounts for particular types of services. While these payment methods do not make allowances for complications, severity of injury or disorder or technical difficulties, they permit estimation of the total amount of funds needed to cover benefits and administrative costs. The combination of controlled fees and benefit limitations allows the carrier to calculate premium rates against measureable and predictable risks.[28]

Historical Development

Most historians trace modern health insurance to riders attached to the casualty policies purchased by travelling businessmen in the mid-19th

[25] Source Book of Health Insurance Data, 1970, p. 59.

[26] Oscar N. Serbein, op. cit., p. 369.

[27] George M. Wheatley, "Voluntary Health Insurance - Progress and Problems" in Fundamentals of Voluntary Health Care, ed. by George B. DeHuszar, p. 404.

[28] Serbein, Loc. cit.

century. Since travel on the nation's newly developed railroad system was very hazardous, passengers sought protection against the loss of income that could result from a transportation mishap. Limited coverage of hospital expenses was made available in response to consumer demand, but it was not until 1903 that surgical benefits were added.

Influence of Unions. Much of the credit for shaping the contemporary insurance pattern belongs to the unions since they were the driving force behind the development of group insurance.[29] Introduced about 1910, early group policies attempted to provide mass coverage to workingmen, most of whom had little or no other insurance protection. Enrolling members and collecting premium payments proved easiest when employers were used as agents of the insurance companies. As welfare bargaining progressed and group insurance became a major part of the negotiated fringe benefit agreements, many employers developed paternalistic attitudes toward their employees.[30] Insurance companies, selling their contracts to employers rather than employees, were management-oriented. The management-insurance company alliance was strong enough to overwhelm any objection by labor to the contents of the insurance plans. Unions generally were forced to accept whatever this alliance made available and were unable to demand the other protection they felt was needed.[31]

As welfare bargaining grew in popularity during the 1920's and 1930's, the basic weaknesses of the prevailing method of selling insurance became apparent. The role of the insurance companies changed from selling the idea of insurance to providing the coverage that had been decided in negotiations. Since insurance agents were paid on a commission basis, some agents tried to bribe the negotiators and fraudulently influence the placement of the policy. Once a policy had been placed, the frequent use of a commission schedule based on claims experience often led the agent to discourage legitimate union claims. Following their poor initial experience, unions were in the forefront of those seeking reforms that would eliminate these abuses.[32]

Union dissatisfaction with insurance companies resulted in two approaches to the health care delivery system. Some unions, notably the United Mine Workers, United Auto Workers and International Ladies' Garment Workers Union turned to self-insurance and prepaid group practice. Most of the others used their political and financial influence to force the insurance carriers to be more responsive to labor's needs. It should be noted that the perceived needs of the unions conflict to a degree with the insurance principles mentioned earlier - infrequency, magnitude and fortuitous occurrence. Union influence, however, was strong enough to change the attitude of many insurers so that today many carriers offer prepayment service plans in addition to cash indemnity insurance.[33]

---

[29]Raymond Munts, Bargaining for Health, (Madison, Wisc.: University of Wisconsin Press, 1967), p. 117.

[30]Ibid.,

[31]Ibid., p. 118.

[32]Ibid., p. 119.

[33]Ibid., p. 125.

Medical Opposition. Another group that strongly influenced the development of health insurance was the organized medical profession. The early attitudes of the medical societies were almost uniformly negative.[34] Physicians believed that high quality care depended on a close personal relationship between the doctor and his patient and that even the existence of a third party would mean that this relationship would be destroyed. In a 1934 statement, the American Medical Association adopted the principle that the costs of medical care should be borne by the patient alone. This position was modified in 1938 when the AMA advocated that if a patient had insurance coverage, benefits should be paid directly to the patient in the form of cash indemnities since cash payments alone would leave the traditional doctor-patient relationship intact. More recent modifications to the AMA policy have removed organized medicine's sanctions against plans that provide services, but the fear of outside control still remains active. One physician who is also affiliated with an insurance company stated:

> The confidence of a patient in his doctor is as
> intangible as the virtues of courage, patience,
> skill, judgment, humanity or integrity. It
> cannot be measured or weighed or tabulated.
> Take all, or any, of these values away, and the
> doctor's usefulness is seriously impaired. The
> doctor fears that the entry of insurance, as a
> third party to this relation, may regiment and
> destroy it. To support and encourage medical-
> care insurance wholeheartedly, he wants to be
> convinced that this will not happen. It may be
> stated with conviction that his fears are as
> much in behalf of his patient as they are for
> himself.[35]

Organized medicine, when opposed to any health care delivery or payment plan, has many weapons at its disposal. These include political lobbying, public relations and propaganda campaigns and disciplinary actions against individuals and against the plans themselves. Political lobbying has resulted in restrictive state laws which effectively prevent insurance carriers from controlling health care delivery. Disciplinary measures include anything "from professional ostracism of participating physicians to intimidation of hospitals and clinics which cooperate with the plans."[36]

In the past four decades, organized medicine's opposition to health care plans has not been directed against the insurance carriers except those

---

[34]Franz Goldmann, op. cit. pp. 55-62.

[35]C. Marshall Lee, "The Challenge of Medical Care Insurance," in Fundamentals of Voluntary Health Care, ed. by George B. DeHuszar, p. 444.

[36]Daniel S. Hirshfield, The Lost Reform, (Cambridge, Mass.: Harvard University Press, 1970), p.97.

involved in providing or influencing services. Faced with the prospect of compulsory federal programs, most doctors have long since accepted insurance as a more attractive alternative. More recent medical opposition has been applied to union plans and to the prepaid group practice plans.[37]

       <u>Physician's Fears</u>. Many physicians fear that any organization which is paying for a service will, sooner or later, try to gain control over the amount, type and timing of medical care. Through their influence with the insurance industry and their powerful political lobbies, they have been able to restrict the role of most carriers to payment. The insurers have generally agreed that they will not interfere with either the practice of medicine or the delivery of health care.[38]

       A number of physicians have felt that health insurance is contrary to the basic American ideal of free enterprise. Insurance companies provide reimbursement of medical expenses on the basis of either fixed or "reasonable and customary" fees, but since no two treatments, even of the same type, are ever exactly alike, the doctors fear that setting arbitrary limits on fees will prevent them from receiving just compensation for the efforts they make in each case. They believe that fees should vary in relation to the complexity of the case, probability of a malpractice suit and intangible value of the services they render.[39]

       Even after they had accepted health insurance as a fact of life, many physicians still had negative attitudes. In a 1954 survey, more than half of the respondents felt that their patients were misled into believing their insurance would cover all doctors' fees in full.[40] Others said that health insurance is suspectible to abuse since doctors sometimes charge a higher fee for an insured patient than for an uninsured one. "Almost half (of the respondents) expressed the belief that the sole reason for such fee raising was an opportunity to obtain more money."[41] It is interesting, however, that most of the respondents felt insurance should cover most but not all medical costs and that many felt that the patient's insurance coverage should be taken into account when setting medical fees.

Growth of Health Insurance

       Pressure from several sources contributed to the growth of health insurance. The general public wanted protection against the high cost of hospital and physician services. Unions, especially during the wage freeze of the Second World War, bargained for broader fringe benefits and greater

---

[37] Somers and Somers, <u>op. cit.</u>, p. 343.

[38] Daniel S. Hirshfield, <u>op. cit.</u>, p. 96.

[39] C. Marshall Lee, <u>op. cit.</u>, pp. 445-450.

[40] George M. Wheatley, <u>op. cit.</u>, p. 406.

[41] <u>Ibid</u>.

health coverage. Doctors saw it as an alternative, albeit unattractive, to socialized medicine. The introduction of group health insurance policies made low-cost coverage possible. Competition between the various carriers gave health insurance greater visibility and led to better coverage. All of these factors contributed to the rapid expansion in the number of persons covered.

By the end of 1969, approximately 88 per cent of the civilian resident population was covered by one or more form of health insurance.[42] Hospital expense insurance, with 175.2 million enrollees, covered more people than any other form of health insurance.[43] In 1955, 105.5 million had this type of protection while in 1940, only 12.3 million were covered. In 1969, 162.1 million people were covered for surgical expense as compared to 88.9 million in 1955 and 5.4 million 15 years earlier. The number covered by regular medical insurance was 134.9 million in 1969, 54.9 million in 1955 and 3.0 million in 1940. Major Medical expense insurance, introduced in its present form in 1954, covered 72.3 million people by 1969.

The majority of the persons having health insurance coverage are enrolled in plans sponsored by insurance companies. The rate of growth of insurance company-provided hospitalization insurance was slightly higher than for all insurers while for surgical expense insurance it was slightly lower. The rate of growth in regular medical protection provided by insurance companies has been significantly higher than that provided by all insurers. Table II - 1 shows the enrollment of each type of health insurance since 1940.

Insurance Trends

A number of significant trends have developed in health insurance during the past three decades. The time limitation on benefit payments in many contracts has been steadily rising to the point that today many policies provide benefits for as long as the policyholder lives. Coverage has become broader, reflecting changes in the medical economics environment. The fixed daily hospital cost benefits and the number of covered hospital days have risen. Some contracts provide coverage for as long as 365 days per illness. Allowances for ancillary services have been increased from $100 or $200 to $500 or more.[44]

The total amount paid for health insurance benefit payments has grown steadily, reaching $14.3 billion in 1969, an increase of almost $2.1 billion or 17 per cent over 1968.[45] Of the 1969 total, $7.6 billion was paid by insurance companies and the balance was paid by Blue Cross, Blue Shield and other Hospital-Medical Plans. Insurance company benefit payments increased only 13 per cent over 1968 while Blue Cross, Blue Shield and the

---

[42] Source Book of Health Insurance Data, 1970, p. 15.

[43] See Table I - 1.

[44] Source Book of Health Insurance Data, 1970, p. 7.

[45] Ibid., p. 31.

TABLE II - I

NUMBER OF PERSONS IN THE UNITED STATES WITH HEALTH INSURANCE PROTECTION BY TYPE OF COVERAGE AND INSURER

(Millions of Persons)

(Index: 1965 = 100)

End of Year	All Insurers		Insurance Companies		All Insurers		Insurance Companies		All Insurers		Insurance Companies		Insurance Companies Only	
	Number	Index	Number	Index	Number	Index	Number	Index	Number	Index	Number	Index	Number	Index
1940	12.3	8.0	3.7	3.9	5.4	3.8	2.3	2.6	3.0	2.7				
1945	32.1	21.0	10.5	11.2	12.9	9.2	7.3	8.3	4.7	4.2	.5	.8		
1950	76.6	50.0	37.0	39.5	54.2	38.6	34.3	39.2	21.6	19.3	8.0	14.0		
1955	105.5	68.9	57.3	61.2	88.9	63.3	53.3	60.9	54.9	49.1	24.4	42.7	5.2	10.0
1960	130.0	84.9	76.7	81.9	117.3	83.5	71.0	81.1	86.9	77.8	40.6	71.1	27.5	53.0
1965	153.1	100.0	93.7	100.0	140.5	100.0	87.5	100.0	111.7	100.0	57.1	100.0	51.9	100.0
1966	158.0	103.2	97.4	103.9	144.7	103.0	90.3	103.2	116.5	104.3	60.8	106.5	56.7	109.2
1967	162.9	106.4	100.3	107.0	150.4	107.0	93.6	107.0	122.6	109.8	64.6	113.1	62.2	119.8
1968	169.5	110.7	104.4	111.4	155.7	110.8	96.1	109.8	129.1	115.6	68.4	119.8	66.9	128.9
1969	175.2	114.4	108.5	115.8	162.1	115.4	99.6	113.8	134.9	120.8	72.3	126.6	72.3	139.3

Note: The data refer to the net number of people covered. Duplication among persons protected by more than one kind of insuring organization or more than one policy providing the same type of coverage has been eliminated. Data presented under "All Insurers" represent coverage provided by insurance companies, Blue Cross, Blue Shield, medical society approved plans and independent plans.

Source: Adapted from Source Book of Health Insurance Data, 1970, New York, N.Y.: Health Insurance Institute, 1970, pp. 17, 18, 20 and 21. Index computations by the author.

other plans increased 21 per cent. Group policies issued by insurance companies paid $6.2 billion in 1969, an increase of 14 per cent over 1968 while individual policy payments, which amounted to $1.4 billion, increased only about 1 per cent.[46]

As health insurance benefits have increased, the proportion of disposable personal income spent for insurance premiums has remained fairly stable. In 1969, a total of $10.2 billion was spent on premiums for policies issued by insurance companies.[47] This represents 1.6 per cent of all disposable income. A year earlier, $9.1 billion or 1.5 per cent of disposable personal income had been spent.

Coverage

There are five general types of health insurance: hospital, surgical, regular medical, major medical and disability income.[48] Hospital insurance covers room and board on a fixed fee per day basis and ancillary services, which are usually compensated on either a co-insurance of fixed fee per day basis. Surgical insurance covers services performed in a hospital by a qualified surgeon and generally contains maximum fees for specified operations. Regular medical insurance usually covers only in-hospital visits by non-surgical physicians. Again, maximum rates are set for specified services. Major Medical covers hospitalization, physician's and surgeon's fees, laboratory work, routine nursing services, and sometimes, drugs. Coverage has very high limits and contracts are written with substantial fixed deductibles or corridor deductibles and with co-insurance factors. The fifth type of health insurance, disability income protection, covers loss of income while the insured is unable to return to work.

Most of the literature on the health care delivery system assumes that everyone desires protection that will pay for "comprehensive" health care. This is usually interpreted to mean full physician care in the home, doctor's office or hospital including preventive, diagnostic, therapeutic and rehabilitative services appropriate to the needs of the individual. Dental care, drugs, appliances, mental illness and special nursing are generally not included in this definition.[49] It is readily apparent that only through a combination of the first four types of health insurance that coverage approaching "comprehensive" care can be realized.

A Health Insurance Institute study of coverage in group plans in 1970 showed that of 359,000 persons in the survey, 40 per cent had basic hospital, surgical or medical expense coverage, 61 per cent were covered for full indemnification for hospital expense of $300 or more, and 33 per cent

---

[46] Ibid., p. 30.

[47] Ibid., p. 41

[48] Franz Goldmann, op. cit., p. 71.

[49] W. P. Dearing, "The Challenge of Comprehensive Health Care," American Journal of Public Health, Vol. 52, (December 1962), p. 2071.

more had full benefits up to a stated maximum. A total of 97 per cent had surgical expense insurance. Of those with basic hospital surgical and medical coverage, 84 per cent had supplementary major medical insurance.[50]

A second study, designed to determine how well medical care costs were covered by group health insurance, involved a sample of more than 40,000 claims. This study showed that the group plans covered 86 per cent of the average policyholder's hospital expenses, 77 per cent of his surgical expenses, 84 per cent of his anesthetist's bill and almost 76 per cent of his X-ray and laboratory charges. Insurance covered more than half of all other medical expenses.[51] These statistics are somewhat misleading however. Insurance companies attempt to keep premiums down through the use of deductibles, co-insurance, exclusions and maximums. In 1968, private health insurance covered only 35.7 per cent of all private personal health care expenditures.[52] The difference presumably reflects amounts for which claims are not submitted because they are not covered by the insurance policy.[53, 54]

Advantages of Health Insurance

Health insurance offers many advantages to subscribers, physicians, hospitals, employers and society as a whole. Those who can afford it have the peace of mind and sense of security that comes from knowing that most, if not all, of their large medical and hospital bills will be paid by insurance if they are injured or become ill. The policyholders feel that even if they require extensive treatment, they will not have to face financial ruin.

Physicians and hospitals benefit from health insurance because they know that payment of a substantial portion of their charges will be guaranteed. Consequently, their losses due to bad debts are minimized and their energies can be devoted to providing health services rather than bill collection.

The medical profession, in keeping with its traditional approach to outside control of the health care delivery system, favors health insurance over other plans because it allows "free choice" of physician by the policyholder.[55] As contrasted with "closed panel" plans, health insurance theoretically permits a patient to choose any physician he desires to provide treatment.

Health insurance provided on a group enrollment basis is attractive to employers since it satisfies the unions, is relatively less expensive than

---

[50]Source Book of Health Insurance Data, 1970, p. 10.

[51]Ibid., p. 11.

[52]U.S. Department of Commerce, Bureau of the Census, Statistical Abstract of the United States, 1970, (Washington, D.C.: Government Printing Office, 1970), p. 64.

[53]W. P. Dearing, op. cit.,

[54]Seymour E. Harris, The Economics of American Medicine, (New York, N.Y.: Macmillan Company, 1964), p. 400.

[55]Ibid., p. 381.

some alternative arrangements and is easy to administer.[56] Since many carriers base their rates on claims experience for particular groups rather than for all persons insured by them, they can offer substantial premium reductions to employers whose employees are rated low risks.

Disadvantages of Health Insurance

Notwithstanding these advantages, health insurance has severe limitations. Most of these are attributable to the separation of financing from health care delivery in contemporary cash indemnity plans and to the philosophy mentioned earlier that insurance should only cover infrequent, substantial and fortuitous medical conditions.[57]

Most health insurance carriers, desiring to eliminate small claims, especially for routine medical services, issue policies which do not cover treatment given in a doctor's office. Consequently, a patient who could be treated without needing hospitalization may be admitted to a hospital only because insurance will pay for it. The decision to hospitalize may be made because the physician sees an opportunity for guaranteeing payment of his bill or because the patient, himself, asks for hospitalization. If a patient's request is denied by his physician, he may threaten to go to another doctor. This type of economic pressure could cause a physician to accede to his patient's desires.[58] Once the decision is made, an insured patient's hospital stay could be prolonged unnecessarily either as a result of delays in processing laboratory tests and reports or because of abuses by the hospital.[59] A hospital may encourage overstays, for example, because the daily cost to the hospital drops rapidly after the first few days or because they have empty beds. Most administrative and diagnostic expenses are incurred soon after the patient is admitted and the hospital usually only recovers these costs after several days have passed.

A second shortcoming of health insurance is that it has few effective controls over professional fees.[60] Since the true value of the care received by a policyholder cannot be accurately determined and since the carriers do not control the health care delivery system, insurance companies have had to select one of four approaches to payment: (1) pay whatever the physician charges; (2) pay the "reasonable and customary" fees; (3) negotiate directly with the physician; or (4) pay an arbitrary amount established by the policy. Clearly, the first alternative could be disastrous. The carrier would have no protection whatever against unreasonably high fees. The disadvantage of the second alternative is that determining the "reasonable and customary" fee is very difficult for all except the simplest and most routine treatments.

---

[56] Ibid., p. 392.

[57] Raymond Munts, op. cit., pp. 124-128.

[58] George M. Wheatley, op. cit., p. 508.

[59] Ibid., p. 408.

[60] Franz Goldmann, op. cit., p. 77.

Direct negotiation is a more attractive alternative in certain respects but would result in prohibitive administrative costs if universally applied to all claims. The last alternative is the easiest from the carrier's point of view but could leave the policyholder with inadequate coverage. Under the terms of indemnity policies, the physician is not required to accept the fee schedule set by contract as full payment for his services.

Another disadvantage of health insurance is that it tends to inflate medical costs.[61] The direct costs of medical care have risen faster than any other item in the Consumer Price Index.[62] Part of this rise may have been caused by physicians including insurance status in their evaluation of their patients' "ability to pay." Some doctors feel that they are justified in charging higher fees of their insured patients than of those who do not have this type of protection.[63]

From a social viewpoint, health insurance has the deficiency of not covering enough of the population. Most of the insurance written today involves group enrollment of industrial workers or enrollment of individuals at relatively high premium rates. Nonindustrial workers, the unemployed and those with low incomes generally do not have adequate coverage. In addition, many policies either exclude dependents completely or only provide partial indemnities.[64]

Since insurance companies simultaneously seek to limit their risks and provide at least partial protection at a reasonable premium rate, they sometimes only insure against specified diseases and conditions and only provide indemnities up to certain specified amounts. Medical bills for other conditions or in amounts exceeding the contractual limits must be paid by the patient. In the event of a major illness, large medical bills could impoverish an insured with inadequate coverage.[65] The insurance companies try to reduce their risks still further through deductibles. A policyholder enrolled under a contract having a deductible clause must pay for all expenses incurred up to a certain amount before coverage starts. Most routine medical bills are relatively small and would normally not exceed the deductible amount. Moreover, on those policies which cover the dependents of the insured, a separate deductible is usually established for each dependent.

Potentially, one of the most severe disadvantages of health insurance is that it may actually encourage needless operations. Any surgery, no matter how minor, involves a certain amount of pain or risk, and no patient should be exposed to it purely because it affords a physician an opportunity

---

[61] George M. Wheatley, op. cit., p. 410.

[62] Source Book of Health Insurance Data, 1970, p. 45.

[63] Seymour E. Harris, op. cit., p. 362.

[64] Goldman, loc. cit.

[65] Ibid.

for profit. Abuses of this kind are rare but could not exist if the insurance plans were also responsible for the quality of care.[66]

A final disadvantage of health insurance, that it ignores preventive medicine, is the result of the philosophy that insurance should cover only large, infrequent, chance losses and should not be used as a budgeting tool.[67] Even though most doctors and carriers agree that preventive medicine can contribute to avoiding costly illnesses in the future, most financing plans do not provide for it, particularly if the treatment is rendered in a physician's office. Since the doctor's fee is an out-of-pocket expense not reimbursable by insurance, patients avoid seeing their physicians until they are seriously ill. In addition to raising the total cost of health care, ignoring preventive medicine increases the risk of poor health.

Major Medical Expense Insurance

Background. Basic hospital, surgical and medical expense insurances, by themselves, fall far short of the definition of "comprehensive" health protection usually used in the insurance industry. This package only approaches comprehensive coverage when major medical insurance is added. Originally called "catastrophic coverage," it is not limited as to the type of expense and covers medical, surgical and hospital costs as well as home and office visits.[68] It is characterized by its deductible and co-insurance features and high dollar limits usually from $5,000 to $25,000.[69] Sometimes the deductible takes the form of a corridor, an excluded amount which is paid by the insured after expiration of basic benefits and before coverage by the major medical policy. The contractual limits may apply to each illness, to each calendar or policy year or to the insured's total lifetime.

Growth. Major Medical was first introduced and aggressively pushed about 20 years ago.[70] Growth was stimulated by union negotiation pressures and by the desire of groups and individuals to reduce the financial impact of prolonged or catastrophic illness. Its greatest attraction was that it would compensate for the inability of basic health insurance to cover the rising cost of care.[71] By 1969, 72,292,000 persons were covered by Major Medical as compared to 66,861,000 in 1968. Of these covered persons, the number enrolled in group policies was 66,630,000 and 61,738,000 respectively.[72]

Benefit Structure. Coverage under Major Medical generally includes all physician, hospital and routine nursing services, drugs, and laboratory fees and excluded expenses covered by other insurance, pregnancy, dental care, cosmetic surgery, alcoholism, narcotics addiction, health examinations and

---

[66] Seymour E. Harris, op. cit., p. 362.

[67] Raymond Munts, op. cit., p. 125.

[68] Somers and Somers, op. cit., p. 250.

[69] Ibid., p. 282.

[70] Ibid., p. 281.

[71] C. Marshall Lee, op. cit., p. 440.

[72] Source Book of Health Insurance Data, 1970, p. 21.

21

treatment in government or other noncharge facilities. There is usually a probation period for preexisting illness.[73]

Cost Controls. The basic premise of major medical is that not insuring small claims leaves more money for larger claims. Small claims are expensive to handle and sharing costs between insured and insurer theoretically regulates utilization through sharing financial responsibility.[74] Insurers attempt to regulate usage through deductibles and co-insurance, but experience has shown that these regulators are not effective.[75] The deductible reduces, but does not eliminate, small claims and co-insurance controls can be bypassed if the doctor or hospital accepts the insurance company's share of the bill as full payment.[76] Moreover, both controls assume that health care consumers have sufficient sophistication to determine if the care they receive is necessary and appropriate. As a practical matter, however, the consumer is usually not knowledgeable and must depend on the advice of his physician.[77]

In addition to deductibles and co-insurance, Major Medical depends on review of flagrant overcharges to control medical fees. This control is inadequate since claims are not reviewed unless they are two or three times the normal fees charged for each treatment. The greatest danger to Major Medical is the addition of smaller increments of 25 per cent to 50 per cent to the bills of those with this type of coverage. All "reasonable and customary" fees are paid and the only recourses against overcharging are direct negotiation with the physician and appeal to local medical societies.[78]

Types of Policies. There are two basic types of Major Medical policies. In the first, all expenses after the fixed deductible are covered. This type of policy covers costs starting with the first dollar after expiration of benefits payable under basic coverage, assuming that the basic is sufficiently large. The second type of Major Medical, featuring a "corridor" deductible, covers costs only after a certain dollar amount past basic benefits has been reached. This type of policy has the obvious disadvantage of not offering protection when it may be needed most.[79]

With the disadvantages mentioned above and the additional disadvantages common to all types of health insurance, it is easy to overlook the advantages that it helps people finance catastrophic illness without charity or government assistance. A combination of Major Medical with basic hospital, surgical and medical expense approaches truly comprehensive coverage.

---

[73]Somers and Somers, op. cit., p. 282.

[74]J. Pollack, "Major Medical Expense Insurance: An Evaluation," American Journal of Public Health, Vol. 47 (March 1957), p. 322.

[75]Ibid., p. 325.

[76]Ibid., p. 330-331.

[77]Ibid., p. 324.

[78]Ibid., p. 332.

[79]Ibid., p. 324.

The Prepayment Service Concept

The most commonly used alternatives to cash indemnity health insurance are the prepayment service organizations, especially Blue Cross and Blue Shield. While indemnity plans make cash payments directly to the insured and completely divorce themselves from the health care delivery system, prepayment service plans, by contracting with hospitals and physicians to provide services, guarantee that these services will be available to their subscribers when needed and, for those with low incomes, without additional cost. Payment is made directly to the providers of services rather than to the subscribers.[80] Since payments up to certain limits are based on actual cost, prepayment premiums rise when health care costs increase.[81] In contrast, health insurance, which provides only fixed indemnities regardless of the actual costs of care, is able to keep premium rates fairly constant. An insurance policyholder must purchase additional coverage if he wants to protect himself from rising costs while a prepayment service subscriber's benefits are periodically raised by the plan without further action by the subscriber.

Blue Cross - Historical Development

The Blue Cross idea originated in Texas in 1929 when a group of Dallas school teachers and Baylor University Hospital negotiated an agreement under which, in exchange for $3.00 per semester, all hospital care within certain limits was to be provided when needed at no charge. Coming as it did at the beginning of the depression, the plan was an instant success. Within ten months after the plan was conceived, approximately 75 per cent of all Dallas school teachers were enrolled.[82]

The Baylor experiment attracted the attention of the rest of the nation and soon other hospitals began offering similar plans. As the number of plans grew, lack of coordination became a serious problem and the need for community-wide arrangements became apparent.[83] The first such plan was organized in 1932 in Sacramento, California and was quickly followed by plans in Newark, New Jersey, Saint Paul, Minnesota and New York City.[84] By 1949, there were 85 member or associate Blue Cross plans covering 33.4 million persons in the United States. In addition, five plans were in operation in

---

[80]Robert M. Cunningham, The Blue Cross Story, (New York, N.Y.: Public Affairs Committee, Inc., 1963, Ninth Edition, Public Affairs Pamphlet No. 101A), p. 3

[81]Ibid., p. 14.

[82]Ibid., p. 4.

[83]Fred J. Cook, The Plot Against the Patient, (Englewood Cliffs, N.J.: Prentice-Hall, Inc., 1967), p. 199.

[84]Ibid.

Canada at that time to serve approximately 2.5 million persons. Since then, some of the plans were consolidated and in 1970 there were 80 Blue Cross Plans including four in Canada, one in Puerto Rico and one in Jamaica.[85]

The development of Blue Cross was strongly influenced by the American Hospital Association.[86] In 1933, having decided to regulate the plans, it issued a series of principles and guidelines which established minimum standards for acceptance by the hospital profession. To be approved, a plan had to be organized as a nonprofit, financially sound, public service covering hospital costs only. Its governing board had to consist of representatives of public, medical and hospital groups; subscribers had to be guaranteed free choice of physicians and hospital and all recognized hospitals in the community had to be eligible to participate in the plan.[87] As a result of this regulation, the plans acquired a hospital orientation which still persists.

Organization

The Blue Cross Plans. The 80 Blue Cross plans are separate, independent community sponsored corporations having separate jurisdictions, separate rate and benefit schedules and separate governing boards. All are nonprofit organizations and most are incorporated under nonprofit charters. In 1970, 44 per cent of the members of the average Blue Cross governing board represented the general public, 42 per cent represented the hospitals and 14 per cent represented the medical profession.[88] The board members serve without compensation and are responsible for deciding corporate policies. Like other corporations, the Blue Cross plans have a paid staff of executive, supervisory and clerical personnel responsible for day-to-day administration. The organizations are usually departmentalized functionally into units responsible for enrollment, contracts, hospital record-keeping, actuarial and statistical data compilation, purchasing, distribution, advertising and personnel.[89]

The Blue Cross Association. Since the Blue Cross plans offer widely differing benefits, it was difficult for national employers to obtain uniform coverage for all their employees under a single contract. To resolve this problem, the Blue Cross Association, a coordinating organization, was established in 1948. It is the responsibility of this organization to determine the type of coverage desired by national employers and then to arrange for suitable contracts to be written by the individual plans serving the areas involved. "Today, the Blue Cross Association is the spokesman for Plans in

---

[85]The Blue Cross and Blue Shield Fact, Book, 1970, (Chicago, Ill.: Blue Cross Association and National Association of Blue Shield Plans, 1970), p. 3.

[86]Somers and Somers, op. cit., p. 292.

[87]Ibid.

[88]The Blue Cross and Blue Shield Fact Book, 1970, p. 2.

[89]Franz Goldmann, op. cit., p. 104.

24

matters of national or regional concern. These include legislation, national advertising, research and the collection and interpretation of statistics, and relationships with other national organizations."[90] The Association represents the plans in negotiations with the government and coordinates benefits for subscribers who are hospitalized in a region other than that covered by their local plan. The Association also operates a subsidiary stock casualty insurance company, Health Services, Inc., which underwrites services desired by national employers and which cannot be obtained from the Blue Cross plans. By contracting with both the Association and Health Services, Inc., national groups are able to equalize benefits throughout the country.[91]

Enrollment Procedures

Blue Cross in 1969 covered 71,090,355 persons in the continental United States and 5,075,274 in Canada, up from 68,577,832 and 4,440,433 in 1968. In the United States and Canada, 58,640,377 persons are enrolled in groups. This represents approximately 87 per cent of total enrollment.[92] Blue Cross plans encourage group enrollment because it prevents people from signing up when they are already sick or expect to need hospitalization and want to have a third party pay the cost. Since groups are enrolled during limited periods, the group members are likely to be representative of the general population and hospitalization rates can be kept down.[93] In addition, by enrolling groups, Blue Cross, like the insurance companies, experiences cost savings and efficiencies through reducing bookkeeping and administration. In 1969, operating expenses were only 5.8 per cent of subscription income for member plans and 10.4 per cent for associate plans.[94]

Basis for Premiums

As originally conceived, Blue Cross premiums were to be based on community rating. All members were to be charged the same rates regardless of risk. Poor risks were to be subsidized by good risks but this method of setting premiums does not allow for competition by insurance companies which can offer them lower rates for the same protection. Although insurance companies limit their exposure through deductibles, corridors, co-insurance and exclusions, these devices are not always perceived as major drawbacks by those in low-risk groups. As a result, Blue Cross could be left with a much higher risk population than it would have otherwise had. The competitive pressure from the insurance companies is partially offset by the tax exemption granted to Blue Cross because of its nonprofit status.[95]

---

[90]Robert M. Cunningham, op. cit., p. 8.

[91]Ibid., p. 10.

[92]The Blue Cross and Blue Shield Fact Book, 1970, pp. 3-5.

[93]Robert M. Cunningham, op. cit., p. 10.

[94]The Blue Cross and Blue Shield Fact Book, 1970, pp. 6-7.

[95]Seymour E. Harris, op. cit., p. 391.

Cost Controls

Hospital costs are influenced by four factors: (1) the direct costs of services, (2) hospitalization rates, (3) average length of stay in the hospital, and (4) the types of services prescribed for each patient. Blue Cross limits the direct costs of services by negotiating fixed fees per bed day with each hospital. The institutions accept these fees as full payment and are then responsible for keeping their costs within these limits. Utilization and length of stay are regulated, at least partially, through encouraging the hospitals to set up committees to review all admissions and by providing some outpatient coverage. Very little except data collection is done to regulate the types of services prescribed for each patient. Blue Cross attempts to control some costs by joining hospital planning groups and backing legislation requiring anyone seeking to build new facilities to prove community need before construction begins. It hopes that by doing this, needless duplication will be eliminated,[96] and the pressure to fill empty beds will not become a dominant factor.

Coverage

Of the 80 separate Blue Cross plans, eight cover New York State through regional offices in Albany, Buffalo, Jamestown, New York City, Rochester, Syracuse, Utica and Watertown. The New York City plan, otherwise known as the Associated Hospital Service of New York, is the largest in the country and covers the Long Island area in addition to the southeastern part of the state.[97] Its benefit structure is typical of most Blue Cross plans.

Two distinctive types of hospitalization plans are offered by Greater New York's Blue Cross. In the 21/180 day plan, the subscriber is covered for full hospital bed costs for 21 days and 50 per cent for the next 180 days in a semi-private room. The costs of room and board are covered as well as the use of equipment, laboratory and X-Ray facilities and drugs provided by the hospital. One hundred dollars is provided for maternity or abortion care. Mental and nervous disorders are covered for 21 full and nine discount days during any 12 month period and pulmonary tuberculosis is covered for 21 days. There is a qualification period of six months before hospitalization for tonsillectomy or adenoidectomy is covered and there is an 11 month qualifying period for pre-existing conditions. Pregnancy is covered only if conception took place while the subscriber was a member of the plan.[98]

The second type of plan is similar in coverage except that full hospital coverage is provided for 120 days except for pulmonary tuberculosis

---

[96]Associated Hospital Service of New York, New Controls on Rising Hospital Costs, (New York, N.Y.: Associated Hospital Service of New York, 1971), pp. 2-9.

[97]The Blue Cross and Blue Shield Fact Book, 1970, p. 4.

[98]Associated Hospital Service of New York, The 21/180 Day Plan, (New York, N.Y.: Associated Hospital Service of New York, 1970), pp. 1-9.

and mental and nervous disorders which are covered for only 20 days. The 120 day plan provides $200 for maternity or abortion hospitalization. Both plans cover dependents to age 19 and exclude workmen's compensation cases, hospitalization in a federal government hospital, convalescent and long-term care, hospitalization for diagnostic studies and ambulance service. Both plans have the same qualifying periods.[99]

As of May 1, 1971, the rates for the 21/180 day plan were $7.00 per month for individuals and $15.80 per month for families when enrolled in groups. For those not enrolled in groups, the rates were $27.30 per quarter for individuals and $56.52 per quarter for families. The rates for the 120 day plan were $10.94 per month for individuals and $24.64 per month for families enrolled in groups. The nongroup rates were $49.17 per quarter and $85.53 per quarter respectively.[100] Much of the difference in rate structure between the group and nongroup subscribers is due to economies in administration and competition from insurance companies.

Advantages

Like health insurance, Blue Cross has the advantages of easing the health care financing problem for patients and of removing some of the financial barriers to hospitalization. As a result, the subscribers are encouraged to use the hospitals before their problems become catastrophic. Another advantage is that hospital costs are kept down as a result of payment guarantees and the incidental saving in bookkeeping and bad debt collection. The patient, of course, derives the benefit of lower charges and improved service while the hospital no longer must contend with bad debts and uncertainty of income.[101]

Disadvantages

Blue Cross shares some important disadvantages with insurance companies. In its role as financing agent, it does not exercise control over the operation of hospital facilities and consequently subsidizes the inefficiencies of these institutions. Like insurance companies, it fails to cover a significant segment of our low income and rural population primarily because they cannot afford to pay the premiums. Blue Cross covers only part of the cost of hospitalization because of discount periods, limits on ancillary services, exclusions, time limitations and, in some plans, reduced benefits for dependents.[102] Finally, like insurance, Blue Cross encourages needless hospitalization.[103]

---

[99]Associated Hospital Service of New York, The 120 Day Hospital Plan of Greater New York's Blue Cross, (New York, N.Y.: Associated Hospital Service of New York, 1970), pp. 3-9.

[100]Rates for the two plans were quoted in the previous two references and reflect the most recent premium changes.

[101]Franz Goldmann, op. cit., pp. 105-111.

[102]Ibid., p. 111.

[103]Fred J. Cook, op. cit., pp. 206-216.

Additional disadvantages, unique to Blue Cross, are the result of the plans' methods of operation, lack of uniformity and loosely knit organizational structure. Reciprocity between member hospitals and nonmember hospitals is weak, payment for services in nonmember facilities is at inadequate levels, and, because each plan is different, a subscriber who becomes ill or is injured in an area other than that covered by his own plan, may not be sufficiently covered.[104] As one study showed, "There was wild confusion between the varying coverages of Blue Cross and Blue Shield plans. Diagnostic procedures covered by Blue Cross in one area were covered by Blue Shield in another; and since there was no reciprocity between Blue Shield plans - and no true reciprocity between Blue Cross plans either for that matter - the unfortunate who thought he was protected by Blue Cross found himself totally unprotected for many items in a Blue Shield area."[105]

A final disadvantage of Blue Cross, the potential lack of responsiveness to public needs, is the result of the historic domination of the plans by hospital representatives and their supporters in the medical profession. Since 42 per cent of the average Blue Cross governing board represents the hospitals and 14 per cent represents the medical profession, the consumer representatives are powerless to oppose their collaborative decisions. The hospital-medical alliance could easily ignore public service in favor of its own interests if it chose to do so.[106]

Blue Shield - Historical Development

The pressures leading to the development of large scale service plans providing physicians' care were felt long before Blue Shield was organized. Blue Cross proved in 1929 that hospital costs could be prepaid and the American health care consumers wanted a mechanism that could cover doctor bills in the same way.[107] In the depression years, few people could afford to pay the high costs associated with major illness.

As the American people became more sophisticated about satisfying their health care needs, they demanded organizations which could provide the fruits of medical progress at a reasonable cost. In fact, as time progressed, high quality health care came to be regarded as a basic right and necessity not to be withheld for purely financial reasons. If no private organization could be set up to satisfy this demand, many felt that a governmental program would be needed. It is probably no coincidence that a year before the first Blue Shield type program was organized, a bill had been introduced in the California legislature which would have provided for compulsory health insurance. As one author suggests:

---

[104] Franz Goldmann, op. cit., p. 112.

[105] Fred J. Cook, op. cit, p. 205.

[106] Ibid., p. 201.

[107] National Association of Blue Shield Plans, Blue Shield, A Helping Hand, (Chicago, Ill.: National Association of Blue Shield Plans, 1968), p. 7.

28

Though this measure got nowhere, it has a scarce effect, and the more perceptive members of the medical profession could see that, if the profession itself did not find a way of providing the public with the protection it needed and wanted, it would have to face an even more grim prospect, intervention by the government and some form of "socialized medicine." The desire to avoid such a calamity became and remained a strong spur to the medical profession in fostering the growth of voluntary programs, and the Blue Shield plans expanded rapidly.[108]

The response of the medical profession to the threat of government intervention was the organization, in 1939, of the California Physicians Service, the first stateside medical service plan. Established by the California Medical Association, it offered complete physicians' services for $1.70 per month to employed persons earning less than $3,000 annually. Participating physicians were compensated directly by the plan.[109] While the coverage offered was comprehensive, it was difficult to sell and was considered financially unsound. Consequently, coverage was limited to certain specific treatments, the plan was offered to persons at many income levels, and a feature was added which permitted the physician to charge anything he wished to subscribers with incomes above a specified amount.[110]

In the same year that the California Physicians Service was organized, other Blue Shield type plans were established in Michigan, Hawaii, and Buffalo, New York. The latter plan was the first to use the Blue Shield name and symbol, but as time progressed, the national Blue Shield Organization restricted the use of these designations to plans which met certain quality standards.[111]

As may be expected in view of the role played by medical practicioners, the establishment and development of Blue Shield was strongly influenced by the American Medical Association. This organization, having endorsed medical service plans in principle, set up a Council on Medical Service and Public Relations in 1943 to review and approve any state or local plans. Renamed the Council on Medical Service in 1946, it devised a series of standards which the plans had to meet to gain AMA approval. Among other things, these standards required that all plans have the approval of the appropriate state and local medical societies, that free choice of physician and patient be unimpaired, that all communication between them remain

[108] Fred J. Cook, op. cit., p. 202.

[109] John W. Castellucci, "The Blue Shield Medical Care Plans," in Fundamentals of Voluntary Health Care, ed. by George B. DeHuszar, p. 388.

[110] Somers and Somers, op. cit., p. 318.

[111] Blue Shield, A Helping Hand, p. 7.

confidential, and that the plans be organized for public service. In addition, the Council required the medical societies to assume responsibility for the quality of the services provided.[112] In 1954, the AMA discontinued these standards for fear of government prosecution under the laws covering restraint of trade, but they had already been adopted by the plans themselves.[113]

In 1946, at the direction of the AMA House of Delegates, another organization, Associated Medical Care Plans, Inc., was established to develop a national health program and coordinate the independent locally administered plans. The organization was renamed the Blue Shield Medical Care Plans in 1950 and was again renamed the National Association of Blue Shield Plans (NABSP) in 1959.[114] Like the Blue Cross Association, the NABSP performs many research, data collection and administrative tasks for the member plans.[115]

As suggested earlier, one of the reasons for the acceptance which the medical profession gave to the medical service plans had been the fear of compulsory health insurance and "socialized medicine." One author has commented:

> Blue Shield has, from the beginning, had a largely defensive coloration. The threats of public health insurance and lay sponsored prepayment plans have been major stimuli to most Blue Shield developments. It has never assumed an unqualified commitment to service benefits.[116]

The lack of wholehearted commitment by the medical profession can be illustrated by its attitude toward paid-in-full service benefits. The typical Blue Shield plan provides that, for those subscribers whose annual income falls below certain limits, the physician must accept the payments specified in the contractual benefit schedule as his full fee. The income limits set by most plans are low (as little as $4,000 for an individual subscriber under one New York plan) and for those above this limit, Blue Shield protection may mean very little additional coverage.[117] In response to consumer demands, several plans in 1957 and 1958 tried to raise their income limits. The Michigan plan, for example, faced with competition for automobile industry business by a prepaid group practice plan sponsored by the United Auto Workers, tried to raise the limit to $7,500. A survey taken by the Michigan State Medical Society had found that the consumers wanted and were willing to pay

---

[112]Somers and Somers, op. cit., p. 319.

[113]Ibid. p. 320.

[114]John W. Castellucci, op. cit., p. 390.

[115]Blue Shield, A Helping Hand, p. 12.

[116]Somers and Somers, op. cit., p. 317.

[117]Ibid., p. 329.

for comprehensive coverage of all medical costs and that most physicians thought Blue Shield limits should be set at $7,500. Although this increase had been approved by the state medical society, dissident doctors, after a lengthy battle, managed to reduce the limit to $6,500, thus making widespread comprehensive coverage impossible. In another example, the Connecticut State Medical Society, bitterly opposing a Blue Shield policy with a high income ceiling, managed to lower the limit from $7,500 to $5,000 and forced the resignation of the plan's president.[118]

Growth

At the end of 1969, there were 74 Blue Shield plans in operation in the United States, Canada and Puerto Rico. During the previous 20 years, the number of plans varied from 65 to 76 as the plans grew and were consolidated.[119] Underwritten enrollment at the end of 1969 was 63,471,684, up from 60,371,013 in 1968 and 57,151,382 the previous year.[120] Blue Shield growth rates parallel those of Blue Cross, not unexpectedly since the two types of plans frequently use common administrative and marketing structures.[121] In addition to the underwritten enrollment shown above, at the end of 1969, Blue Shield served 16,121,361 nonunderwritten persons, chiefly recipients of Medicare and Medicaid. Coverage for these people represent a significant attempt to assist those who would never before have had medical protection.[122]

Organization and Methods of Operation

National Organization. Like Blue Cross, the Blue Shield plans are members of a nationwide organization, the National Association of Blue Shield Plans (NABSP). This body was established in 1946 at the direction of the AMA and is the coordinator of the 74 member plans. The 33 members of its board of directors, most of whom are physicians, are responsible for setting Blue Shield's national policies but do not control the member plans or design contracts. The principal task of the NABSP is to hold meetings to discuss accounting procedures, claim processing techniques, record keeping, data collection, enrollment methods, market research, and office management. These meetings are the plans' primary means of sharing experiences and developing standardized operating procedures.

In addition to acting as a clearing house for the interchange of ideas, the Association is Blue Shield's national public relations spokesman and is responsible for setting minimum standards for plan membership. Like those applied by the AMA Council on Medical Service, the NABSP standards

---

[118]Ibid., pp. 329-332.

[119]Blue Cross and Blue Shield Fact Book, 1970, p. 13.

[120]Ibid.

[121]Somers and Somers, op. cit., p. 321.

[122]Blue Cross and Blue Shield Fact Book, 1970, pp. 14-15.

require that the plans have local physician support, that they be nonprofit organizations, that free choice of physicians be unimpaired, that they have some type of utilization review mechanism, and that normal coverage must meet medical costs for the majority of the subscribers. The NABSP also imposes certain reporting and financial restrictions on the plans.[123] The administration and functions of the national organization are financed through dues levied on the individual plans in proportion to their membership.[124]

State and Local Plans. The state and local plans, being autonomous of the NABSP, set their own policies, write their own subscriber contracts, and negotiate and administer agreements with local participating physicians. While the internal organizations of each plan differ, all have an unpaid board of directors responsible for setting local policy, committees for the supervision and control of medical matters and a paid administrative staff which handles actuarial and routine corporate functions.

Some plans share the same corporate structures as Blue Cross, while others are separate corporations controlled directly by the local medical societies. Most plans are administratively associated with the Blue Cross plans operating in the same areas. The relationship between the two types of plans is so close, in fact, that frequently the membership of the separate boards of directors includes the same individuals, and a shared staff may be responsible for sales, billing and bookkeeping.[125] When Blue Cross and Blue Shield are so closely interrelated, with Blue Cross doing most of the administrative operating work, it is difficult to understand why Blue Shield's operating expenses are relatively so much greater than those incurred by Blue Cross.[126] In 1969, Blue Shield member plans' operating expenses were 11.0 per cent of earned subscription income while Blue Cross member plans spent only 5.8 per cent.[127] All Blue Cross and Blue Shield plans and the national organizations are computer linked through a telecommunications center located in the Blue Cross Association headquarters in Chicago. This network, approximately 39,000 miles long, permits rapid communications between the plans and is useful in the processing of inter-territory claims.[128]

The Blue Shield/Physician Relationship. The relationship between Blue Shield plans and the local physicians is interesting since unlike closed panel prepayment plans, Blue Shield stresses the consumer's free choice of any physician willing to provide the services he wants. Because the doctors are free to sign or to refuse to sign the Blue Shield participation contract,

---

[123] Blue Shield, A Helping Hand, pp. 12-13.

[124] John W. Castellucci, op. cit., p. 393.

[125] Somers and Somers, op. cit., p. 324.

[126] Ibid., p. 327.

[127] Blue Cross and Blue Shield Fact Book, 1970, pp. 6, 18.

[128] Ibid., p. 12.

the plans frequently pay for the services rendered by nonparticipating physicians. The distinction between participation and nonparticipation is important since the participating doctor agrees to accept the schedule of fees if the subscriber's income is below certain limits, while the nonparticipant is free to charge anything he wishes. Another distinction is that a participant agrees to abide by the Blue Shield corporate rules and to submit any disputes to arbitration while a nonparticipant obviously need not do so. Blue Shield's processing of claims differs also since payment is made directly to a participating doctor and directly to the patient if he is treated by a nonparticipant. Since the payment made by Blue Shield is the same in either case, it would, at first, seem that there is no reason for physicians to participate, but most doctors have found participation to be good business. Participating doctors need not worry about collection of their fees while nonparticipants do not have the same assurance that they will be paid by their patients.[129]

Coverage

The largest Blue Shield plan in the United States is the Greater New York plan, otherwise known as the United Medical Service of New York. Like most Blue Shield plans, United Medical Service offers a mixture of pre-payment service and indemnity protection. Three plans are offered which feature substantially the same types of coverage but with different maximum benefit allowances. Two of the three plans offer a paid-in-full service provision and the third is a pure indemnity plan.

The three plans, known as the Two Star, Three Star and Executive Indemnity or Four Star plans offer routine care benefits to cover the physician's visits to the hospital up to a maximum of either 201 or 365 days. Intensive care benefits are provided for an additional five days if the illness issufficiently severe to warrant such care. Care of premature infants weighing five pounds or less is provided for a maximum of five weeks. Thirty additional days of care are covered if the subscriber is afflicted with pulmonary tuberculosis or a nervous or mental condition or requires physical therapy and rehabilitation. Complications of pregnancy are covered under the same fee schedule as routine care. One in-hospital consultation in each specialty is provided for which the maximum fee payment varies from $20.00 to $50.00 depending on the plan. Assisting surgeon's services are covered if they were required in the performance of a regular Blue Shield procedure for which an allowance of $100.00 or more is provided and if no suitable assisting surgeon employed by the hospital is available. The plans also provide allowances for obstetrical and surgical-maternity services in connection with a delivery, miscarriage or abortion provided conception took place while the subscriber was covered by Blue Shield.

In addition to the in-hospital services mentioned above, Blue Shield provides up to 21 days of home care in any contract year for certain specified illnesses if hospitalization is not feasible. Other covered treatment outside the hospital includes an allowance for visiting nurse service by an accredited agency and emergency first aid rendered by a physician within 24 hours after injury. The plans also provide allowances for surgery and treatment of

---

[129]
Somers and Somers, op. cit., pp. 325-326.

fractures and dislocations performed in a hospital, doctor's office or any other location and for diagnostic services, including X-Rays and laboratory tests, for which a $20.00 deductible is imposed. A summary of the benefit allowances for selected items under each of the three plans appears in Table II - 2.

All three plans apply the same exclusions. These include, but are not limited to, Workmen's Compensation cases, care paid for under a federal, state or local law, services by practitioners other than those licensed to provide them, services included in the hospital's bill, cosmetic surgery, routine care of the newborn, routine eye examinations and routine care of teeth and feet.

The Two Star and Three Star plans provide paid-in-full service benefits to those who are treated by a participating physician and whose annual income do not exceed certain limits. The maximums under the Two Star plan are $4,000.00 under an individual contract or $7,000.00 under a family contract. The limits under the Three Star plan are $6,000.00 and $8,500.00 respectively. For those whose incomes exceed these limits, the plans are primarily indemnity policies.

The subscription rates for individual contract holders under the Two Star plan are $1.75 per month when enrolled in a group or $8.40 per quarter when not a participant in a group plan. The corresponding rates for family contract holders are $6.00 per month and $21.72 per quarter respectively. The rates for individuals holding Three Star certificates are $2.50 per month with group enrollment or a nongroup rate of $10.08 per quarter and the corresponding family contract rates are $7.50 per month and $26.52 per quarter. Executive Indemnity or Four Star rates are $2.80 per month and $11.76 per quarter for individual contract holders and $8.60 per month and $31.68 per quarter for those holding family contracts.[130]

Advantages

Blue Shield shares with health insurance the features of free choice of physician and minimum interference with the doctor-patient relationship. These features benefit both the subscriber and the physician since the selection of any qualified practitioner willing to provide treatment is unimpaired and, once a selection has been made, a close relationship of trust and confidence can be set up. This is frequently not true of closed panel practice as the patient may not be assured of receiving the services of the physician he has selected.

In addition to these shared advantages, Blue Shield, unlike health insurance, has had a marked influence in raising the quality of the medical care received by its subscribers. All Blue Shield plans exclude from reimbursement services rendered by nonmedical practitioners or practitioners whose treatment exceeded the limits of their licenses. To be assured that all services will be covered, a patient must be treated by a qualified physician, thereby reducing the chance of receiving substandard care.

---

[130]Rates for the three Blue Shield plans were quoted in the following pamphlets, all published by United Medical Service, Inc., 1971: The New Two Star Better Benefits Plan, The New Three Star Better Benefits Plan, and The New Executive Indemnity Plan.

TABLE I - 2

COMPARISON OF BLUE SHIELD BENEFIT SCHEDULES

Selected Benefits

	Two Star		Three Star		Executive Indemnity	
Days of Routine Care-In-Hospital	201		365		365	
Allowance Per Day - Doctor's Visits	1st - 7th	$7.00	1st	$15.00	1st	$25.00
	8th-14th	6.00	2nd	10.00	2nd- 7th	12.00
			3rd- 7th	7.50	8th-70th	10.00
			8th-21st	7.00	71st-365th	7.00
			22nd-365th	6.00		
Intensive Care Allowance - Up to Five Additional days	$13.00		$15.00		$20.00	
In-Hospital Consultation Including Full Examination and Report	20.00		35.00		50.00	
Premature Infants	100.00		125.00		175.00	
Surgical Allowances for Selected Treatments						
Brain	500.00		750.00		1,500.00	
Heart	500.00		750.00		1,500.00	
Lung	500.00		550.00		1,000.00	
Eye (Cateract Extraction)	275.00		425.00		575.00	
Obstetric Service - Delivery	100.00		150.00		250.00	
Anesthesia - 20% of Medical or Surgical Fee. Minimum payment.	20.00		25.00		35.00	
Assisting Surgeon's Services	50.00		150.00		300.00	

Sources: United Medical Service, The New Two Star Better Benefits Plan, New York:
United Medical Service, Inc. 1971.
United Medical Serfice, The New Three Star Better Benefits Plan, New York:
United Medical Service, Inc., 1971.
United Medical Service, The New Executive Indemnity Plan, New York:
United Medical Service, Inc., 1971.

Note: All dollar amounts shown above are maximum limits except where noted.

Disadvantages

Among the most frequently voiced complaints about Blue Shield is the fact that coverage, except for the poor, is far from comprehensive.[131] Those plans offering paid-in-full service benefits usually set the income limit for qualification so low that most subscribers do not qualify. For middle-income contract holders, a Blue Shield policy alone is totally inadequate protection against the high cost of physicians' services. The critics frequently voice the complaint that, "unless one was virtually impoverished ..., the physician was permitted to charge any fee he saw fit in addition to his Blue Shield allotment, a provision that, in practice in many areas, has largely vitiated any benefit that may be derived from a Blue Shield policy."[132] The United Medical Service Two Star Plan, for example, provides an allowance of only $500.00 for the excision of a cyst from the brain, but a highly qualified surgeon may charge several times that amount for this procedure.[133]

A second disadvantage, confusion about whether or not an illness is covered, is common to both Blue Shield and health insurance. Both types of protection cover pre-existing conditions only after a waiting period, but since under group enrollment, no medical examination is usually required, there may be doubt about the validity of a claim submitted by a newly enrolled subscriber. A physician rendering treatment to a Blue Shield contract holder normally would not know if his policy was in force early enough to cover some conditions, and a patient, believing his ailments are covered by his Blue Shield contract, may find himself without protection.[134]

Finally, like Blue Cross, Blue Shield has been criticized for its failure to respond to the needs of the public. The historic domination and control of the plans by organized medicine has led to the complaint. that consumer demands may be ignored. The bitter fights in Michigan and Connecticut can be cited as examples. In both cases, the local medical societies were able to prevent the plans from raising their income limitations on service benefits despite the desires of the subscribers.

Prepayment Service Plans in Perspective

The prepayment service plans, notwithstanding their limitations, represented a significant advance from cash-indemnity health insurance. As the first attempts to provide comprehensive health benefits to at least part of the population, they were a radical departure from the usual insurance philosophy that protection should be offered only against large, infrequent, and fortuitous health hazards. As pioneers of the prepayment concept, they paved the way for other types of organizations that come closer to making comprehensive coverage a reality.

---

[131] Cook, loc. cit.

[132] Ibid., p. 202.

[133] Ibid., p. 217.

[134] Franz Goldmann, op. cit., p. 125.

36

Introduction

The inadequacies of cash-indemnity health insurance and the prepay-ment service plans resulted in a critical reevaluation of the health care delivery system by the public, organized labor, and certain members of the medical profession. Both insurance and the service plans are financial mechanisms oriented toward private, fee-for-service, solo-practice and are divorced for the actual delivery of health care. Both assumed that if sufficient funds were made available, consumers could buy any health services they needed and that the predominant form of organization could supply them. With the growing complexity of medical treatments, however, the need for a reorganization of the delivery system became apparent and large scale group medical practice came into being.[135]

Group Practice Plans - Overview

Definition. Group practice has been defined in a study by McNamara and Todd as: "The application of medical services by three or more physicians formally organized to provide medical care, consultation, diagnosis and/or treatment through the joint use of equipment and personnel and with the income from medical practice distributed in accordance with methods previously determined by members of the group."[136] In March 1969, a total of 6,371 of the organizations listed in the records of the American Medical Association met these criteria.[137]

Specialty and Size. Group practice organizations may be categorized as either single specialty, general practice or multi-specialty. Of the groups surveyed in the 1970 study, 3,169 were single specialty, 784 were engaged exclusively in general practice and 2,418 were multi-specialty.[138] Although the average size of all group practice plans responding to the survey was 6.3 physicians, they ranged in size from three to more than 850. The average size of the single specialty groups was 4.1 physicians while general practice groups averaged 3.4 physicians. Multi-specialty groups averaged 10.1 physicians but this number is biased upward by the inclusion of the two giant multi-specialty groups, New York's Health Insurance Plan and the Kaiser-Permanente organization which operates on the West Coast.[139]

---

[135] C.C. Cutting, Features of Prepaid Group Practice, (Oakland, Calif.: Kaiser/Permanente Medical Care Program, 1970), p. 3.

[136] M.E. McNamara and C. Todd, "A Survey of Group Practice in the United States, 1969," American Journal of Public Health, Vol. 60, (July 1970), p. 1304

[137] Ibid., p. 1303.

[138] Ibid.

[139] Ibid., p. 1306.

Most of the single specialty and general practice groups surveyed had from three to five physicians each. Approximately 86.4 per cent of the single specialty groups and 97.7 per cent of the general practice groups fell into this size category. Of the multi-specialty groups, 45.2 per cent reported more than five physicians.[140]

Of the 40,093 physicians practicing in the groups surveyed, 7,162 were general practitioners, 6,458 practiced internal medicine, 3,708 were general surgeons, 3,499 were radiologists and 3,211 were obstetricians or gynecologists.[141] These specialists comprised 60.0 per cent of the total and, with the exception of radiologists, most commonly practiced in multi-specialty groups.

Prepayment. Of all responding groups, the survey identified 396 which provided care at least partially on a prepaid basis. Of these, 58.6 per cent were multi-specialty groups.[142] Geographically, most were located in the Middle Atlantic, South Atlantic or Pacific regions with California, New York and Washington having the heaviest concentration. Like the other groups, the prepaid groups are organized as single-ownerships, partnerships, corporations, associations or foundations. The survey found that partnerships and corporations are the most common organizational forms and that the percentage of each is approximately the same for the prepaid organizations as for all groups.[143]

Prepaid Group Practice

Group practice, by itself, is only part of the reorganization taking place in the American health care delivery system. To make health care affordable, some form of budgeting technique is needed. By adding prepayment to group practice, this requirement is satisfied. It is easy to understand, therefore, why this form of organization is increasingly being singled out as the solution to the contemporary health care delivery crisis.[144]

Definition. Prepaid group practice is the combination of a prepayment financing plan with an administrative structure that will deliver medical services to a defined population.[145] It is usually characterized by its guarantee that comprehensive services will be available when needed, by the

---

[140]Ibid., p. 1305.

[141]Ibid., p. 1308.

[142]Ibid., p. 1309.

[143]Ibid., p. 1310.

[144]See for example L.F. Swan, "Group Approach to Medical Care," Nursing Outlook, (January 1970, p. 57, D.M. Landay, "Trends in Negotiated Health Plans; Broader Coverage, Higher Quality Care," p. 7 and S.R. Garfield, "The Delivery of Medical Care," Scientific American, Vol. 222, (April 1970), p. 15.

[145]I.G. Greenberg and M.L. Rodburg, "The Role of Prepaid Group Practice in Relieving the Medical Care Crisis," Harvard Law Review, Vol. 84, (February 1971), p. 901.

prepayment of these services by subscribers on the basis of fixed periodic payments, by the use of physicians practicing in multi-specialty groups and the compensation of physicians through a method other than fee-for-service.

The availability of services when needed is usually guaranteed through direct ownership or lease of facilities and through contractual arrangements with groups of physicians.[146] Most of the comprehensive plans provide a compensation arrangement to cover services rendered by nonplan physicians if these services are not available within the plan. The value of this provision becomes evident when the services of a particular specialist are required or if an accident or illness strikes while the subscriber is temporarily away from the area served by the plan.[147] As an alternative to insurance prepayment allows for the budgeting of most medical expenses whether or not they are large, infrequent or fortuitous. Subscribers usually pay the plans directly on a monthly, quarterly or annual basis or indirectly through payroll deductions made by their employers.[148]

Physician Compensation. The methods of compensating physicians under a prepaid group practice plan deserve particular mention because they have been at the root of organized medicine's opposition to any new form of health care delivery system. The prepaid group practice plans pay their physicians on either a fixed salary or a capitation basis. Under a capitation arrangement, the group is paid a fixed sum per subscriber and is then free to determine each physician's share of the pooled funds. While the sharing agreements vary among the plans from the simple to the complex, all such arrangements share the common characteristic that there is little or no direct relationship between the compensation received by the physician and the quantity of services which he renders.[149]

Medical Opposition. Official medical opposition to salary and capitation arrangements has softened considerably in the last several decades but still remains a potent force in inhibiting the growth of the prepayment plans. Voicing the misgivings of organized medicine, Dr. Milford O. Rouse, a past president of the AMA, has said:

> The fact ... remains that most physicians providing
> patient care respond better to the incentive of fee-
> for-service than they do to salary. Payment for the
> service rendered stimulates the professional by

---

[146] Ibid., p. 902.

[147] Health Insurance Plan of Greater New York (H.I.P.) for example, provides up to $350.00 for treatment outside its service area. Report of the President, Twenty-Fourth Annual Meeting, Health Insurance Plan of Greater New York, May 4, 1971, p. 8 (hereinafter referred to as H.I.P. Annual Report, 1970).

[148] Greenberg and Rodburg, op. cit., p. 903.

[149] Ibid., p. 907.

providing a reward related to the service. Salary
too often invites lethargy and reduces the level
of performance.[150]

Clearly there are pros and cons to this argument. The advocates of
fee-for-service compensation claim that salary or capitation destroys the
close relationship between physician and patient while the supporters of
prepaid group practice assert that by removing the direct relationship between
compensation and service, the financial barriers to quality care are eliminated
and that the physician can concentrate on medical rather than administrative
matters.

Voluntary Enrollment. Many prepaid group practice plans feature
voluntary enrollment. Typically this involves the requirement that prior
to deciding to subscribe to a prepaid group practice plan, a potential
enrollee must be offered an alternative plan, usually one featuring cash
indemnity. Once having enrolled, the subscriber is offered the option to
change to the alternative plan after a specified time interval. Known as
dual choice, the prepaid group plan advocates believe this arrangement is
instrumental in reducing the amount of consumer dissatisfaction.[151]

Sponsorship

Plans incorporating group practice can be classified as either
physician or consumer sponsored.[152] The latter classification includes consumer cooperatives such as Group Health Association of Washington, D. C. and
Group Health Cooperative of Puget Sound in Washington State, community plans
typified by Kaiser-Permanente on the West Coast and the Health Insurance Plan
of Greater New York (HIP) and industry or union plans such as Community Health
Association of Detroit, Michigan and the United Mine Workers Welfare and
Retirement Fund.

Similarities. Consumer and physician sponsored group practice plans
share certain common characteristics. Both types of plans, with the exception
of the two giant community plans and a few union plans, place little emphasis
on health education or on the evaluation of the care provided in their clinics.
Both types of plans perceive treatment of diseases as their prime function and
assume that all services rendered by their participating physicians meet the
standards expected of a professional. In addition, both types of plans, due
to common origins and shared consumer demands, have similar basic coverage.
The majority of the group plans of either type can be traced historically to
clinics established before World War I to serve industrial workers. Many of
today's plans were shaped by the thinking of the service oriented physicians
who founded these clinics.[153]

---

[150]M.O. Rouse, "Organizing and Delivering Health Care, Part 4," Journal of the
American Medical Association, Vol. 202, (Nov. 27, 1967), p. 901.

[151]Greenberg and Rodburg, op. cit., p. 908.

[152]J.L. Schwartz, "Consumer Sponsorship and Physician Sponsorship of Prepaid
Group Health Plans: Some Similarities and Differences," American Journal
of Public Health, Vol. 55, (January 1965), p. 94.

[153]Ibid., pp. 95-96.

Differences. There are a number of significant differences between the two types of plans which can be traced directly to their sponsorship. Enrollment criteria, for example, differ markedly since most physician sponsored plans enroll groups only while consumer plans also accept individuals subject to a medical review or examination. The two types of plans also differ somewhat in the amount of benefits offered beyond the minimum office, hospital or home treatment for sickness or accidents, diagnostic services and maternity care. Consumer sponsored plans frequently provide for eye examinations, home nursing, dental care or the services of psychologists while physician sponsored plans rarely include these benefits. Another difference is that complaint mechanisms, which are usually well developed in consumer plans, are almost nonexistent in physician plans. The consumer plans have always stressed their procedures for handling grievances while the physician plans have emphasized the professionalism and collected skills of their doctors. Finally, the two types of plans differ in their profit objectives. Consumer plans are usually nonprofit while physician plans are not.[154]

The Ross-Loos Medical Group - A Physician Sponsored Plan

The Ross-Loos Medical Group, started in 1929 by Doctors Ronald Ross and Clifford Loos to provide low-cost prepaid medical services to some 400 employees of the Los Angeles Water and Supply Department, is the oldest and largest active physician-controlled plan.[155] With this modest enrollment and a staff consisting of the two partners and one hired physician, the plan started to grow to the point that, today, it has an enrollment of approximately 120,000 including 36,000 individual subscribers and has a staff of 45 partners and 75 other full-time doctors.[156] While the plan emphasizes group enrollment, the number of individual enrollees attests to the fact that guaranteed lifetime coverage, even though at a higher subscription rate than the group rate, is attractive to a great many people.

The group is organized as a partnership with an elected executive committee and an executive partner who serves as administrator. Partners are selected on the basis of age, location and personal qualifications. In addition to medical personnel, the plan has a staff of laymen responsible for all administrative functions such as accounting, subscriber relations, purchasing and building operations.

All partners are on a drawing account and receive a share of the profits. General staff members are given a salary and since they are not permitted to engage in private practice, they are given a 50 per cent share of the fees charged those who are not members of the prepayment plan. Approximately six per cent of those treated are charged on a fee-for-service basis.

---

[154] Ibid., pp. 96-98.

[155] Somers and Somers, op. cit., p. 357.

[156] Letter from M. W. Shearer, Assistant Administrator, Ross-Loos Medical Group, November 15, 1971.

The Group operates an outpatient clinic in Los Angeles and a number of branches in outlying suburbs.[157] All branch physicians share in any savings resulting from underrunning the budget established by the plan.[158]

The arrangement which the plan has set up to deal with its group subscribers is one of its most unique organizational features. Whenever a large group of subscribers enrolls in the plan, a committee is selected to negotiate the details of the contract and to serve as a medium for the processing of complaints and suggestions. The committee helps ease tensions and enables the plan to become sensitive to the needs of consumers.[159]

The staff of the Ross-Loos Group represents a number of medical specialties including allergy, anesthesiology, dermatology, general medicine, general surgery, internal medicine, neurology, neurosurgery, obstetrics, opthomology, orthopedics, otolaryngology, optometry, pathology, pediatrics, proctology, psychology, radiology and urology.[160] All physicians are permitted to use any hospital with which they may be affiliated but most, for reasons of convenience, use their staff privileges in Queen-of-Angels Hospital. The plan did not own its own hospital, but expected to break ground for one in April 1972.[161]

Recognizing that the treatment of minor ailments is easier and less costly than the treatment of severe and complicated disorders, the plan, unlike other physician-sponsored organizations, stresses the importance of preventive care. It encourages its subscribers to have regular check-ups and to seek help when early disease symptoms appear. Consequently, the rate of physician services is higher than most plans, but the average cost per contact is lower.[162]

Coverage in the Ross-Loos plan includes comprehensive service in the doctor's office, house calls within 15 miles of the clinic or any of its branches, surgery, anesthesia, pre-and post-operative care, eye examinations, obstetrics, laboratory and X-Ray work and physiotherapy. The plan does not cover mental illness, alcoholism, self-induced abortion, drug addiction, dental care, cosmetic surgery, blood transfusions, eyeglasses or drugs. Hospitalization is provided through a supplementary mandatory hospitalization insurance sold by the group. A small charge is made for surgical care rendered to dependents of the subscriber.[163]

---

[157]Ibid.

[158]A. Deutsch, "Group Medicine, Part 2: The Ross-Loos Clinic, New York's H.I.P.," Consumer Reports, (February 1957), p. 84.

[159]Ibid., pp. 83-84. The group has also delegated responsibility for handling complaints to an individual in charge of "Special Situations." A meeting of all individuals involved in the processing of complaints is held weekly by the Administrator. Letter from M.W. Shearer, November 15, 1971.

[160]Letter from M.W. Shearer, November 15, 1971.

[161]Ibid.

[162]A. Deutsch, op. cit.,

[163]Ibid.

42

Group Health Association of Washington D. C. - A Consumer Sponsored Cooperative Plan

The Group Health Association of Washington, D. C. (GHA), a typical consumer cooperative, was chartered in 1937 as a nonprofit corporation.[164] Founded in response to pressures by government employees for an economical means of meeting medical costs, the organization grew rapidly in its first few years until further growth was hampered by opposition from the American Medical Association and by the restrictive legal climate in neighboring Virginia. The organization is important historically since it won a legal battle against the AMA in 1939 under the antitrust laws, thus it paved the way for the future growth of closed-panel, prepaid practice plans. In a precedent setting decision, the courts ruled that organized medicine could not legally prevent the plan from hiring qualified physicians or restrict the use of any hospital or other facility.[165]

Despite the legal victory, GHA remained relatively small until 1959 when the Washington Transit Workers Union enrolled 10,000 of its members. With increased size, the plan built the Labor-Management Health Center, a clinic, which later was transferred to the Transit Workers Welfare Fund.[166]

Basic coverage under the GHA plan is similar to that provided by the Ross-Loos Medical Group. Routine medical and surgical procedures are included except brain and nerve surgery, cosmetic surgery, chiropody and radiation therapy. Treatment for tuberculosis, mental diseases, drug addiction, and alcoholism are also excluded. The plan provides coverage both with and without hospitalization and offers prescribed drugs, medicines, supplies and eyeglasses at reduced cost.[167]

Policy decisions are made by a board of trustees elected by the membership. All board members serve without pay. The plan also employs a paid staff responsible for day-to-day administration.[168] Although the organization owns its own clinics, the medical staff also utilizes any available facilities in the community hospitals.[169]

The Health Insurance Plan of Greater New York - A Consumer Sponsored Community Plan

The Health Insurance Plan of Greater New York (HIP), which covered 766,315 people including approximately 55,000 Medicare recipients and 75,000

---

[164]Franz Goldmann, op. cit., p. 169.

[165]Daniel S. Hirshfield, op. cit., p. 88.

[166]Somers and Somers, op. cit., p. 349.

[167]Franz Goldmann, op. cit., p. 170.

[168]Ibid., p. 172.

[169]Ibid., p. 171.

43

Medicaid eligibles by the end of 1970, is the second largest prepaid group practice plan in the United States.[170] As such, it has influenced the thinking of those legislators who see this type of organization as an integral part of the proposed national health insurance program.[171]

The plan was organized under the direction of former New York City Mayor Fiorello LaGuardia as the solution to the health care financing problem of his municipal employees. Finding that many city workers could not remain solvent when they incurred large medical bills and that they frequently were forced to deal with loan sharks, LaGuardia appointed a panel of 16 people in April 1943, to investigate the possibility of organizing an insurance plan that could provide comprehensive coverage at reasonable cost. The panel, composed of representatives of the medical profession, consumer groups and the general public, after many months of careful deliberation, recommended that a prepaid group practice plan featuring capitation reimbursement and group enrollment be established.[172]

Two obstacles had to be overcome before such a plan could begin operating. The first, the recruiting of a medical staff, was easily surmounted. With the end of the Second World War, there were many highly qualified physicians available. Many of these physicians had served in the military in organizational structures which were very similar to prepaid group practice and, therefore, did not have the strong antipathy to this form of organization that their fee-for-service, solo-practice colleagues had. The second obstacle was much more difficult to overcome. The legal climate in New York State was inhospitable to prepaid group practice. LaGuardia's panel worked more than two years to remove the legal barriers which effectively prohibited any form of health care financing mechanism other than an indemnity or prepayment service plan from operating. After incorporation proceedings were finally completed, the plan organized 20 medical groups with 472 physicians and, on March 1, 1947, began enrolling subscribers.[173]

H.I.P. is a nonprofit corporation operating under section 9-C of the New York State Insurance Law and is regulated by the state Insurance Department, and state and city health departments and departments of social services.[174] It is governed by an unpaid board of 30 directors representing the community. The H.I.P. parent organization is an administrative body responsible for planning, research and statistics, data processing, enrollment, public relations and legal matters. Medical services are provided by

---

[170]H.I.P. Annual Report, 1970, pp. 5, 29.

[171]Ibid., p. 2.

[172]Committee for the Special Research Project in the Health Insurance Plan of Greater New York, Health and Medical Care in New York City, (Cambridge, Mass.: Harvard University Press, 1957), p. 4.

[173]Ibid., p. 4.

[174]H.I.P. Annual Report, 1970, p. 4.

30 independent medical partnerships. The plan operates a chain of 30 medical centers and ten sub-centers.[175] In 1968, it bought its first hospital, LaGuardia in Queens, and currently plans to build another in the Bronx.[176] H.I.P. and its medical groups share control of a centralized laboratory and an Emergency Service Program. The plan also operates the H.I.P. Drug Plan, a subsidiary corporation which furnishes prescription drugs through the plan's central pharmacy to those who exercised their drug plan option.[177] Most of the plan's physicians are engaged on a part-time basis and, therefore, are permitted to retain their private, fee-for-service practices.[178]

H.I.P. benefits include general medical, specialist and surgical care, obstetrics, laboratory procedures, periodic health examinations, immunizations, therapeutic services, use of blood facilities, eye refractions, prescribed nursing care and ambulance service. Emergency care for accidents or injuries outside the H.I.P. service area is covered on an indemnity basis up to $350. Since the plan does not provide for hospitalization, all subscribers are required to carry Blue Cross or equivalent indemnity coverage.

H.I.P. benefits exclude services provided under government legislation such as Workmen's Compensation, treatment for alcoholism, drug addiction, tuberculosis when the use of a sanatarium or special hospital is required, cosmetic surgery, dental service, drugs, prosthetic appliances and eyeglasses.[179] The plan has a two-step rate structure. Basic coverage at the normal premium is provided for those whose incomes fall below certain levels. Other subscribers are charged a higher premium.[180]

Advantages of Group Practice Plans
_____

Group practice plans, whether or not they involve prepayment, share a number of advantages. Because of their unique organizational characteristics, they offer their doctors, their patients and society as a whole benefits not found in the solo-practice/indemnity insurance combination.

To a physician, perhaps the greatest advantage offered by group practice is the elimination of all or most of his administrative burden, thereby allowing him to devote his full attention to treating patients. Obviously, the prime concern of a medical professional should be the practice of medicine, not the collection of fees, the purchase of equipment and supplies or the processing of voluminous paperwork. In solo-practice, on the

_____

[175]Ibid., p. 6.

[176]Ibid., p. 10.

[177]Ibid., p. 6.

[178]A. Deutsch, op. cit., p. 86.

[179]E.F. Daily, "Medical Care Under the Health Insurance Plan of Greater New York," Journal of the American Medical Association, Vol. 170, (May 16, 1959), p. 273.

[180]A. Deutsch, op. cit., p. 85.

other hand, the doctor usually must handle these details alone, or, at best, with the assistance of a nurse or a small office staff. Adding administrative responsibilities to the average physician's already heavy workload could seriously reduce his efficiency.[181]

Another advantage derived by group physicians is the intellectual stimulation gained from working with other professionals. Because many solo-practitioners live in medical isolation, they are not subject to the criticism of other physicians and, therefore, lose the opportunity to gain from their knowledge. When successful, group practice affords all participating physicians the means of learning from one another.[182]

Group doctors also enjoy the benefits of regular working hours, planned vacations and scheduled nonduty time which can be used for study and professional development. Frequently, solo practitioners find that they are so busy that they have no time for their families and private lives. Many also fear that their patients will be unattended or lost if they take time off for vacations or professional meetings and seminars.[183]

Finally, group practice relieves the physician of the fear that patients may be lost through referral to specialists. "In solo-practice, the general physician often hesitates to refer a patient to a specialist, even when he knows he is not adequately equipped to handle the case himself. There are two main reasons for this reluctance: the doctor may fear the reputation of being 'one who is always sending you to a specialist, so he is probably ignorant himself,' or he may fear the loss of the patient (and the resulting fees) to a specialist."[184] Since more than 60 per cent of all group physicians practice in multi-specialty groups, the skills needed are frequently found within the doctor's own organization.

To the patient, the primary advantage of group practice is that he enjoys better care as a result of quality control and the availability of pooled skill and equipment. All of the larger group plans and most of the smaller ones have some mechanism for insuring that the care rendered meets recognized standards, but the mere fact of working closely with one another raises quality. While a solo-practitioner may be able to hide his errors, a group physician cannot. Moreover, a kind of quality synergism takes place because ready access to all members of the group encourages uninhibited consultation whenever doubts about diagnosis or treatment arise. The combined knowledge of the group is greater than the knowledge of any single physician.[185]

---

[181]Greenberg and Rodburg, op. cit., p. 947.

[182]Raymond Munts, op. cit., p. 207.

[183]A. Deutsch, "Group Medicine, Part 3: The Kaiser Health Plan," Consumer Reports, (March 1957), p. 138.

[184]Ibid.

[185]Ibid.

The patient also reaps the benefits of the cost savings that result from the common use of staff and equipment and from group administration and purchasing. If each physician in the group had his own practice in his own facility, a great deal of needless expense would be incurred which would be passed on to the patient. Sharing buildings, administrative and nursing personnel and equipment is a more efficient use of resources than is possible in solo-practice.[186]

A further advantage to the patient is the reduction of fragmentation in the delivery system. Under group practice, most specialists are located in the same facility, thereby eliminating the constant need to travel from one physician's office to another.[187] Medical histories are usually kept in a centralized place accessible to all physicians. As a result, needless duplication of tests and X-Rays and the possibility of conflicting treatments are eliminated. Each physician knows what treatment has been rendered in the past and, therefore, can better judge what new treatment is needed.[188]

Group practice plans have a great potential for serving society as a whole because they could be democratically controlled by both the medical profession and consumer groups through representation on governing boards[189] and because they could be advantageously used to provide better medical care for the poor.[190] While a solo-practitioner is free to disregard the needs of society, a group practice plan that is democratically controlled may not be. If the controlling board contains enough consumer representation, the plan would probably be more responsive to their needs.

Besides the benefits mentioned above, group practice plans that operate on a prepayment basis share some additional advantages. Like insurance, prepayment reduces the economic barriers to health care, but unlike indemnity plans, the prepaid group practice organizations offer comprehensive coverage without deductibles or co-insurance and frequently without any additional charges.

One significant feature of prepaid group practice plans is that they can provide quality care at less cost by reducing hospitalization rates and eliminating unnecessary surgery.[191] As Fred J. Cook, a critic of the prevailing health care delivery system, states: "...in group practice, where doctors are on salary and fee is not a consideration, there are a lot less appendectomies, tonsillectomies and hysterectomies than there are in private fee

---

[186] Ibid.

[187] Deutsch, loc. cit.

[188] Greenberg and Rodburg, op. cit., pp. 900-901.

[189] E.R. Weinerman, "An Appraisal of Medical Care in Group Health Centers," American Journal of Public Health, Vol. 46, (March 1956), p. 301.

[190] L. F. Swan, op. cit. p. 57.

[191] Greenberg and Rodburg, op. cit., pp. 922-924.

practice where the decision to yank out an organ is too often based on the physicians' desire to extract some extra money from the patient."[192]   Compensating physicians by a means other than fee-for-service removes all financial incentives to hospitalize or provide undeeded treatment and, in fact, pays them to keep the patient healthy. The costs of unnecessary hospitalization or treatment reduce each physician's bonus or share of the plan's capitation funds.[193]

At first glance, the inverse relationship between the doctor's income and the number and types of treatments he renders would seem to encourage under-treatment and over-economizing. This does not seem to have occurred because of consumer pressures, peer reviews, the threat of malpractice suits, and in some plans, built-in financial incentives.[194]

Another advantage of prepaid group practice plans is their ability to plan and build facilities for the treatment of moderately complex disorders. A solo-practitioner may find that he does not have the equipment needed to treat illnesses of this complexity and that he must, therefore, send his patients to a general hospital. This, however, is a wasteful and inefficient use of highly sophisticated facilities. If he had access to an intermediate level facility, he could treat his patients at far less cost than he could in a general hospital. Since prepaid group practice plans pay the costs of all services, they generally approach this problem by building their facilities to the level of sophistication needed.[195]

Disadvantages of Group Practice Plans

Notwithstanding the numerous advantages cited above, group practice can have serious drawbacks. Most of these relate to the potentially impersonal treatment that patients may receive when they see group physicians.

Although many groups, particularly the larger ones, have taken steps to eliminate clinic-like unresponsiveness to the needs of the patient, most of the complaints which they receive concern the breakdown of the doctor/ patient relationship. It is this breakdown which has caused the misgivings of many physicians who are genuinely interested in improving the quality of health care. As one critic has stated, "Science is not enough in medical care; the rapport between patient and doctor - the patient's feeling that his doctor has a personal interest in his health - is a vital factor. This rapport is particularly important in the treatment of common ailments in which emotional and social factors play an important role, and in the treatment of such chronic disorders as heart disease, arthritis, peptic ulcers and asthma."[196]   That a close relationship is helpful in the treatment of disease

---

[192]Fred J. Cook, op. cit., p. 257.

[193]Greenberg and Rodburg, op. cit., pp. 924-925.

[194]Ibid., p. 926.

[195]Ibid., p. 927.

[196]A. Deutsch, op. cit., p. 137.

cannot be doubted, particularly in the light of the efforts expended by some of the groups to dispel the "mass medicine" stigma that has been applied to this form of organization.[197]

Size alone frequently causes dissatisfaction with group practice. Groups that are too large tend to give impersonal service, become over-departmentalized, and lose the benefits found in informal consultation.[198] Groups that are too small tend to experience excessive queuing and waiting time[199] and frequently do not have a sufficient number of specialists within their own organization to handle moderately complex treatments.

In many groups, care is provided by part-time physicians. Since these doctors have both group and private-fee patients, their attention and time is split, usually to the disadvantage of the group patient. This is especially true if their compensation by the group is in the form of a salary or a share of the capitation funds. Although many groups encourage their patients to choose a "family doctor" from among their physicians, part-timing makes this practice difficult, if not impossible. It is almost inevitable that the patient will find his chosen physician occupied with other duties when he is needed most.[200] Another size-related disadvantage of group practice is that most groups do not employ auxiliary health workers such as dentists, nutritionists or health educators.[201] Consequently, much of the potential for preventive health care is lost. Many major problems could be avoided by encouraging patients to practice good health habits.[202]

Quality Control in Prepaid Group Practice Plans

While many complaints have been lodged against group practice, there has been little criticism of the quality of the care rendered.[203] All competent group physicians are concerned that the treatment which they and their colleagues dispense should be above minimum standards but when their incomes depend on the qualifications and abilities of the other members of their group, their concern becomes a personal one. In a prepaid group practice plan, the incompetence of any member physician shows up in reduced earnings for all. Incompetence and excessive hospitalization or treatment are costly and are paid for out of the same funds that are used to pay bonuses or capitation shares.[204]

---

[197]Greenberg and Rodburg, op. cit., p. 940.

[198]E. R. Weinerman, op. cit., p. 306.

[199]G. Baehr, "Prepaid Group Practice: Its Strength and Weaknesses, and Its Future," American Journal of Public Health, Vol. 56, (November 1966),p. 1899.

[200]Weinerman, loc. cit.

[201]J. L. Schwartz, op. cit., pp. 101-102.

[202]G. Rosen, "Health Education and Preventive Medicine - 'New' Horizons in Medical Care," American Journal of Public Health, Vol. 42, (June 1952),p.693.

[203]Greenberg and Rodburg, op. cit., p. 928.

[204]Ibid.

As in all groups, quality care in prepaid group practice plans is assured by allowing only qualified physicians to become members. Most plans require their entering physicians to be board certified or board eligible. Even though there is a national shortage of doctors, the plans, by offering only a limited number of positions each year, are able to maintain their selectivity and thus can maintain their high quality standards.

The increased use of consultations is a second factor influencing the quality of care rendered in a prepaid group practice plan. Since there are no financial barriers to the free flow of ideas, plan physicians seek out the advice of specialists within the organization whenever they are in doubt about any case. It is obviously less expensive for staff specialists to give a confirming opinion than for the group to defend itself if a patient initiates a malpractice suit against a plan physician who gave a treatment without a consultation.[205]

Another factor contributing to high quality in prepaid group practice plans is the widespread use of unitary medical records. With such records, all medical histories are kept in a centralized location accessible to all plan physicians. When a doctor reviews these records, continuity of care is assured. In addition, when records are available for review by any plan physician, the doctor writing the medical history tends to use extra care to insure accuracy.[206]

Most of the larger prepaid group practice plans also maintain their quality standards through the use of peer-review mechanisms. Most often these take the form of regular meetings in which each doctor critically analyzes the performance of the others, but some plans have their physicians audited by outside doctors or, if large enough, by doctors from another branch of the same plan. Patients treated by solo-practitioners do not receive the benefits of such review mechanisms since these doctors view any attempt to criticize or rate their work with suspicion or hostility.[207]

Finally, good management of a physician's time contributes to high quality care. Prepaid group practice physicians work shorter, more regular hours than solo-practitioners and therefore suffer less from fatigue. In addition, many prepaid plans budget time for "state of the art" medical education. In the prevailing delivery system, solo-practitioners either cannot leave their offices because no other physician is available to care for their patients while they are away, or will not leave for fear of losing patients to other physicians.[208]

Dual Choice Arrangements in Prepaid Group Practice Plans

Many prepaid group practice plans have taken steps to reduce complaints about their impersonal treatment of patients and the lack of free

---

[205]Ibid., p. 929.

[206]Ibid.

[207]Ibid., pp. 930-931.

[208]Ibid., pp. 929-930.

choice of physician in closed panel arrangements. Some plans, particularly
the larger ones, have required that before group enrollment is permitted,
prospective subscribers must be offered a choice between an indemnity plan
or prepayment plan and the prepaid group practice plan. Known as "dual
choice," this type of arrangement was developed because the plan managers
felt many subscribers would object to being enrolled, as a result of collective
bargaining agreements, in plans which they did not choose. If afforded the
opportunity to select the types of plans desired from among reasonable alternatives, the subscribers should, at least in theory, be more satisfied with
their choices than they would have been otherwise.[209]

The first step in the establishment of a dual choice arrangement is
the selection of alternative plans by the leaders of the group that is seeking enrollment, usually the trustees of a union welfare fund. Descriptive
information about each alternative plan is distributed to each of the
prospective enrollees who must then apply for membership in the plans they
desire. All of the alternative plans agree, at the time of their selection
by the leaders of the enrolling group, that they will accept applicants
without restrictions. After they become members of a plan, the subscribers
are given the opportunity annually to change to an alternative plan.[210]

Studies have shown that, when the members of a group who are already
enrolled in a health plan are offered dual choice for the first time, they
usually favor the incumbent plan, but if dual choice is offered from the
beginning, the percentage choosing each type of plan is approximately even.[211]
Significantly, these studies have also shown that the reasons given for
choosing one plan over another by those offered dual choice are rarely related
to structural differences between the plans. They are, instead, influenced
by the comprehensiveness of coverage, the accessibility of physicians and
facilities, the experience of the enrollees, the cost of the coverage and by
cultural pressures. A prepaid group practice plan, for example, may be chosen
because it offers broader benefits at less cost while an indemnity plan may be
selected as a result of ties to a personal physician or for prestige
reasons.[212]

Since subscribers are given the opportunity each year to reconsider
their choices, the rate of change from one type of plan to another could
theoretically be a measure of consumer satisfaction. In reality, however,

---

[209] A. Yedidia, "Dual Choice Programs," American Journal of Public Health,
Vol. 49, (November 1959), p. 1476.

[210] Ibid.

[211] E.R. Weinerman, "Patients' Perceptions of Group Medical Care," American
Journal of Public Health, Vol. 54, (June 1964), pp. 881-882.

[212] Ibid.

studies which attempt to establish a direct relationship between satisfaction and the rate of change have been inconclusive.[213]

The Adaptability of Prepaid Group Practice
Plans to the Medicare Program

Prior to 1965, the elderly frequently found themselves without protection of any kind against the high costs of medical services. Both indemnity and prepaid group practice plans were generally unwilling to accept them as individual subscribers because they had substantially higher health risks than the rest of the population. With the advent of Medicare, however, these risks were substantially underwritten by the federal government and it became possible to enroll them at only moderately higher premiums than were paid by other subscribers.[214]

As originally conceived, organizations providing services to those covered by Medicare were to be reimbursed on the basis of 80 per cent of the reasonable cost of those services. This arrangement was easily accommodated by the indemnity plans but was inconsistent with the accounting philosophy of the prepaid group practice plans. In these organizations, each subscriber pays a portion of the total costs of the services rendered to all subscribers. The actual cost of any single treatment is difficult if not impossible to compute. Accordingly, agreements have been made with the government that provide for the payment of 80 per cent of the Medicare recipient's share of the total allowable costs of services provided to all subscribers.[215] In addition, the agreements made provision for the differences in utilization between Medicare and regular subscribers so that the aged are not subsidized by the young, and set up arrangements under which the co-insurance and deductible requirements of the Social Security Act can be satisfied.[216] While cumbersome, these agreements are workable and, therefore, permit the aged to receive care from prepaid groups.[217]

THE KAISER-PERMANENTE PLAN

Introduction

The Kaiser-Permanente Medical Care Program is a nonprofit, self-sustaining, hospital based, group practice plan featuring voluntary enrollment,

---

[213]Weinerman states that "The data on choice and change of group health services require a broad social perspective in interpretation. In large part, they reflect the pattern of the culture rather than only the mechanics of the program." Ibid., p.887.

[214]H.F. Newman, "The Impact of Medicare on Group Practice Prepayment Plans," American Journal of Public Health, Vol. 59, (April 1969), p. 630.

[215]H. West, "Group Practice Prepayment Plans in the Medicare Program," American Journal of Public Health, Vol. 59, (April 1969), p. 624.

[216]Ibid., pp. 626–628.

[217]Ibid., p. 624.

capitation prepayment, integrated health care facilities, comprehensive benefits and emphasis on preventive medical care.[218] As the largest of the community health plans in the United States, it shares many of the same characteristics as other similar organizations but, because of its size, and its unique organizational structure, it is often used as a model for the development of other closed panel plans.[219] Although not originally designed as a challenge to the conventional fee-for-service, solo-practice mode of health care delivery, it gradually evolved as the acknowledged leader in the prepaid group practice field and established a series of operating principles which other plans frequently emulate.

History

The giant Kaiser-Permanente organization had its origins in the early construction activities of Henry J. Kaiser's building company.[220] In 1933, the firm employed more than 5,000 men in the digging of a fresh water canal from the Colorado River to Los Angeles. Among the many hardships faced by these construction workers was the total absence of medical care near the digging site and sick or injured workmen sometimes had to cross more than 200 miles of desert to get to a physician. The need for more accessible medical care attracted the attention of a young physician, Dr. Sidney Garfield, who recruited a small team of doctors and, with a $2,500 investment, set up an on-site 12 bed hospital. Payment was originally made on a fee-for-service basis but the inadequacies of this method were soon apparent. As a replacement for this arrangement, an agreement was made with an insurance company whereby 15 per cent of the insurance premium would be paid directly to the hospital each month in exchange for treatment of all industrially related conditions. A voluntary supplementary plan was organized which would cover nonindustrial ailments in return for five cents per man day collected through payroll deductions. Dr. Garfield felt that quality care at a low price without charity or tax support was possible and that a large enough capital surplus could be accumulated to build more hospital facilities and buy equipment. The plan was highly successful but, in 1938, when the Colorado River Canal digging operation was completed, Kaiser closed the labor camps and Dr. Garfield returned to his private practice in Los Angeles.

Shortly after the desert operations were completed, Kaiser's construction company successfully bid on a contract to build the Grand Coulee Dam. A privately owned hospital was already in existence at the site but, in response to union dissatisfaction with its operation, Kaiser persuaded his partners to help him reorganize it. Dr. Garfield was recalled from his

---

[218]G. Williams, "Kaiser: What Is It? How Does It Work? Why Does it Work?," Modern Hospital, (February 1971), p. 76.

[219]Ibid., p. 67.

[220]Historical information taken from Kaiser Industries Corporation, The Kaiser Story (Oakland, Calif.: Kaiser Industries Corporation, 1968), pp. 55-59, and E.F. Kaiser, "One Industry's Involvement in Health Care," Journal of Medical Education, Vol. 45, (February 1970), pp. 88-90.

private practice and arrangements similar to those in the earlier plans, were made to provide low cost medical care to the construction workers and their families. The Grand Coulee plan, which stressed the principles of prepayment, multi-specialty group practice, integrated facilities and preventive medical care, became the prototype for the present organization.

In 1941, as the Grand Coulee project was nearing completion, Kaiser started building shipyards in the San Franciso Bay area. After the attack on Pearl Harbor, the company employed more than 200,000 people, far too many for the local medical facilities to handle adequately. The doctors who had been involved with the Grand Coulee project were brought in and the Permanente Foundation was organized to build, finance and staff four new hospitals in the area. Although the plan was highly successful, when the war and ship-building activity plan ended, membership dropped to a low of only 32,000. Because of personal experiences with the cost of medical care, pressure from ex-employees and a feeling that a workable solution to the health care delivery problem had been found, Kaiser decided to keep the plan in operation. Membership rose during the next two decades and by December 1970, it had grown to 2,166,305 members.[221]

As in the case of many other prepaid group practice plans, growth was not easy. The first problem was the opposition of organized medicine to closed-panel practice. Participating physicians were ostracized by local medical societies and were kept from using community hospitals. Some medical organizations, through contacts in the military induction system, even succeeded in having Kaiser's doctors procured for the Armed Forces. This opposition continued until 1959, when the American Medical Association finally approved the plan.[222]

The second major problem faced by the plan was the conflict in the relationship between medical and industrial management. Since the plan originated under the sponsorship of Henry Kaiser, it was not surprising that he and his associates assumed positions of leadership in the organization. Even after the plan was reorganized into partnerships known as Permanente Medical Groups, the participating physicians viewed Kaiser's role as lay domination. The conflict was resolved in a series of conferences at Lake Tahoe, Nevada. These meetings were used to establish an advisory council which would develop guidelines to be used in determining spheres of respon-sibility. In effect, the council recognized that patient care is a medical matter, but that industry, through its willingness to take risks and its administrative ability, could make a valuable contribution. The successful resolution of this problem has contributed greatly to allowing the plan to operate, as it does today, in Northern and Southern California, Oregon, Hawaii, Colorado and Ohio without fear of internal disintegration.[223]

---

[221] Kaiser Foundation Health Plan, Inc., and Kaiser Foundation Medical Care Program, 1970, (Oakland, Calif.: Kaiser Foundation Health Plan, Inc. and Kaiser Foundation Hospitals, Inc.) (Hereinafter referred to as Kaiser Foundation Annual Report, 1970), p. 23.

[222] G. Williams, op. cit., p. 70.

[223] Ibid., p. 71.

Organization

Kaiser-Permanente can be divided organizationally into three main structures. The first of these, the Kaiser Foundation Health Plan, is basically an administrative unit. The second structure, Kaiser Hospitals, is a functional unit responsible for the management all medical facilities. The third structure, the Permanente Medical Group, is responsible for providing physician services to the plan's subscribers.[224] These three structures are duplicated in each of the six Kaiser-Permanente regions.[225]

Kaiser Foundation Health Plan. The Kaiser Foundation Health Plan is a nonprofit corporation with a self-perpetuating board of directors. As originally organized, it had eight directors including two members of the Kaiser family, two Kaiser lawyers and four Kaiser Industries executives.[226] The current board of 12 members includes some outsiders but as of 1970 was still dominated by Kaiser executives.[227]

The responsibilities of the Health Plan are primarily administrative and include the enrollment of groups and individuals and the coordination of activities of the other two major units. It is responsible for negotiating capitation payment agreements with the medical groups.[228] In addition, it runs a research institute, a nursing school and a rehabilitation center and owns Dapite, Inc. a subsidiary which prepackages medicines under their generic names. These are sold at slightly above cost to the hospitals and medical groups.

Kaiser Hospitals. Kaiser Hospitals is a separate organization, administratively related to Health Plan. The boards of directors of these two organizations have common members and both organizations share regional offices in each of the six areas served by Kaiser-Permanente. Each regional office has its own manager, hospital administrator, health planner and controller and is responsible for central purchasing, budgeting, cost control and recruiting of nonphysician personnel. The organization does not make policy decisions or control expansion. Financial control is maintained through the use of budgets and any surplus funds are reinvested internally. All medical services performed in the hospitals are rendered by the Permanente Groups.[229]

---

[224] Greenberg and Rodburg, op. cit., p. 911.

[225] G. Williams, op. cit., p.73.

[226] Somers and Somers, op. cit., p. 350.

[227] Kaiser Foundation Annual Report 1970, p. 24.

[228] G. Williams, op. cit., pp. 71-73.

[229] Peter S. Bing, et al., Report of the National Advisory Committee on Health Manpower, Vol. II, Appendix IV, (Washington, D.C.: Government Printing Office, November 1967), p. 198.

Permanente Medical Groups. The Permanente Medical Groups are
partnerships or associations which are autonomous of each other and of the
Health Plan. The relationships of the groups and the Health Plan is
financial; the groups retain control over professional matters and control
their own rate of expansion. There are six Permanente Groups, one for each
of the regions served by the plan. Each group controls its own clinics
which are usually run by a physician specializing in internal medicine.
Surplus funds resulting from underrunning the groups' budget are distributed
to the participating physicians according to a contractual formula.[230]

Inter-Relationship of the Three Structures. Notwithstanding their
separate organizational structures, the three organizations are very closely
related. The members of each organization realize that both financial and
professional success depend upon mutual cooperation. "The strength of the
Kaiser-Permanente program lies in the hyphen and active efforts to preserve
and strengthen the hyphen."[231] Much of this strength has come from the
establishment in 1967 of the Kaiser-Permanente Committee, which is composed
of representatives from each of the units and which is responsible for
advising the various governing boards of the needs and thoughts of the
individual hospitals and medical groups.[232]

Membership

The Kaiser-Permanente Plan had 2,166,000 members in 1970, of which
about 1,800,000 are residents of California. Roughly 40 per cent of the
membership is enrolled in groups sponsored by various union welfare funds
and 42 per cent are employees of the local, state and federal governments.[233]
Although usually thought of as a blue-collar plan, less than half of the
membership falls into this category. The plan's membership is slightly
younger than the general population. Only three per cent to seven per cent
of the enrollees in each region are more than 65 years old. The plan also
serves a small number of persons whose incomes are below poverty levels under
subsidy arrangements with the Office of Economic Opportunity.[234] Most of the
recent growth of the plan has been due to increasing the numbers covered in
existing contracts and to opening new locations in the established regions.
Further growth has been hampered by the plan's limited capacity to plan,
finance, build and staff new facilities. One region has even had to close
membership to the outside public for more than two years because the existing
personnel and facilities would be inadequate to care for additional subscribers.[235]

---

[230]Ibid., p. 200.

[231]G. Williams, op. cit. p. 74.

[232]Ibid.

[233]Ibid.

[234]Ibid., p. 74-75.

[235]Ibid. p. 81.

Personnel

The plan employs the equivalent of 2,000 full and part-time physicians, of whom about two-thirds are partners in the Permanente groups.[236] New physicians become partners after a three year probationary period, during which there is a 13.6 per cent attrition rate. Once partnership status has been achieved, less than one per cent of the physicians withdraw from the organization annually.[237] All physicians applying for employment by the plan must be certified or certifiable by an American medical specialty board, must express an interest in group practice and must be undeterred by salary limitations. While Permanente salaries are comparable to the national average, they rarely reach the level attained by some specialists in private, fee-for-service practice.[238]

Kaiser-Permanente physicians are supported by approximately 14,000 allied health workers of whom about 4,000 are nurses. While the national ratio of physicians to other health workers is roughly ten to one, the plan's ratio is only seven to one.[239] This would suggest that either patients are not receiving the quality of care which they should be getting or that nurses and paramedics are being used more efficiently than in other delivery systems. The first alternative has repeatedly been proven false; care under the Kaiser-Permanente plan has consistently been proven to be of high quality.[240] The second alternative seems to be the correct one. Even though the delivery system has been organized in a very traditional manner, efforts have been made to free nurses and paramedics from their routine clerical duties, thus making better use of their specialized training.[241]

Facilities

As a hospital based plan, Kaiser-Permanente owns its own facilities. In 1970, 21 hospitals with a total of 4,280 beds and 54 clinics for ambulatory care were in operation.[242] When the plan expands into new areas, it builds its own facilities because those already in existence generally lack a unified staff and record keeping system and because control is easier when both hospitals and physicians are affiliates of the same organization. All hospitals are approved by the Joint Commission on Accreditation of Hospitals.[243]

---

[236]Ibid. p. 75.

[237]Northern California Group Rate. Bing, et al., p. 200.

[238]Williams, loc. cit.

[239]Ibid. p. 90.

[240]Peter S. Bing, op. cit., pp. 203-206.

[241]G. Williams, op. cit., p.90.

[242]Kaiser Foundation Annual Report 1970, p. 21.

[243]G. Williams, op. cit., p. 78.

Kaiser hospitals differ from the ordinary community hospitals in several important respects. They differ in construction and layout since they were designed to separate internal and external traffic flow and to handle large numbers of ambulatory patients in outpatient areas. They also operate nearer to capacity than most community hospitals since they were built to accommodate only seriously ill patients on an in-patient basis. In addition, patient turnover is faster because the average hospital stay is shorter. The medical staff continuously reviews patient lists to determine who can be sent home or to extended-care facilities.[244]

Criteria for Expansion Into New Areas

Kaiser-Permanente has developed several criteria for the selection of new locations. An area must have a minimum population base of 250,000 to 300,000 to provide the 50,000 members which the plan feels are needed to support an efficient medical center. In addition, the area must be capable of supplying one physician and seven to eight allied health workers including nurses and paramedics. The plan also estimates that 1.85 hospital beds and $130,000 in capital investment are needed for each 1,000 persons enrolled.[245] Once established, all such new locations are expected to achieve financial stability within three years. These criteria are not always rigidly adhered to. When the Northern California Region was established, for example, the plan invested only $83,000 per 1,000 enrollees.[246] It is obvious, however, that even at that rate, opening a new area is enormously expensive.

Coverage and Rates

Kaiser-Permanente health care coverage is comprehensive. The typical plan covers an unlimited number of office, clinic, or hospital visits for general, emergency or specialized care, unlimited health checkups, 111 to 365 days of hospital care at no charge except for a flat fee for maternity, all in-patient services including drugs and special nursing when prescribed by a physician and free ambulance service. In addition, the plan provides for reimbursement of up to $3,000 for medical expense incurred while travelling in any area not served by Kaiser-Permanente. Optional supplemental benefits are available to cover outpatient prescription drugs and short-term psychiatric care.[247]

Like the other prepaid group practice plans, Kaiser-Permanente does not cover all medical expenses. Tuberculosis, custodial or convalescent care,

---

[244]Ibid., pp. 78-79

[245]Daniel O. Wagster, Kaiser Foundation Health Plan: A Study in Growth, (Oakland, Calif.: Kaiser Foundation Medical Care Program, 1969), p. 8.

[246]Ibid., p. 6.

[247]See Williams, p. 80, E. K. Faltermayer, "Better Care at Less Cost Without Miracles," Fortune, (January 1970), p. 82, and Kaiser Foundation Annual Report 1970, p. 9.

drug addiction, cosmetic surgery, corrective appliances, eyeglasses and dental work are excluded. Pre-existing conditions can be covered at a higher premium.

Typical Kaiser-Permanente plans have a three-step rate structure. An individual subscriber is enrolled for $11.05 to $14.20 per month, a subscriber and his spouse for $22.10 to $28.40 per month and a family for $31.75 to $40.30 per month. In 1970, the average annual Kaiser-Permanente rates were $150.00 per member and $450.00 per family. The Oregon, Northern California and Hawaii regions charge $1.00 per office or clinic visit while there is no fee in Southern California, Ohio and Colorado. Northern California charges a fixed rate of $3.50 for each day house call and $5.00 for house calls made at night.[248]

Economies of Operation

As many studies have pointed out, one of Kaiser-Permanente's most striking features is that its rates are far lower than those of other plans offering similar coverage and that its rate of increase in premium rates is lower than the United States average. The major source of economies is control over the type of care rendered and where it is provided. For example, there is no financial incentive to hospitalize a patient who could receive adequate treatment in an out-patient clinic or doctor's office. On the contrary, such hospitalization would reduce each physician's share of the available capitation funds and, therefore, would reduce his total annual income. It should be emphasized that lower cost is not due to lower quality care, lower levels of service, or unusually good health of the subscribers. Many studies have shown that the health care received through Kaiser-Permanente is equal to or superior to that found elsewhere in the same areas. Some subscribers do use nonplan medical services occasionally and the proportion of indigents and older persons is lower than regional averages but neither of these factors is responsible for the plan's massive economies.[249] Lower costs are primarily the result of lower hospitalization rates which, in turn, result in fewer hospitals and fewer beds being needed.[250]

Additional savings are to be found through shared facilities, equipment and personnel, savings theoretically available to all group practice plans.[251] Moreover, since the plans are financially self-sufficient and do not depend on charity or government assistance, they are able to plan and build more efficient facilities and equipment than are generally found in the United States and, therefore, are able to achieve savings.

---

[248] G. Williams, *op. cit.*, p. 80.

[249] Peter S. Bing, *op. cit.*, pp. 206-7, 215-220.

[250] G. Williams, *op. cit.*, p. 84.

[251] E.W. Saward, "The Relevance of Prepaid Group Practice to the Effective Delivery of Health Services," (Paper presented at the 18th Annual Group Health Institute, Saulte Ste. Marie, Ontario, Canada, June 18, 1969), pp. 10, 16.

Advantages and Disadvantages

Kaiser-Permanente, like other prepaid group practice plans, eliminates the financial barriers to care, and offers a wide range of physician skills and easy access to the health care system. In addition, it features a well developed quality control mechanism, good record management and low hospitalization rates. It offers physicians all of the advantages of prepaid group practice and gives added financial incentives for efficiency.[252]

The plan also has a number of deficiencies, the most important of which is the potential breakdown of the physician-patient relationship.[253] This is the most commonly voiced complaint about the plan and one which Kaiser-Permanente has taken steps to correct. The plan attempts to get subscribers to choose a "family doctor" from among the group's physicians, schedules time for "squeeze in" appointments and operates a central appointment system so that patients can see the physicians they prefer.[254]

Other disadvantages include lack of adequate community representation on the boards of directors,[255] some inefficiences in the use of facilities and personnel[256] and the lack of priority systems for the treatment of "sick, early sick, worried well and well" subscribers.[257] This last deficiency, the result of removing the financial barriers of health care, is partially overcome through computerized multiphasic screening.[258]

HEALTH CARE DELIVERY AND FINANCING SYSTEMS -
SUMMARY AND CONCLUSIONS

Review of Organizational Forms

Comprehensive protection against the costs of health care, though long desired, is a relatively recent development. Little more than a hundred years ago, there was no mechanisms other than "passing the hat" which could help sick or injured people defray medical expenses. In the latter half of the 19th century, fraternal or mutual aid plans were organized by employers, fraternal organizations or consumer groups. These plans, funded through

---

[252] E. K. Faltermayer, op. cit., pp. 82-83.

[253] G. Williams, op. cit., p. 86.

[254] Ibid., p. 85.

[255] A. Deutsch, op. cit., p. 136.

[256] Bing, loc. cit.

[257] S. R. Garfield, op. cit., p. 19.

[258] Ibid., p. 20.

regular membership contributions, sometimes were directly involved in the actual provision of health services but most frequently provided coverage through cash indemnity payments. At about the same time, some union health and welfare funds were established but their impact on the health care delivery system was minor until the Second World War.

From an organizational viewpoint, the most significant events shaping the contemporary health care delivery system occurred in the first half of this century. Although casualty insurance covering some hospital expenses was already in existence, surgical benefits did not appear until 1903. Seven years later, the first group policies were written and the first medical expense insurance was introduced. In 1929, with health insurance well established, two new types of organizations were developed. The first of these was the Baylor University agreement which later became known as Blue Cross. A prepayment service plan, its members received the services provided in the enrollment agreement rather than cash indemnities. The second organizational development was the establishment of the Ross-Loos Medical Group which, today, is the oldest and largest active physician-sponsored prepaid group practice plan. As contrasted with health insurance and the prepayment service plans, both of which are purely financing mechanisms, this organization actually provided medical services for its subscribers. The Ross-Loos experience paved the way for the establishment in the next two decades of the two giant community-sponsored prepaid group practice plans, the Health Insurance Plan of Greater New York and the Kaiser-Permanente Medical Care Program. These plans, particularly the latter, have been used as models in recent legislative proposals for a national health insurance program.

Health insurance, the most common form of protection against the financial hazards of illness or accidental injury, provides cash benefits to the insured. Designed to cover large, infrequent and fortuitous risks, it offers policyholders freedom from the fear that a sudden illness could result in financial catastrophe. It benefits the hospitals and medical profession by minimizing the risk of financial loss due to inability of the patient to pay for the services rendered. It removes the financial barriers to treatment and, at the same time, permits "free choice" of physician by the policyholder. Health insurance does, however, have some serious deficiencies. Since small claims and expenses for preventive care are generally excluded and ceilings are placed on those treatments that are covered, the policyholder still must pay a large portion of his medical expenses. Health insurance has few controls over fees or over hospitalization rates because it is divorced from the actual delivery of care. It tends to be inflationary since many physicians feel justified in charging their insured patients higher fees other than patients. The rising cost of medical care forces policyholders to purchase additional coverage but when they do, medical fees rise still further. Finally, health insurance is susceptible to abuses by unscrupulous physicians who may perform needless surgery purely to obtain a higher fee.

The prepayment service plans, typified by Blue Cross and Blue Shield, contract with hospitals and physicians to provide certain specified services to their subscribers. These providers are paid directly by the plans rather than by their patients. The plans share the advantages and disadvantages of health insurance but have additional drawbacks which result from their loosely knit organizational structures and historic domination by the medical and hospital professions. The plans were originally conceived as autonomous local or regional organizations and consequently failed to develope workable reciprocity agreements. A subscriber from one area may find that his coverage is inadequate if he requires treatment while in another area. A second disadvantage is that the plans failed to provide adequate consumer representation on their boards of directors and, therefore, could easily ignore the needs and desires of the public.

The greatest potential for reforming the traditional health care delivery system lies in the prepaid group practice plans, especially those patterned after the Kaiser-Permanente model. Analysis of these plans has shown that high quality medical care can be rendered at less cost than in the traditional system. The administrative burdens of the physicians have been reduced, group organization is conducive to professional development, workable quality control mechanisms have been introduced, the potential for greater use of preventive health techniques and for greater democratic control is enhanced, and good control of hospitalization rates and the sharing of staff and equipment has resulted in lower costs.

Barriers to the Growth of Prepaid Group Practice

Despite their appeal, the prepaid group practice plans have not grown as rapidly as might have been expected. One wonders why, in view of their many advantages, the plans have been unable to expand their membership to more than a few million people, most of whom live in New York or on the West Coast. Those who have studied their development have advanced a number of reasons for their slow growth, most of which are related to the opposition of the medical profession, internal organizational problems, and environmental factors.

Medical Opposition. One of the earliest factors hindering the growth of prepaid group practice plans was the hostility of organized medicine. This hostility has lessened in the last decade but is still instrumental in maintaining the plans' undesirable "impersonal mass medicine" image.[259] Furthermore, local medical societies still look unfavorably upon group doctors. "The power or organized medical opposition (now lessening) can be accurately assessed only by those who understand the economic and professional handicaps faced by the practicing physician who is denied membership in the medical society and is ostracized by his local colleagues."[260]

Medical opposition to closed panel practice sometimes stems from purely mercenary sources. Some solo-practitioners fear that they would be

---

[259]"The apprehensiveness of the medical profession toward prepaid group practice is crucial, and probably stems from a fear that it is only the beginning of full-fledged socialized medicine. Opposition from organized medicine may have played a significant role in shaping an undesirable image of group practice in the eyes of the public." R. L. Bashshur, C.A. Metzner and C. Worden, "Consumer Satisfaction With Group Practice, The CHA Case," American Journal of Public Health, Vol. 57, (November 1967), p. 1991.

[260]Deutsch, loc. cit.

unable to compete on equal terms with massive organizations which have large financial resources while others claim that prepaid group practice could lead to socialized medicine.[261] There are many physicians, however, who resist closed panel practice on purely ethical grounds. They contend that a patient should be free to choose the services of any physician he desires. While recognizing that, even in fee-for-service arrangements, the patient's choice may be limited by reason of economics, accessibility or lack of knowledge, they feel that further impediments would deprive him of his democratic rights.[262]

Another factor preventing medical endorsement of prepaid group practice plans is the strong conservatism of the medical profession. As guardians of public health, physicians have an obligation to view all new developments in the health field with skepticism. Frequently, however, this skepticism leads to resistance to new delivery systems that are both practical and necessary.[263]

Legal Barriers. Political lobbying against prepaid group practice plans is one of the most potent weapons in organized medicine's arsenal. At the recommendation of the state medical societies, a number of states have passed the so-called "Blue Shield Laws" which require that any plan which delivers medical services must be sponsored, approved or controlled by the medical society or that all physicians be permitted to participate or that the majority of physicians in the area must participate. Many other states restrict closed panel plans by subjecting them to regulation by their insurance departments. Still other states have "Corporate Practice Rules" which prohibit corporations from engaging in a profession. In recent years, a number of restrictive laws have been successfully challenged or have been circumvented through the use of legal fictions and accommodations with state legislatures but the overall legal climate in the United States is still unfavorable to prepaid group practice plans.[264]

Internal Problems. The growth of closed panel plans has also been hindered by administrative and organizational problems including peer rivalries and lack of ability to work together as a team. The tradition of independence among physicians is a long one. Group practice plans, like most other organizations, cannot tolerate the same level of individuality as solo-practice without being torn apart from within. Each participating physician must subordinate some of his desires for independence for the survival of the organization.[265]

---

[261] Greenberg and Rodburg, op. cit., p. 956.

[262] Ibid., pp. 938-939.

[263] Deutsch, loc. cit.

[264] Greenberg and Rodburg, op. cit., pp. 960-975.

[265] Deutsch, loc. cit.

Financial Problems. Once a competent team of medical professionals capable of working in unison has been found, the prepaid group practice plan frequently faces financial problems. Although even established plans sometimes have difficulty raising money, funding problems are particularly acute for fledgling organizations. The start-up costs for even a moderately equipped and housed group are enormous and labor costs may far exceed income during the first few years. Sources of investment capital must be found and, after the plan is in operation, sound management must be applied to keep it in financial health. The slow growth of the prepaid group practice plans is an indication that both of these factors are in short supply.[266]

Personnel Problems. The prepaid group practice plans have also suffered from the nationwide shortage of doctors, particularly since outstanding physicians can earn more in private fee-for-service practice. While this does not mean that inferior doctors are employed by the prepaid group practice plans, it is clear that they cannot compete with the virtually unlimited compensation available to the best private solo-practitioners.[267]

Societal Barriers. Growth has also been hampered by public ignorance of the advantages of prepaid group practice and by the inadequate support generally given by organized labor and the government. Large numbers of people have been enrolled only in areas where massive attempts to inform the public of the features of this type of organization have been made. In large areas of the United States, many people are completely unaware that an alternative to indemnity insurance and fee-for-service practice exists.[268]

Finally, rapid growth has been hindered by traditional cultural patterns. In general, people seek the medical services of those who they have come to know and trust. The intimate doctor/patient relationship touted so vociferously by organized medicine is indeed a potent force with which the prepaid group practice plans must contend. Many such plans, however, have been unable to set up any mechanism which could successfully take the place of this close relationship. As a result, for most people, the traditional pattern remains undisturbed.[269]

If a new health maintenance organization is to be established in any area, these barriers to growth must be carefully evaluated and overcome. Only then can the lessons learned from the organizational and operational experiences of the various delivery systems already in existence be applied.

---

[266] Greenberg and Rodburg, op. cit., pp. 949-953.

[267] A. Deutsch, op. cit., pp.137-138.

[268] Ibid., p. 138. See also Williams, p. 93, Weinerman, June 1964, pp. 881-882 and Weinerman, March 1956, pp. 301-302.

[269] E. R. Weinerman, op. cit., p. 304.

BIBLIOGRAPHY

Books

Bing, Peter S. et al., <u>Report of the National Advisory Commission on Health
    Manpower</u>. Vol. II app. IV. Washington, D. C.: U. S. Government
    Printing Office, 1967.

Castellucci, John W. "The Blue Shield Medical Care Plans," <u>Fundamentals of
    Voluntary Health Care</u>. Edited by George B. De Huszar. Caldwell,
    Idaho: Caxton Printers, Ltd., 1962.

Committee for the Special Research Project in the Health Insurance Plan of
    Greater New York. <u>Health and Medical Care in New York City</u>.
    Cambridge, Mass.: Harvard University Press, 1957.

Cook, Fred J. <u>The Plot Against the Patient</u>. Englewood, N.J.: Prentice-
    Hall Inc., 1967.

Faulkner, Edwin J. <u>Health Insurance</u>. New York, N.Y.: McGraw-Hill Book Co.,
    1960.

Goldmann, Franz. <u>Voluntary Medical Care Insurance in the United States</u>.
    New York, N.Y.: Columbia University Press, 1948.

Harris, Seymour E. <u>The Economics of American Medicine</u>. New York, N.Y.:
    MacMillan Co., 1964.

Hirshfield, Daniel S. <u>The Lost Reform</u>. Cambridge, Mass.: Harvard University
    Press, 1970.

Kaiser Industries Corporation. <u>The Kaiser Story</u>. Oakland, Calif.: Kaiser
    Industries Corporation, 1968.

Lee, C. Marshall. "The Challenge of Medical Care Insurance," <u>Fundamentals
    of Voluntary Health Care</u>. Edited by George B. De Huszar.
    Caldwell, Idaho: Caxton Printers, Ltd., 1962.

Munts, Raymond. <u>Bargaining for Health</u>. Madison, Wisc.: University of
    Wisconsin Press, 1967.

Serbein, Oscar N. "The Nature of Prepayment Plans," <u>Fundamentals of
    Voluntary Health Care</u>. Edited by George B. De Huszar. Caldwell,
    . Idaho: Caxton Printers, Ltd., 1962.

Somers, Herman M. and Somers, Anne R. <u>Doctors, Patients and Health Insurance</u>.
    Washington, D.C.: Brookings Institution, 1961.

Wheatley, George M. "Voluntary Health Insurance - Progress and Problems,"
    <u>Fundamental of Voluntary Health Care</u>. Edited by George B. De Huszar.
    Caldwell, Idaho: Caxton Printers, Ltd., 1962.

65

Articles

Baehr, G. "Prepaid Group Practice: Its Strength and Weakness and Its Future," _American Journal of Public Health_, Vol. 56, November 1966, pp. 1,898-1,903.

Bashshur, R. L., Metzner, D. A. and Worden, C. "Consumer Satisfaction with Group Practice, the CHA Case," _American Journal of Public Health_, Vol. 57, November 1967, pp. 1,991-1,999.

Daily, E. F. "Medical Care Under the Health Insurance Plan of Greater New York," _Journal of the American Medical Association_, Vol. 170, No. 3, May 16, 1959, pp. 272-276.

Dearing, W. P. "The Challenge of Comprehensive Health Care," _American Journal of Public Health_, Vol. 52, December 1962, pp. 2,071-2,079.

Deutsch, A. "Group Medicine, Part 2: The Ross-Loos Clinic, New York's H.I.P.," _Consumer Reports_, February 1957, pp. 83-86.

_____. "Group Medicine, Part 3: The Kaiser Health Plan," _Consumer Reports_, March 1957, pp. 135-138.

Falk, I. S. "Beyond Medicare," _American Journal of Public Health_, Vol. 59, April 1969, pp. 608-623.

Faltermayer, E. K. "Better Care at Less Cost Without Miracles," _Fortune_, January 1970, pp. 80-130.

Garfield, S. R. "The Delivery of Medical Care," _Scientific American_, Vol. 222, No. 4, April 1970, pp. 15-23.

Greenberg, I. G. and Rodburg, M. L. "The Role of Prepaid Group Practice in Relieving the Medical Care Crisis," _Harvard Law Review_, Vol. 84, February 1971, pp.887-1,001.

Kaiser, E. F. "One Industry's Involvement in Health Care," _Journal of Medical Education_, Vol. 45, February 1970, pp. 88-95.

Landay, D. M. "Trends in Negotiated Health Plans; Broader Coverage, Higher Quality Care," _Monthly Labor Review_, May 1969, pp. 3-10.

McNamara, M. E. and Todd, C. "A Survey of Group Practice in the United States, 1969," _American Journal of Public Health_, Vol. 60, July 1970, pp. 1,303-1,313.

Newman, H. F. "The Impact of Medicare on Group Practice Prepayment Plans," _American Journal of Public Health_, Vol. 59, April 1969, pp. 629-634.

Pollack, J. "Major Medical Expense Insurance: An Evaluation," _American Journal of Public Health_, Vol. 47, March 1957, pp. 322-334.

Rosen, G. "Health Education and Preventive Medicine - 'New' Horizons in Medical Care," _American Journal of Public Health_, Vol. 42, June 1952, pp. 687-693.

Rouse, M.O. "Organizing and Delivering Health Care - Part 4," Journal of the American Medical Association, Vol. 202, No. 9, November 27, 1967, p. 135.

Saward, E. W. "The Relevance of the Kaiser-Permanente Experience to the Health Services of the Eastern United States," Bulletin of the New York Academy of Medicine, Second Series, Vol. 46, No. 9, September 1970, pp. 707-717.

Schwartz, J. L. "Consumer Sponsorship and Physician Sponsorship of Prepaid Group Practice Health Plans: Some Similarities and Differences," American Journal of Public Health, Vol. 55, January 1965, pp. 94-102.

Swan, L. F. "Group Approach to Medical Care," Nursing Outlook, January 1970, pp. 56-57.

Weinerman, E. R. "An Appraisal of Medical Care in Group Health Centers," American Journal of Public Health, Vol. 46, March 1956, pp. 300-309.

_____. "Patients' Perceptions of Group Medical Care," American Journal of Public Health, Vol. 54, June 1964, pp. 880-889.

West, H. "Group Practice Prepayment Plans in the Medicare Program," American Journal of Public Health, Vol. 59, April 1969, pp. 624-629.

Williams, G. "Kaiser: What Is It? How Does It Work? Why Does It Work?" Modern Hospital, February 1971, pp. 67-95.

Yedidia, A. "Dual Choice Programs," American Journal of Public Health, Vol. 49, November 1959, pp. 1,475-1,479.

Pamphlets

Associated Hospital Service of New York. New Controls on Rising Hospital Costs, New York, N.Y.: Associated Hospital Service of New York, 1971.

Associated Hospital Service of New York. The 21/180 Day Plan. New York, N.Y.: Associated Hospital Service of New York, 1970.

Associated Hospital Service of New York. The 120 Day Hospital Plan of Greater New York's Blue Cross, New York, N.Y.: Associated Hospital Service of New York, 1970.

Blue Cross Association and National Association of Blue Shield Plans. The Blue Cross and Blue Shield Fact Book, 1970. Chicago, Ill.: Blue Cross Association and National Association of Blue Shield Plans, 1970.

Cunningham, Robert M. The Blue Cross Story, New York, N.Y.: Public Affairs Pamphlet No. 101A, 1963.

Cutting, C. C. Features of Prepaid Group Practice, Oakland, Calif.: Kaiser-Permanente Medical Care Program, 1970.

Health Insurance Institute. Source Book of Health Insurance Data, 1970, New York, N.Y.: Health Insurance Institute.

National Association of Blue Shield Plans. Blue Shield, A Helping Hand, Chicago, Ill.: National Association of Blue Shield Plans, 1968.

United Medical Service, Inc. The New Two Star Better Benefits Plan, New York, N.Y.: United Medical Service, Inc., 1971.

United Medical Service, Inc. The New Three Star Better Benefits Plan, New York, N.Y.: United Medical Service, Inc., 1971.

United Medical Service, Inc. The New Executive Indemnity Plan, New York, N.Y.: United Medical Service, Inc., 1971.

Wagster, Daniel O. Kaiser Foundation Health Plan: A Study in Growth, Oakland, Calif.: Kaiser Foundation Medical Care Program, 1969.

Miscellaneous

Health Insurance Plan of Greater New York. Report of the President, Twenty-Fourth Annual Meeting, Health Insurance Plan of Greater New York, May 4, 1971. New York, N.Y.: Health Insurance Plan of Greater New York, 1971.

Kaiser Foundation Health Plan, Inc. and Kaiser Foundation Hospitals, Inc. Kaiser Foundation Medical Care Program, 1970. Oakland, Calif.: Kaiser Foundation Health Plan, Inc. and Kaiser Foundation Hospitals, Inc.

Saward, Ernest W. "The Relevance of Prepaid Group Practice to the Effective Delivery of Health Services," Paper presented at the 18th Annual Group Health Institute, Saulte Ste. Marie, Ontario, Canada, June 18, 1969

Shearer, M. W. Personal Correspondence, November 15, 1971.

United States Department of Commerce, Bureau of the Census. Statistical Abstract of the United States, 1970, Washington, D.C.: Government Printing Office.

CHAPTER II

AN ORGANIZATION PLAN FOR THE H.M.O.

Richard Seuss

INTRODUCTION

Many critics hold that the American system of medical care has failed to respond to the needs of the people in spite of the many highly publicized advances in medical science. They offer convincing evidence that this country has failed to develop a system which would equitably deliver high quality medical care to the citizenry.[1]

The system is chaotic and erratic. In some places the finest medical care is readily available, in other communities it is impossible to find even one doctor.[2]

Moreover, medical costs are out of control. The affluent and middle classes of Americans watch in awe as the size of their medical bills soars; the poor in our country, struggle sometimes unsuccessfully to obtain the minimum medical care needed for survival.[3]

As the author of Chapter I (A Survey of Health Care Financing and Delivery Systems) suggests, the individual who is not a subscriber of a system similar to the Kaiser-Permanente program finds comprehensive medical insurance either very expensive or impossible to obtain. If he does not subscribe to such an organization, he must purchase major medical insurance or a combination of two or more lesser policies in order to assure comprehensive coverage. Both of these alternatives may be costly. The subscriber to the Kaiser-Permanente Health Plan obtains benefits at costs lower than has been possible from community hospitals or most insurance plans.[4]

---

[1] Peter Rogatz, Robert Bruner, Donald Meyers, Organization and Quality of Health Services, Report presented at Fairleigh Dickinson, January 15, 1970, p. 3. (Mimeographed).

[2] Ibid. p. 4.

[3] "Lid on the Fastest Riser?" The Christian Science Monitor, October 3, 1971, p. 12.

[4] "Prepaid Medical Care: Nation's Biggest Private Plan," Time, September 14, 1962, p. 64.

In 1965, in his health message to the Congress, President Johnson said:

> Our first concern must be to assure that the
> advance of medical knowledge leaves none
> behind. We can - and we must - strive now
> to assure the availability of, and accessibility
> to, the best health care by all Americans,
> regardless of age or geographic status.[5]

In this same year Congress enacted the Medicare and Medicaid legislation and thereby recognized the citizen's right to some minimum level of health care. But instead of achieving this socially worthwhile goal, the new programs brought higher prices without improving the methods for delivery of services.

As recently as November 1967, a report of the National Advisory Commission on Health Manpower, stated:

> There is a crisis in American health care.
> The intuition of the average citizen has
> foundation in fact. He senses the contra-
> diction of increasing employment of health
> manpower and decreasing personal attention
> to patients. The crisis, however, is not
> simply one of numbers. It is true that sub-
> stantially increased numbers of health man-
> power will be needed over time. But if
> additional personnel are employed in the
> present manner and within the present
> patterns and 'systems' of care, they will
> not avert, or even perhaps alleviate, the
> crisis. Unless we improve the system through
> which health care is provided, care will
> continue to become less satisfactory, even
> though there are massive increases in the
> cost and in numbers of health personnel.[6]

My objective in this chapter is to present an organization plan for a medical care entity, a Health Maintenance Organization, (HMO) which could both control costs and provide comprehensive medical care for all segments of the community. The principles of the plan are applicable to many places in the country if suitable modifications are made.

---

[5] *Annual Report of the Kaiser Foundation Medical Care Program, 1967.*
(Oakland, California: The Henry J. Kaiser Foundation, 1967), p. 11.

[6] *Ibid.*, p. 23.

THE HEALTH MAINTENANCE ORGANIZATION

This chapter contains a plan of organization for a Health Maintenance Organization (abbreviated H.M.O.) as the major part of a system of
health care delivery which would perform the dual role of controlling costs
and providing high quality comprehensive medical care at reasonable rates.
A Health Maintenance Organization is:

> A legislative term for a group practice
> prepayment plan intended to offer com-
> prehensive coverage of doctor-office as
> well as hospital services and including
> periodic health check-ups, immunization,
> eye refractions, and other services
> emphasizing prevention, rehabilitation
> and continuity of medical care.[7]

The Department of Health, Education and Welfare in response to the
questions put forth by Senator Long's Committee on Finance in the U. S. Senate
concerning H.M.O.'s, stated that the effective management of total health
care needs can be accomplished under a variety of organizational structures.
H.E.W. does not attempt to predict the degree to which one organizational
structure will predominate over another.[8]

But this publication of the Department of H.E.W. states that:

> In general, these structures can be char-
> acterized in terms of two major dimensions:
> (1) the degree of centralization and control
> to the extent of owning and operating all or
> most facilities directly; and (2) the degree
> of commitment to prepayment, in terms of
> relative proportion of services devoted to
> the enrollment prepaying population versus
> also using resources for fee-for-service
> practice.[9]

The Kaiser Foundation Health Plan and the Group Health Cooperative
of Puget Sound represent H.M.O. types which are highly centralized and highly
committed to prepaid group practice. The H.I.P. model and the Group Health
Association in Washington, D. C. exhibit lesser degrees of centralization
(i.e., use of community hospitals) and lesser degrees of commitment (i.e.,
some use of physician groups which have significant fee-for-service practice

---

[7]Greer Williams, Kaiser-Permanente Health Plan Why It Works. (Oakland, Calif.:
The Henry J. Kaiser Foundation, 1971), p. 11.

[8]Committee on Finance - United States Senate, Health Maintenance Organizations-
Staff Questions With Responses of the Department of Health, Education, and
Welfare, (Washington: U.S. Government Printing Office, Sept. 27,1971), p. 3.

[9]Ibid. p. 4.

and/or relatively high use of part-time consulting specialists). Finally, the Medical Society Foundation model exhibits a high degree of decentralization among facilities and sources providing the services with prepayment commitments generally limited to specific beneficiary groups having specifically itemized benefit packages.[10]

The organizational structure of the Kaiser-Permanente Health Care System is used as the starting point for the H.M.O. described in this chapter, although there will be many differences. This system was chosen because it accepts the responsibility for organizing and delivering medical care adequate to most of the needs of a defined population - its members. Under this total system, responsibilities for costs, manpower, facilities and other considerations are readily perceivable to the community served. Furthermore, it is a one class system. Each member is entitled to necessary medical care of the same quality, and in the same place, irrespective of income, race, religion, or age.[11]

This Health Maintenance Organization would consist of four main components: (1) the Health Maintenance Organization Foundation, Inc.; (2) the H.M.O. Foundation Hospital (Medical Center) Inc.; (3) the Regional Medical Groups; (4) the H.M.O. Services, Inc. (See Figure III - 1 for the Organization of these components in this H.M.O.).[12]

THE H.M.O. COMPONENTS

Health Maintenance Organization Foundation, Inc.

The operation of this component is similar to that of the Kaiser Foundation or to the H.M.O. in Rochester, N.Y. This foundation is the parent organization of the subject H.M.O. It will be a nonprofit, tax-exempt corporation which would make arrangements for medical, hospital and related services for voluntary subscribers and their dependents.[13]

This Foundation would contract with such provider organizations as: the H.M.O. Hospitals, Inc., (Medical Center), the H.M.O. Services, Inc., and the Regional Medical Groups to provide the necessary services for its subscribers.[14]

The Foundation would raise capital and receive subscribers payments and would retain from its revenues only those amounts needed to cover administrative costs and to provide a nominal surplus. The balance of its

---

[10]Ibid.

[11]Annual Report of the Kaiser Foundation Medical Care Program, 1970, (Oakland, California: Henry J. Kaiser Foundation, 1970), p. 5.

[12]Annual Report of the Kaiser Foundation Medical Care Program, 1965, (Oakland, California: Henry J. Kaiser Foundation, 1965), p. 4.

[13]Ibid., p. 5.

[14]Ibid.

FIGURE II - 1

COMPONENTS OF A HEALTH MAINTENANCE ORGANIZATION

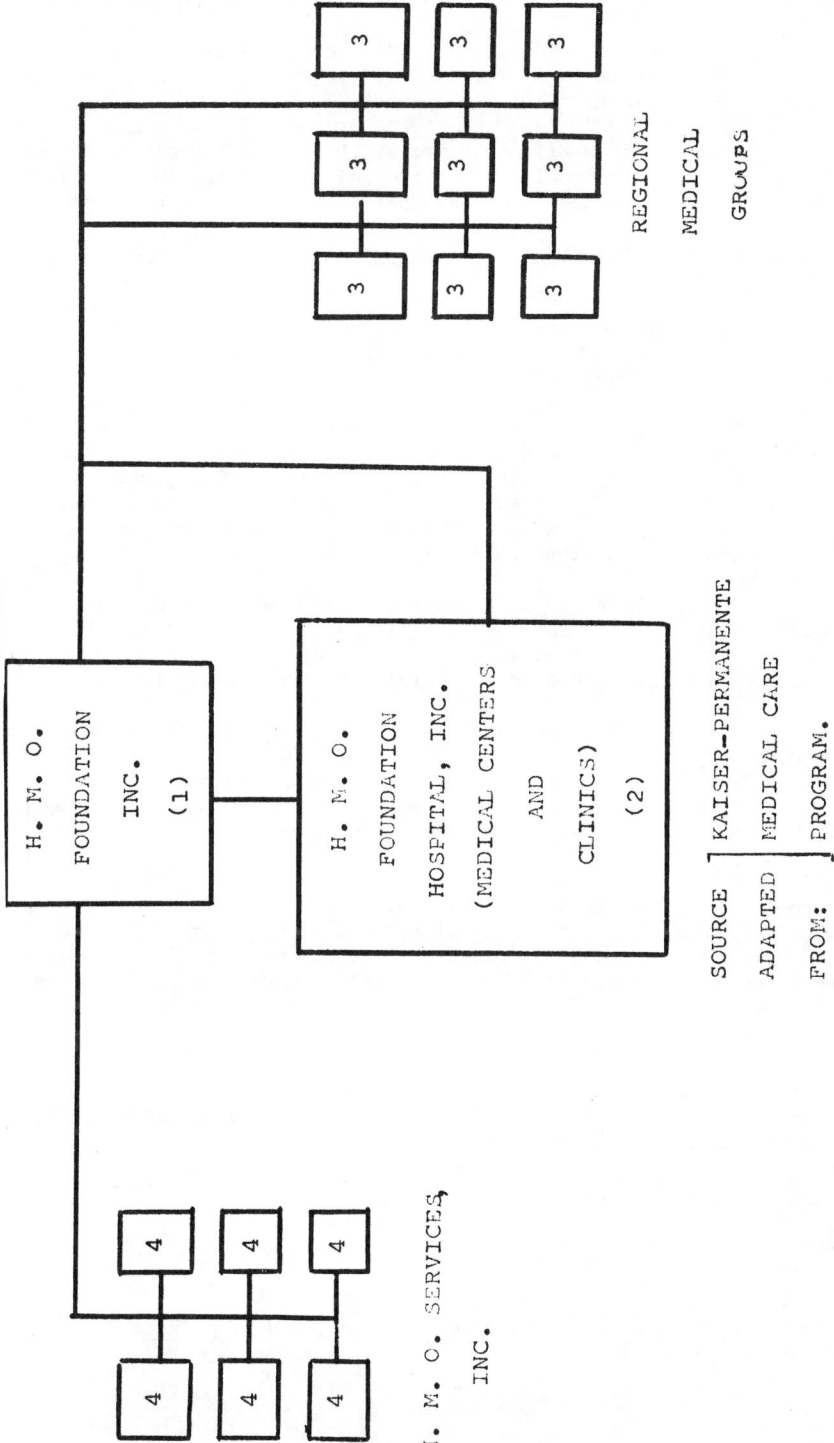

SOURCE
ADAPTED   KAISER-PERMANENTE MEDICAL CARE
FROM: PROGRAM.

73

operating income would be distributed to the providers of its services in accordance with the terms of the contracts between the parent organization and the provider organizational components.

However, from time to time, additional monies may be raised and retained for the purpose of debt retirement, investment in facilities and additional working capital as determined by the Board of the Foundation.[15]

The Organizational Structure of the H.M.O. Foundation, Inc.

The corporate leadership would consist of at least a Board of Directors, a President, Vice-President for Marketing, a Vice-President for Finance and other lower-level executives.

The Board of Directors (1) would consist of at least the following: a Chairman of the Board, a Vice-Chairman of the Board, the President and Chief Executive Officer of the H.M.O., an Executive Vice-President for Regional Groups, the Vice-President for Finance, the Executive Vice-President of the H.M.O. Services, Inc., and other outside directors. Figure II - 2 shows a chart of this organization.[16]

The President of the Foundation (2) would be appointed by the Board. He would be responsible for the marketing of the H.M.O. Health Care Service and for the disbursement of all income according to the contractual agreements. In effect he would be the Chief Executive of the entire H.M.O.

The Vice-President for Marketing (4) would be responsible for obtaining subscribers for the H.M.O.'s Health Services. Of course, this would include the coordination of the marketing effort in the various regions. He would assist the President in the selection of the regions into which the Health Plan may expand.[17] See Chapter IV for details of the marketing plan.

The Vice-President for Finance (3) would be the Supervisor of the financial function for the Controllers of all other H.M.O. components. This would enable him to have a first-hand view of the system's revenues and expenditures. He would also be responsible for the financial forecasting and the appraisal of the effectiveness and use of the funds in the various parts of the H.M.O.[18]

---

[15]Herbert L. Fish, Paul E. Holden, Hubert Z. Smith, Top - Management Organization and Control, Vol. 84, No. 4, (February 1971), p. 217.

[16]Ibid., p. 220.

[17]Philip Kotler, Marketing Management, (New Jersey: Prentice - Hall, 1967), p. 142.

[18]Pearson Hunt, Charles M. Williams, Gordon Donaldson, Basic Business Finance, (Illinois: Richard D. Irwin, Inc., 1966), p. 6.

FIGURE II - 2

THE ORGANIZATION CHART FOR THE HMO FOUNDATION, INC.

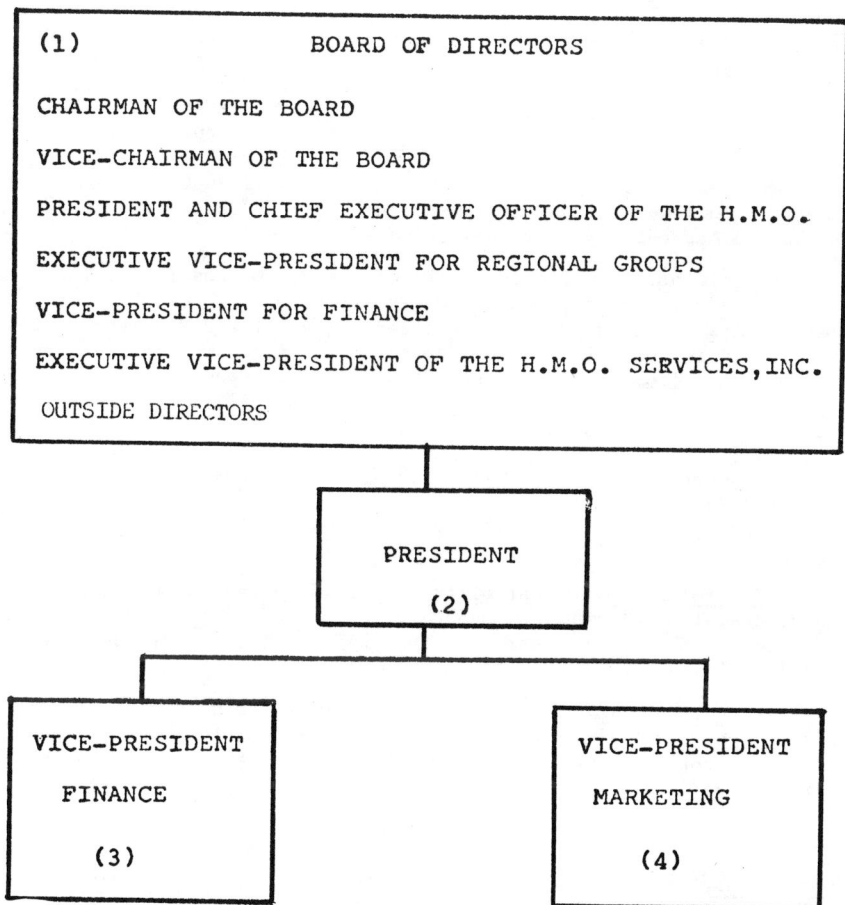

```
+-----------------------------------------------------------+
| (1)                    BOARD OF DIRECTORS                 |
|                                                           |
| CHAIRMAN OF THE BOARD                                      |
|                                                           |
| VICE-CHAIRMAN OF THE BOARD                                 |
|                                                           |
| PRESIDENT AND CHIEF EXECUTIVE OFFICER OF THE H.M.O.        |
|                                                           |
| EXECUTIVE VICE-PRESIDENT FOR REGIONAL GROUPS              |
|                                                           |
| VICE-PRESIDENT FOR FINANCE                                 |
|                                                           |
| EXECUTIVE VICE-PRESIDENT OF THE H.M.O. SERVICES,INC.       |
|                                                           |
| OUTSIDE DIRECTORS                                          |
+-----------------------------------------------------------+
                          |
               +---------------------+
               |     PRESIDENT       |
               |        (2)          |
               +---------------------+
                    |           |
      +-----------------+   +-----------------+
      | VICE-PRESIDENT  |   | VICE-PRESIDENT  |
      |    FINANCE      |   |    MARKETING    |
      |      (3)        |   |      (4)        |
      +-----------------+   +-----------------+
```

The H.M.O. Hospitals, Inc. (Medical Center)

This would be a nonprofit corporation. It would own, operate and staff one or more of the community hospital facilities, and it would sponsor activities for education and research.[19]

All loans for this organizational component, which would be necessary in the building and operating of its hospitals and clinics, would be guaranteed by the H.M.O. Foundation, Inc.[20]

Structure of the H.M.O. Hospitals, Inc.

Board of Directors. The composition and members of the Board of Directors (Figure II - 3) of this component would be the same as that for the H.M.O. Foundation, Inc. This would facilitate the coordination of the two components.[21]

In their capacity, the Board of Directors of the H.M.O. Hospital, Inc. would establish the standards for patient care in the hospitals and the clinics of the system. These standards must comply with those standards prescribed by such accrediting agencies as: the American College of Surgeons, the American College of Physicians, and the American Specialty Boards (Joint Commission on Accreditation of Hospitals).[22]

President. The President (2) of the H.M.O. Hospitals, Inc. would also initially hold the office of Vice-President of the Health Maintenance Medical Centers in the H.M.O. As President of all the H.M.O. Foundation's Hospitals, his responsibility would be to see that the medical centers and clinics operate according to the standards of performance established by the Board, and he would also be responsible for the overall planning of the future expansion of the services of this organization.

Vice-President and Manager. (8) As Vice-President and Manager, he would be responsible for the operation of all the medical centers and clinics in one particular region. Ultimately there could be as many Vice-Presidents as regions.

Controller. The Controller (4) would be responsible for the entire financial operation of this component. Regional Controllers of the H.M.O. (if any) would assist the Controller and the Administrator in budgetary and financial auditing.

Industrial Relations. Pigors and Myers, Authors of Personnel Administration, state that the Vice-President of Industrial Relations (7) should be responsible for establishing the policies and guidelines for the recruitment, selection and placement of personnel on the regional and local level.[23]

---

[19]Annual Report of the Kaiser Foundation Medical Care Program, 1965, (Oakland, California: Henry J. Kaiser Foundation, 1965), p. 6.

[20]Ibid., p. 28.

[21]Time, loc. cit.

[22]Interview with Barry Zeman Planning Council, Planning Council, Long Island Jewish Hospital, November 22, 1971.

[23]Paul Pigors, and Charles A. Myers, Personnel Administration, (New York: McGraw-Hill Book Co. 1969), p. 32.

FIGURE II - 3

THE ORGANIZATION CHART FOR THE HMO HOSPITALS, INC.

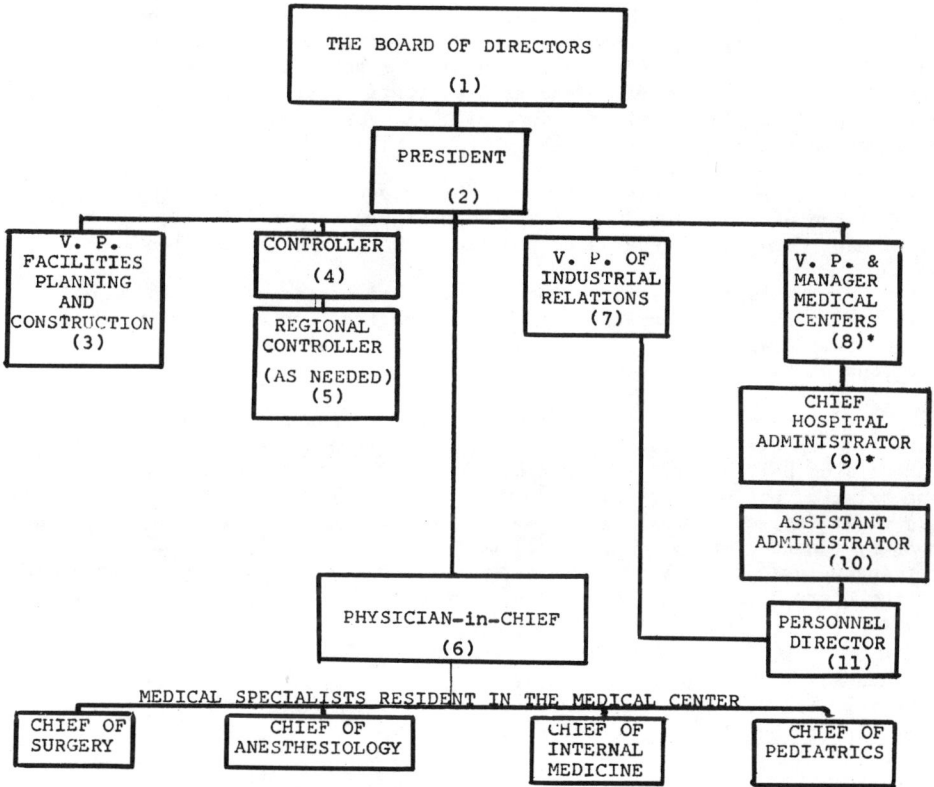

```
                    ┌─────────────────────────┐
                    │  THE BOARD OF DIRECTORS  │
                    │           (1)            │
                    └─────────────────────────┘
                                │
                         ┌──────────────┐
                         │  PRESIDENT   │
                         │     (2)      │
                         └──────────────┘
```

V. P. FACILITIES PLANNING AND CONSTRUCTION (3)	CONTROLLER (4)	V. P. OF INDUSTRIAL RELATIONS (7)	V. P. & MANAGER MEDICAL CENTERS (8)*

	REGIONAL CONTROLLER (AS NEEDED) (5)		CHIEF HOSPITAL ADMINISTRATOR (9)*

ASSISTANT ADMINISTRATOR (10)

PHYSICIAN-in-CHIEF (6)

PERSONNEL DIRECTOR (11)

MEDICAL SPECIALISTS RESIDENT IN THE MEDICAL CENTER

CHIEF OF SURGERY	CHIEF OF ANESTHESIOLOGY	CHIEF OF INTERNAL MEDICINE	CHIEF OF PEDIATRICS

* POSITIONS 8 AND 9 MAY BE OCCUPIED BY THE SAME PERSON IN A SMALL HOSPITAL

It would be the duty and responsibility of the Personnel Director (11) of each medical center and clinic to implement these policies.

The Personnel Director, in each medical center and clinic, would work with the Administrator of the hospital in establishing personnel policies and in wage and salary administration.

Professional Staffing. The professional medical staffing of the hospital would be performed by the Physician-in-Chief and the Medical Center Administrator aided by the heads of the various medical specialties resident in the medical centers.

A Physician-in-Chief (6) of a facility would correspond to the Chief-of-Staff of a community hospital, and he would serve in this capacity. In addition, a Physician-in-Chief would be responsible for the operation of the clinical facility within the medical center, the activities of the Chiefs-of-Service, the various committee activities which would occur in any community hospital, and for the appointment of physicians to the staff of the clinical facility. The recommendation of staff privileges would be made by him to the Executive Committee concerning all physicians who would like to practice in the hospital.[24]

The Physician-in-Chief would be responsible for insuring that the care of the patients would be of the highest professional level, and that it would meet with the standards prescribed by the Executive Committee.[25]

The local administration of a medical center would be a joint effort with the Physician-in-Chief and the Medical Center Administrator. The Administrator would have several assistants who would supervise specific sections of the medical center.

Some of the Medical Center Administrator's (9) responsibilities, as stated in the Job Descriptions and Organizational Analysis for Hospitals and Related Health Services would be as follows: (1) to review and evaluate the existing policy procedures and work methods by means of periodic studies; (2) to arrange an administrative management organization which would include budget, finance, and personnel; (3) to meet with the various department heads for the purpose of solving administrative problems; (4) to make recommendations to the Board of Directors concerning a fee schedule for patients' services; (5) to approve the budget for patients' meals.[26]

---

[24]Letter from Jack Chapman, Director of Public Relations, Kaiser-Permanente Health Plan, October 15, 1971.

[25]Ibid.

[26]United States Employment Service, Job Descriptions and Organizational Analysis for Hospitals and Related Health Services, (Washington, D. C.: United States Printing Office, 1952), pp. 23-24.

Interrelationships. The Physician-in-Chief and the Administrator
would be responsible for the following: (1) to co-ordinate and integrate the
functional phases of the total medical center, clinics and group practice
activities on the local level; (2) to prepare a yearly budget for the control of expenditures in the medical center, based on past experience, knowledge of market trends, and other financial considerations; (3) to make
periodic reports to the Regional Committee and to the Medical Groups which
operate within this center, concerning the various phases of the hospital
operation and its financial condition; (4) to coordinate the activities of
the hospital staff in order to prevent the overlapping or duplication of
functions, responsibilities or supervision.[27]

In cooperation with the Physician-in-Chief, the medical staff, the
department heads, and the administrator would develop and maintain a teaching
program.[28]

The H.M.O.'s clinics (if any) would be operated jointly between
the Physician-in-Chief and the Administrator. The clinic's organization would
be similar to the general hospital operation. (Chiefs-of-Service is defined
as the chief of each specialty. For example: Chief of Surgery, Chief of
Pediatrics, etc.)[29]

A difference, according to Greer Williams, in the operation of
these medical centers would be in the use of centralized services, such as
accounting, purchasing, auditing, storeroom and warehousing and business
offices. There would not be any secondary billing of patients since this
service would be performed by a centralized business office. Food service
would also be quite different because the medical center would not have the
customary kitchen. All food would be catered. This would include special
diets. Local, privately operated launderies could also be used. In the
case of maintenance and engineering, many services of this type would be
provided through a Facilities Planning and Properties and Construction
Division of the H.M.O. Hospitals, Inc.[30]

The local administration within a medical center would be a
coordinating committee which would consist of the Physicians-in-Chief, the
Administrator of the hospital and the Manager of the H.M.O. Services, Inc.

Facilities. The Vice-President (3) in charge of Facilities Planning,
Properties and Construction, would aid the H.M.O. in the engineering, design
and maintenance of all the medical centers and clinics.

---

[27]
Letters from Jack Chapman, Director of Public Relations, Kaiser -
Permanente Health Plan, October 15, 1971.

[28]
Ibid.

[29]
Ibid.

[30]
Williams, loc. cit.

79

Miscellaneous Services. As indicated in the book, Hospital Organization and Management by Malcolm T. MacEachern, the following services could be provided by the medical center (a detailed description of each is in Chapter X of this book): multiphasical testing services, central services department, nursing services, outpatient and inpatient services, ambulatory services, radiology-nuclear machine services, social services department clinical laboratories, (in conjunction with the research institute if there is one), dietetic department and medical library.[31]

The H.M.O. Services, Inc.

This organization would be jointly owned by the H.M.O. Hospitals, Inc. and by the H.M.O. Foundation, Inc.

As a service organization in every region of this H.M.O., it could perform the centralized business and administrative services for the Foundation Hospitals, and possibly the Medical Groups, and could operate all prescriptions pharmacies at hospital and nonhospital locations. This would include all the billing of customers, bookkeeping, purchasing, public relations, storage of medical records for member and nonmember patients on the computers. (See Figure III - 4 for a table of organization for this component.)[32]

The Organization of the H.M.O. Services, Inc.

The Board of Directors of the H.M.O. Foundation, Inc. and the H.M.O. Hospitals, Inc. (1), would elect the president (2) of this organization. It would be his responsibility that it would provide the quality service as stipulated in the contractual agreement with all H.M.O. component organizations.

The following is a description of the various departments which might constitute this organization:

Department of Finance. This department would be headed by a controller (3), and its purpose would be to operate a centralized business office for the medical centers, clinics, and medical groups in this region. Such a service would include a centralized system of billing and bookkeeping. If there should be a large number of subscribers in a particular region, these services may be computerized. The possibility of such a computer is discussed in another section of this chapter. (See Chapter VII for greater detail on the financial operation of the H.M.O.)

The controller would also be responsible for the financial budgeting and operation of the H.M.O. Services, Inc. Budgets would have to be established for each service provided by this organization. With these budgets, the

---

[31] Malcolm T. MacEachern, Hospital Organization and Management,(Illinois: Physicians Record Co., 1962), p. 321.

[32] Annual Report of the Kaiser Foundation Medical Care Program, 1968, (Oakland, California: Henry J. Kaiser Foundation, 1968), p. 25.

FIGURE II - 4

ORGANIZATION CHART FOR HMO SERVICES, INC.

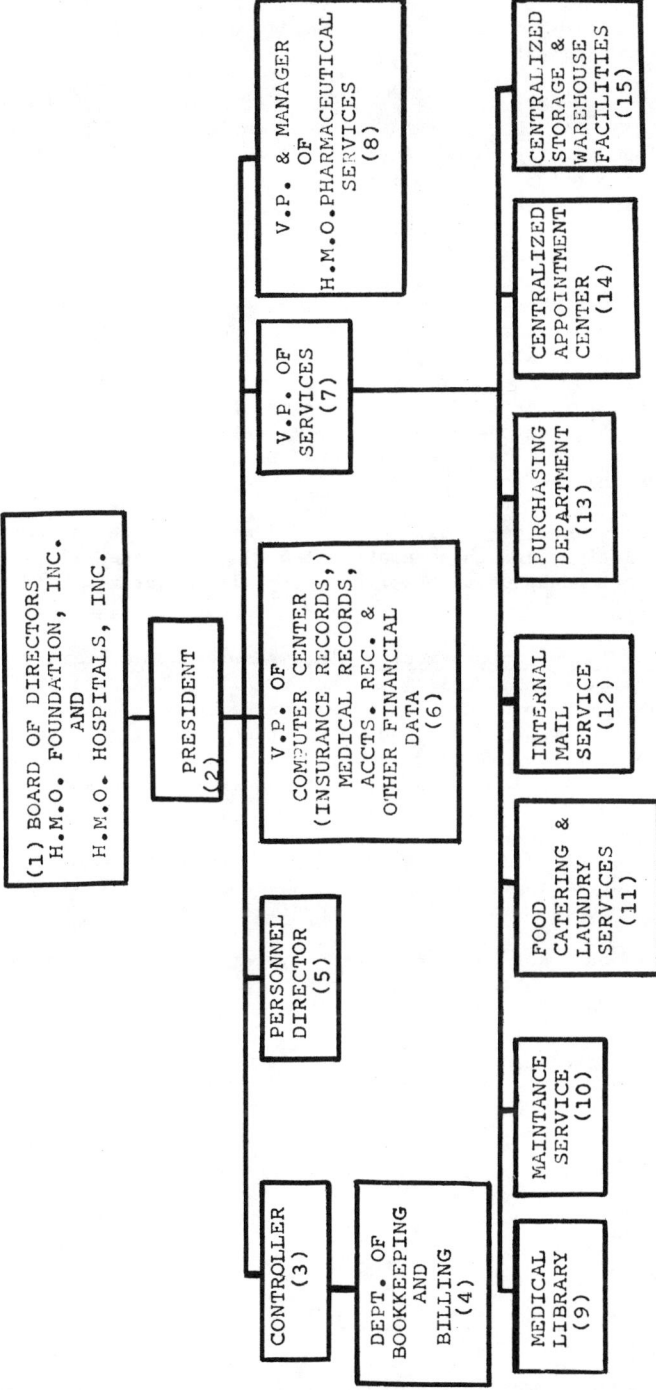

president of this organization would be able to negotiate an equitable contract with the parent organization.

Service Department. This department would be headed by the Vice-President of Services (7). This department would provide such common services as food catering and laundry services (11), medical library (9), purchase department (13), centralized storage and warehouse services (15), a centralized appointment center in the medical center (14), maintenance services (10), and an internal mail service (12).

Meals and Laundry Purchases. Each patient in the medical center would be allowed to choose his meals from a menu for the following day. All meals would be supplied and delivered by this department because the food would not be prepared at the medical center premises as is the case in most community hospitals. The next day, the prepared food would be delivered to the hospital and refrigerated. At meal time, the food would be heated in micro-wave or infra-red ovens. If for some reason the patient would be unable to eat at this time, his meal could be quickly heated at any time convenient for the patient.[33]

Laundry services would be provided according to the arrangements by this organization, and this department would also make all purchases for the H.M.O. and it would provide for the centralized warehouse and storeroom facilities.

Subscribers' Appointments. This service would operate a centralized appointment system in the medical center for all the medical offices of the H.M.O. similar to the one used by the Kaiser-Permanente Health Plan. In this system, eight to 24 women, schooled in courteous handling of telephone calls, would sit at one or two circular tables. In the center of the table there would be a turntable which would hold the appointment books for each doctor of the Health Plan.[34]

When a patient would call, he would speak to the first available operator. She would inquire into his needs and she would give him the first opening with any doctor the caller so specifies.[35]

This would not be an emergency system. Urgent calls would be referred to another number. However, one of these operators in the appointment center, could dispatch an ambulance in a true emergency.[36]

In the process of making an appointment, a subscriber would be encouraged to select his doctor from among the internists, pediatricians,

[33] Williams, loc. cit.

[34] Williams, loc. cit.

[35] Williams, loc. cit.

[36] Williams, loc. cit.

obstetricians and gynecologists available, and then to make an appointment between nine in the morning until five in the afternoon.

The reason for providing such a service would be to avoid what other health plans have experienced. In those systems, which lacked a centralized appointment, it is reported that the doctors' telephones had been kept perpetually busy during office hours. In many instances, patients had been kept waiting as long as thirty minutes on the telephone trying to make an appointment.[37]

In scheduling appointments for each physician, the operator would have to keep in mind that new appointments for a physician's examination would last about 30 minutes and return appointments would only last 15 minutes.[38]

The waiting time for appointments would vary. In the experience of the Kaiser-Permanente System, the waiting time for appointments varies from three to six weeks.

The principle of the "squeeze-in" appointments would be incorporated in this appointment center. Each doctor would set aside an hour or more each day just for the purpose of meeting his regular patients in instances of emergency.[39]

Mail. In very large regions (200,000 subscribers and over), this department would be responsible for the internal mail services of the region. In a small region, this service would be handled by the medical center itself.

Maintenance. The Maintenance Services sector of the Regional Services Department would provide the following services: (1) maintenance services for all clinics, hospitals and medical offices; (2) the maintenance and protection of all buildings, equipment and fixtures; (3) the maintenance of adequate sanitary conditions; (4) the continuous supply of utilities, refrigeration, linens, steam and air-conditioning; (5) a housekeeping program which would meet the needs of the facilities of the H.M.O.

The Computer Department. The Vice-President and Manager of this department would operate these facilities in cooperation with the department of the Controller, the Director of Marketing and with the Multiphasical Screening Service, (if any) in the medical centers.[40]

---

[37]Williams, loc. cit.

[38]Williams, loc. cit.

[39]Williams, loc. cit.

[40]Annual Report of the Kaiser Foundation Medical Care Program, 1968, (Oakland, California: Henry J. Kaiser Foundation, 1968), p. 13.

Pharmaceutical Service. This department would prepackage medicines under their generic name. It would supply the medicine to all of the Health Plan's subscribers at rates which could be much cheaper than the brand name prescription equivalents.[41]

In achieving effective distribution of its product to all subscribers of the H.M.O., this department could establish a mail order service and several local pharmacies which would be strategically located for its customers' convenience. (See Chapter X for greater detail on the Pharmaceutical Plan.)

The Regional Medical Groups

A Regional Medical Group (RMG) would be a partnership of physicians. An R.M.G. would contract the the H.M.O. Foundation, Inc. to render medical care to the Health Plan members at a negotiated per capita fee. Non-Health Plan members could also be accepted as patients on a fee-for-service basis.[42]

The Medical Group would operate on a cost-reimbursement basis. This would mean that their net income would not increase because of greater hospital utilization of hospital services. Stating it another way, their income would not depend on illness.[43]

When a doctor is first hired by a Group, he would serve as an apprentice for a two-year period. At the end of this trial period, if he has met the standards of the H.M.O. and if he has the approval of the physicians-in-chief, he may become a participant in the association. This would entitle him to participate up to a certain percentage in the profits of the Group. At the end of the third year, he is eligible to be elected to the partnership by the membership.[44]

In practice, a Regional Medical Group would work as follows: (1) All working policies and procedures would be established by an Executive Committee which would be elected by the partners ; (2) The day-to-day administration of the Group would be delegated to an Executive Director, a physician, who would be appointed by the Executive Committee subject to the ratification of the partnership; (3) In addition, business meetings of all Regional Medical Groups would be held quarterly.

Primary Care

This is care rendered at the first point of contact. In this H.M.O., this service would be rendered by the paramedical staff which operates under the supervision of the Regional Medical Groups in the clinics.

---

[41]Letters from Edd B. Bell, Director of Employee Relations, Kaiser-Permanente Health Plan, May 5, 1971.

[42]Annual Report of the Kaiser - Foundation Medical Care Program, 1963, (Oakland, California: Henry J. Kaiser Foundation, 1963), p. 5.

[43]Ibid., p. 7.

[44]Ibid., p. 12.

Definitive diagnosis and treatment would not be available at this level of care. The patient would be referred to the Medical Center or the doctor's office.[45]

Secondary Care

This care consists of diagnostic or therapeutic services beyond the capabilities of the sources of primary care for which the Regional Medical Groups are directly responsible.[46]

Tertiary Care

Tertiary Care would include the more complex diagnostic and therapeutic services not provided for in this system of care. Cases which require special services would be farmed out on an individual basis by the medical group to major hospitals and medical centers which are equipped to perform such services. Such services at this level of care would include: nuclear machines, super-voltage radiotherapy, cardiovascular surgery, organ transplantation, etc.[47]

Quality of Medical Care

In the R.M.G., an audit of the medical care would be performed by the Executive Committee. This committee would serve as a peer review board for all of the doctors in the group. In addition to this peer review board, a unified medical record would be kept on all of the services performed by the Group.[48]

Education and Research

Most H.M.O. groups throughout the country encourage the continuation of the education and clinical research by its members. To achieve this the work week is 40 hours long, so as to allow each physician at least one-half day per week which he would use for continuing his self-education or working in the laboratory.

To encourage the physician's personal involvement in clinical research, financial support could be provided by the H.M.O. Foundation or Foundation Hospitals.[49]

---

[45]Rogatz, Bruner, Meyers, loc. cit.

[46]Rogatz, loc. cit.

[47]Rogatz, loc. cit.

[48]Letter from Jack Chapman, Director of Public Relations, Kaiser - Permanente Health Plan, September 13, 1971.

[49]Annual Report of the Kaiser - Foundation Medical Care Program, 1963, (Oakland, California: Henry J. Kaiser Foundation, 1963), p. 13.

Principles of a Health Maintenance Organization

Ernest W. Saward, Medical Director of the Permanente Clinic in
Portland, Oregon, in his article "The Relevance of the Kaiser-Permanente
Experience To The Health Services of the Eastern United States" states the
fundamental principles underlying this type of H.M.O. They are: (1) The
organization should be self-sustaining. Grants may be necessary to get
such a program started, but the grants should be amortized by the health
plan once the program has matured. Membership payments for certain groups
may have to come from federal programs, but this would in no way impair
the concept of the program as self-sustaining. (2) There would be prepayment of monthly dues to mutualize the cost of the medical care with
community rating. There would be many ways in which to finance the payment
of dues. Medicare, Medicaid and the Office of Economic Opportunity (OEO)
groups may be adapted to the program with relative convenience for the
members. (3) The coverage and the services which would be provided must be
comprehensive. (4) Group practice, as described earlier, must be used.
(5) The Health Plan must have medical-center facilities. This would include
one or more hospitals and ambulatory clinical centers. These centers would
be coordinated with neighborhood primary-care clinics which could be situated
in the peripheral areas of the region. All facilities must use unified
medical records as described earlier coupled with centralized administrative
services. (6) The Health Care program must use a system of capitation
payment.[50]

Difficulty of Establishing A
Health Maintenance Organization

Legal Obstacles

Before a Health Maintenance Organization can operate in the East,
it is essential that certain legislative and regulatory difficulties be overcome.

With the passage of the Non-Profit Medical Corporation Act, or
New York State Legislation 5704-A, or the Lombardi Law, physician groups may
be formed. Health service corporations are now enabled to use their assets
to organize prepaid comprehensive medical groups.[51]

The preamble of the Lombardi Law states:

The legislature hereby finds and declares that:
improving the present method of delivering

---

[50]Ernest W. Saward, "The Relevance of the Kaiser - Permanente Experience to
the Health Services of the Eastern United States," Bulletin, New York
Academy of Medicine, Vol. 46, No. 9, (September 1970), p. 715.

[51]"The Non-Profit Medical Corporation Act," Newsletter-Medical Society's
Reference Committee, November 1970, p. 2.

health care services is a matter of vital
state concern. Without improving the present
system, increased health insurance and other
benefits will continue to drive up the cost
of medical care and overload the delivery
system. 'Prepaid comprehensive health care
plans', the preamble continues, wherein
the consumer receives comprehensive health
services for a periodic charge and the
providers are paid on a fixed per capita
basis, represent a promising system for
delivering a full-range of health care
services at a reasonable cost.[52]

In addition to this law, the public health law was amended by
adding a new article which serves to encourage the formation of H.M.O.'s.[53]

Section 4401 states that "comprehensive health services" means all
those health services which a reasonably defined population might require in
order to be maintained in good health, and shall include, at least, emergency
care, inpatient hospital and physician care, ambulatory health care and outpatient preventive medical services.[54]

On the federal level, at the time this chapter was written, Congress
had not as yet taken action on a bill which would implement the national
development of H.M.O.'s. However, Secretary Richardson has the authority
and means to funnel funds through H.E.W. channels into the activation of
state approved prototype H.M.O. programs.[55]

In the State of Pennsylvania, only within the last two years, the
State has allowed a prepaid group practice program to operate in a restricted
manner.[56] Prepaid group plans have been allowed to operate in New Jersey
since the State Supreme Court struck down the restrictive regulations in the
law a few years ago.[57] The State of Connecticut, only recently, has permitted a certain type of H.M.O. to operate.[58] In the State of Ohio, the
restrictions for the operation of prepaid group practice were removed ten
years ago. This action permitted the Community Health Foundation Program to
function.[59]

---

[52]Ibid.

[53]"New York's Approach to Prepaid Comprehensive Group Practice," Newsletter-
Medical Society's Reference Committee, November 1970, p. 4.

[54]Ibid.

[55]"The Non-Profit Medical Corporation Act," loc. cit.

[56]Saward, loc. cit.

[57]Saward, loc. cit.

[58]Saward, loc. cit.

[59]Saward, loc. cit.

Manpower Obstacles

Edward Dolinsky, Chief, Office for Group Practice Development, H.E.W., Rockville, Md., believes that there is a nationwide professional manpower shortage.[60] There is a highly inflationary sellers' market for physicians' professional services. However, there are a number of specialties in medicine for which the annual supply seems to bear little relation to demand. This imbalance in the supply of the various medical specialties has resulted in a significant handicap for the organization of comprehensive services.[61]

As Albert Deutsch mentions in his "Group Medicine" in The Health and Medicine Magazine, that the doctors in a group practice are required to work together in professional harmony. These physicians must be convinced of its usefulness, and they must be able to accommodate themselves to patterns which differ from those of solo practice. In a medical environment in which is embedded the long-standing tradition of solo practice, where the virtuoso role is set up as an ideal and where few are content to be team members, where men display the frailties as well as the strength of human beings, the qualities that make for a successful group-work are difficult to find.[62]

According to the article "Prepaid Group Practice" by Mr. Finch and Mr. Egeberg in the Harvard Law Review, H.M.O.'s encounter difficulties in the hiring of physicians because of the relatively high initial investment in establishing a group practice. This problem is especially acute when there is no outside financial backing (as there is in the Kaiser Plan) or a ready-made patient following (as there is in HIP). Young physicians, who would be interested in participating in a group as a result of their training in modern medicine, are least able to afford the expense of becoming a partner in a newly formed group. Furthermore, the established doctor in solo practice would be hesitant about giving up a lucrative private practice and gambling on the noble adventure of setting up a group practice.[63]

Membership Obstacles

The enrollment of a membership-base for a Health Maintenance Organization is initially a very slow process. The Harvard H.M.O. and the Rhode Island Group Health Association have found attracting sufficient subscribers painfully slow.[64]

---

[60] R. Egeberg, R. Finch, "Prepaid Group Practice," Harvard Law Review, Vol. 84, No. 4, (February 1971), p. 953.

[61] Annual Report of the Kaiser - Foundation Medical Care Program, 1967, (Oakland, California: Henry J. Kaiser Foundation, 1967), p. 4.

[62] Albert Deutsch, "Group Medicine - Part 3: The Kaiser Health Plan," Health and Medicine, (March 1957), p. 137.

[63] Egeberg, Finch, loc. cit.

[64] "The Blue Sheet," Drug Research Reports, October 13, 1971, p.4. Interview With Leo Pettitt, Administrator and Director of Operations of the Rhode Island Group Health Association, November 5, 1971.

The creation of the kind of integrated facilities, hospital-based with outlying neighborhood centers and staffed by a broad range of specialists required the support of a large membership. Small memberships might not support such a H.M.O. except at higher costs. An enrollment campaign that overcomes this prolonged period of insufficient membership would be necessary for survival.[65]

For example, The Drug Research Report of October 18, 1971, refers to the enrollment problems encountered by the Harvard H.M.O. It states:

> Gaining members was a prime problem. The
> people in the Boston area most in need of
> care were the unemployed or marginally-
> employed and could not be reached by going
> through the traditional health insurance
> mechanism; they did not belong.[66]

Dr. Joseph Doresy, H.C.H.P. Medical Planning Director, told a Senate Health Subcommittee on October 6, 1971:

> initial resistance to enrolling in a new
> H.M.O. reaches across all classes of our
> society.[67]

A Proposal for an Enrollment Mechanism. Ernest W. Saward, Medical Director of the Permanente Clinic, believes that an enrollment mechanism based upon an existing health insurance such as Blue Cross is necessary. Subscribers to Blue Cross would be permitted to choose between the H.M.O. or any of the current organizations of health care delivery with which Blue Cross is affiliated. The national Blue Cross organization has been receptive to this idea, but to date it is handicapped by restrictive regulations.[68]

Saward states that in place of Blue Cross, a national health insur-ance could conceivably be created in a form which would encourage enrollment into H.M.O.'s. This national health insurance could use the Federal Employees Health Benefits Act as a prototype. But this national insurance plan could not be of help to the H.M.O. if it is written in the form of the Medicare Law. The Title Eighteen regulations take little cognizance of the peculiar-ities of prepaid group practice and its budgetary system of payment.[69]

---

[65]Interview with Barry Zeman, Hospital Planning Board, Long Island Jewish Hospital, November 22, 1971.

[66]"The Blue Sheet," loc. cit.

[67]"The Blue Sheet," loc. cit.

[68]Saward, loc. cit.

[69]Saward, loc. cit.

Financial Obstacles

Group practice prepayment plans have encountered difficulties in obtaining capital for both the initiation and expansion of their operation.[70]

In the pre-operational phase, the H.M.O. would need funds for initial outlays for plant, equipment, personnel, and to sustain the system during the first several years of inevitable operating losses. Unless some outside source of funds is found, a fledgling H.M.O. may be doomed to failure. The experience of the Community Health Foundation of Cleveland bears this out. It was the first prepaid group practice plan without initial support from the outside and its financial position became so precarious, that within several years Kaiser was invited to participate financially and managerially in the operation of the plan to rescue it from disaster.[71]

Once in operation, a self-supporting plan must become sufficiently large enough to achieve economies of scale. The management of the Kaiser-Permanente Program estimates that at least 50,000 - 70,000 subscribers would be needed just to break-even with reasonable membership fees. This Health Plan has shown the ability to enroll from ten to 20 per cent of the population. This means that a community population of at least 250,000 to 300,000 would appear necessary to attain the minimum enrollment required to break-even.[72]

Capital investment, too, seems to be a major obstacle for new and established plans. For example, even Kaiser has been unable to finance expansion sufficiently to meet demand. (See Chapter IV for a detailed discussion of capital funding of the H.M.O.)[73]

Managerial Obstacles

There are many difficulties which are encountered in recruiting management of the H.M.O.'s. There is an insufficient number of persons with expertise in the organization and management of group practice prepayment plans to support substantial expansion over the next several years. This problem is most acute in the start-up phase of the organization. Many plans, after seeking the necessary technical advisers, have found their fees beyond the financial capability of the plan.[74]

Even when group practices have been able to overcome initial hurdles, they have difficulty in finding a sufficient number of qualified administrators.[75]

---

[70]Interview with Leo Pettit, Administrator and Director of Operations of the Rhode Island Group Health Association, November 5, 1971.

[71]Egeberg, Finch, loc. cit.

[72]Williams, loc. cit.

[73]Egeberg, Finch, loc. cit.

[74]Deutsch, loc. cit.

[75]Egeberg, Finch, loc. cit.

One possible solution to this problem might be on-the-job training financed by the Federal Government except that: (1) There are few plans in which to train the numbers of managers who would be needed for expansion (2) There would be no incentive to train additional managers unless expansion of H.M.O.'s appears clearly feasible. (3) The Federal Government has made very few resources available and is likely to continue the same posture toward H.M.O.'s until this form of health care grows in importance.[76]

Facilities and Physicians Needed for the Health Maintenance Organization

The Medical Center

This is a fundamental part of the H.M.O. There are several reasons why it would be necessary for the system to own and operate its own medical center: (1) The organization must completely control and operate the center in the interests of the consumer and the organizations which comprise the system. (2) Ownership of the center allows the organization to have optimum operation of the integrated outpatient and inpatient services which would require a hospital base with a unified staff and medical records as well as administrative control of available beds. (3) The most important reason for having and owning a medical center would be for the purpose of controlling operational costs.[77]

It has been the experience of the Kaiser-Permanente System, that 1.8 beds per 1,000 subscribers would be necessary for the successful oper-ation.[78] Therefore, with a probable break-even of 50,000 members, a 100 bed hospital would be sufficient in the initiation phase. It has also been estimated that it would cost roughly $50. - $120. a bed a day to operate a medical center, depending on the region.[79] Hospital admissions run about 8.5 per hundred enrollees per year in such H.M.O.'s as the Kaiser-Permanente Organization, H.I.P., and the Group Health Cooperative of Puget Sound.[80]

---

[76] Egeberg, Finch, loc. cit.

[77] Herbert C. Klarman, "Economic Aspects of Health Maintenance Organizations - Their Impact on Hospitals," Report Presented at the annual Meeting of Greater New York Hospital Association, April 28, 1971, pp. 4, 5, 6. and E. Richard Weinerman, "An Appraisal of Medical Care in Group Health Centers," American Journal of Public Health, Vol. 46, (March 1956), pp. 305 - 306.

[78] Williams, loc. cit.

[79] Interview with Eugene Burger, Hospital Administrator, Park East Hospital, N.Y., August 25, 1971.

[80] Annual Report of the Kaiser - Foundation Medical Care Program, 1963, (Oakland, California: Henry J. Kaiser Foundation, 1963), p. 57.

The Medical Office and Physicians

The Kaiser-Permanente experience suggests that no Regional Medical Group office should be farther than a 30 minute drive from a medical center. Such an office would include a consultation room reserved for the physicians and at least two examing rooms or treatment rooms.[81]

Dr. Paul Ellwood, Executive Director of the American Rehabilitation Association and one of the originators of the current H.M.O. concept, told a Senate Health Sub-Committee on October 8, 1971, that H.M.O.'s should have:

1.2 M.D.'s /1,000 enrollees, 3.2 acute hospital beds/1,000 enrollees, 2.9 nurses/M.D., .14 general surgeons and .04 orthopedic surgeons/1,000 enrollees.[82]

Computer Costs

A computer could be used for recording the patients' medical history, accounts receivable, summary of the tests in the multiphasical screening, and the various insurance policies of the subscribers.

According to the Kaiser-Permanente Testing Programs for September 1967 to August 1968, based on a patient load of 47,404, the total cost for operating the multiphasic screening system that year was $1,010,653 which amounted to $21.32 per examinee.[83]

Processing of the Patients

The Garfield Method[84] can be used to process the members of the H.M.O. In this procedure, when each subscriber first joins the system, he would go through a series of health tests (multiphasical screening) which would be either computer assisted or performed manually. These tests would include: mammography, electrocardiography, tonometry, chest x-ray film, blood pressure, respirometry, visual acuity, audiometry, ankle reflex, hemoglobin (men), hemoglobin (women), white cell count, serum glucose (1 hour), serum cholesterol, serum uric acid, serum albumin, serum total protein, serum calcium, serum creatinine, serum transaminase, VDRL, urine culture (men), urine culture (women), urine glucose, urine protein.[85]

---

[81]Annual Report of the Kaiser Foundation Medical Care Program, 1963, (Oakland, California: Henry J. Kaiser Foundation, 1963), p. 7.

[82]"The Blue Sheet," loc. cit.

[83]"Multiphasic Testing, 1971," Socio - Economic Report, Vol. XI, No. 1, January 1971, p. 11.

[84]Sidney R. Garfield, "The Delivery of Medical Care," Scientific American, Volume 222, Number 4, (April 1970), pp. 15- 23.

[85]Health Insurance Plan of Greater New York, 1970 Annual Report - "Tomorrow's Medical Care Today," Report of the President at the 24th annual meeting of H.I.P. of Greater New York, May 4, 1971, p. 26.

After these tests have been performed, and the results have been analyzed, the subscriber would be placed in one of four categories, which would be: well, sick, early sick, worried well and would be directed to the appropriated medical facility for further treatment as necessary.[86]

The patient would be transferred among the services (Health - Care Center, Health Testing and Referral Service, Sick - Care Center, and the Preventive Maintenance Service) as his condition changed. A computer center would regulate the flow of patients and information among the units, coordinating the entire system. (See Figure II - 5 for an illustration of the Delivery System.)

The Organizational Structure of the Health Maintenance Organization At Zero to 50,000 Membership Level

In the initial phase of this Health Plan, it is recommended that this organization purchase a medical center and that it expand from this base.

At this stage of development, the Hospital Administrator would be responsible, in addition to those already mentioned, for the following: internal mail; appointment center; operation of internal communications; maintenance; preparation of meals; laundry services; purchases of supplies and warehouse facilities; the operation of the medical library; provision for an administrative organization of the hospital which would include the budget and finance departments, personnel department, purchase and supply departments, building and grounds maintenance department, and housekeeping department. He would, also, with the cooperation of the Physician-in-Chief, provide for the integration of these services with the functional phases of the total medical center and group practice activities in the Health Plan.[87]

The only function of the H.M.O. Services, Inc., at this phase of development, would be to provide a Central Business Office, to prepackage the medicine, to provide a single medical record file for all the subscribers, and to provide a record of all the insurance policies of each subscriber.

As noted in Figure II - 6, the organizational structure of the Health Plan would be very simple at this level of development.

The Organizational Structure of the Health Maintenance Organization at the 50,000 - 100,000 Membership Level

As the membership of this organization expanded from the 50,000 to 100,000 level, 100 doctors would be needed at the 100,000 subscriber level along with 180 beds in the medical center.[88] Exactly what facilities would be needed would depend upon the situation of the Health Plan. If the Health

---

[86]Garfield, loc. cit.

[87]Letter from Jack Chapman, Director of Public Relations, Kaiser - Permanente Health Plan, October 15, 1971.

[88]Williams, loc. cit. "The Blue Sheet," loc. cit.
These figures were calculated from the ratios found in the above articles.

FIGURE II - 5

THE GARFIELD DELIVERY SYSTEM

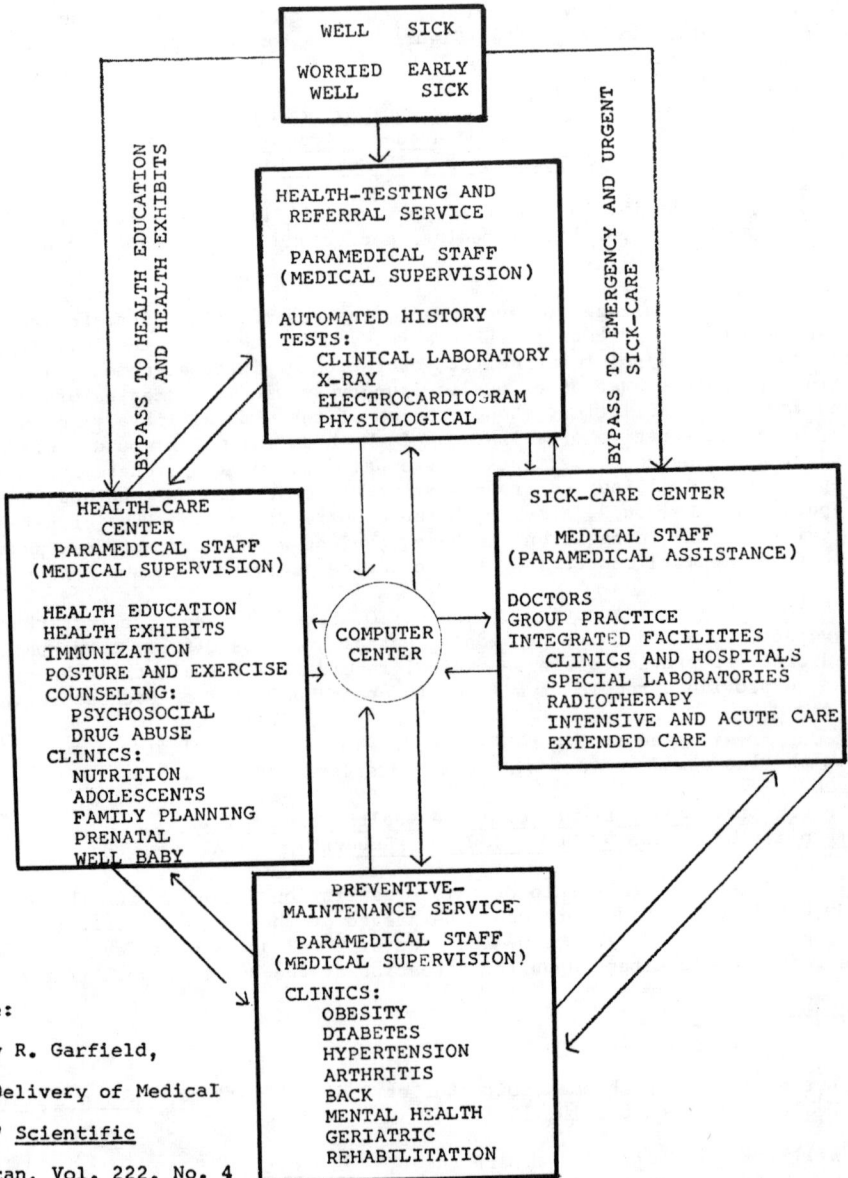

Source:

Sidney R. Garfield,

"The Delivery of Medical

Care," Scientific

American, Vol. 222, No. 4

(April, 1970), p.22.

94

FIGURE II - 6

COMPONENTS OF A HEALTH MAINTENANCE ORGANIZATION
AT THE ZERO TO FIFTY THOUSAND MEMBER LEVEL

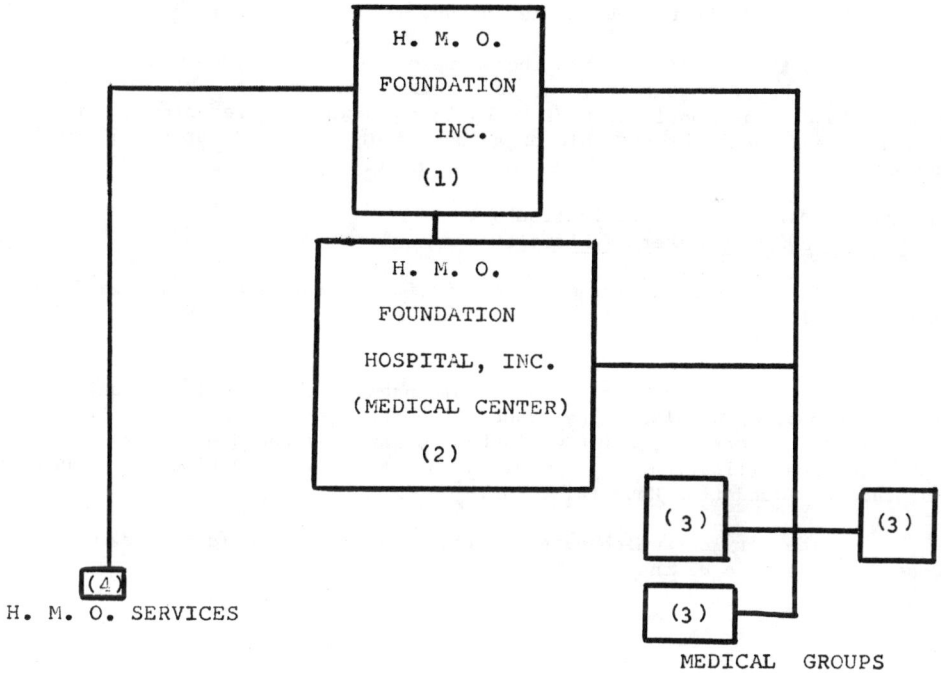

H. M. O. SERVICES

MEDICAL   GROUPS

SOURCE ADAPTED FROM: THE KAISER-PERMANENTE MEDICAL CARE PROGRAM

Plan has originally purchased a hospital with approximately 150 to 180 beds, the only change that would occur would be in an increase in the number of medical groups. If the Health Plan has purchased a 100 bed hospital, then it would have to purchase another hospital wherever suitable for the H.M.O. Figure II - 7 shows the organizational structure of the Health Plan at the 100,000 membership level.

The Organizational Structure of the Health Maintenance
Organization at the 150,000 - 500,000 Membership Level

This organization of the Health Plan would require the following facilities and doctors at these specific levels of membership: 150 doctors and 270 beds would be required at the 150,000 membership level; 200 doctors and 360 beds would be needed at the 200,000 membership level; 300 doctors and 540 beds would be needed at the 300,000 membership level; 400 doctors and 720 beds would be needed at the 400,000 membership level; and 500 doctors and 900 beds would be needed at the 500,000 membership level.[89]

As the number of subscribers approached the 500,000 membership level, it is hoped that the H.M.O. Hospitals, Inc. would be able to acquire federal funds which would be used to build and operate a research institute.[90] Figure II - 8 shows the possible organization of the H.M.O. at the 500,000 membership.

The Health Maintenance Organization
Beyond the 500,000 Membership Level

As the organization would expand,it would be hoped that the H.M.O. would be able to add a nursing school and a rehabilitation center to the system.

The H.M.O. Hospitals, Inc. would promote the rehabilitation center and the school of nursing. The school of nursing would be a nonprofit educational corporation, which would be sponsored by the H.M.O. Hospitals, Inc. The rehabilitation center would be operated as a division of the Health Maintenance Foundation Hospitals, Inc.[91]

The services which each Service Organization would provide would depend on the size of the Health Plan in each region.

---

[89]
Williams, loc. cit.
"The Blue Sheet," loc. cit.
Calculations made in the same manner as footnote 88.

[90]
Annual Report of the Kaiser Foundation Medical Care Program, 1961, (Oakland, California: Henry J. Kaiser Foundation, 1961), pp. 15- 16.

[91]
Annual Report of the Kaiser Foundation Medical Care Program, 1965, loc. cit.

FIGURE II - 7

COMPONENTS OF AN HMO AT THE 100,000 MEMBER LEVEL

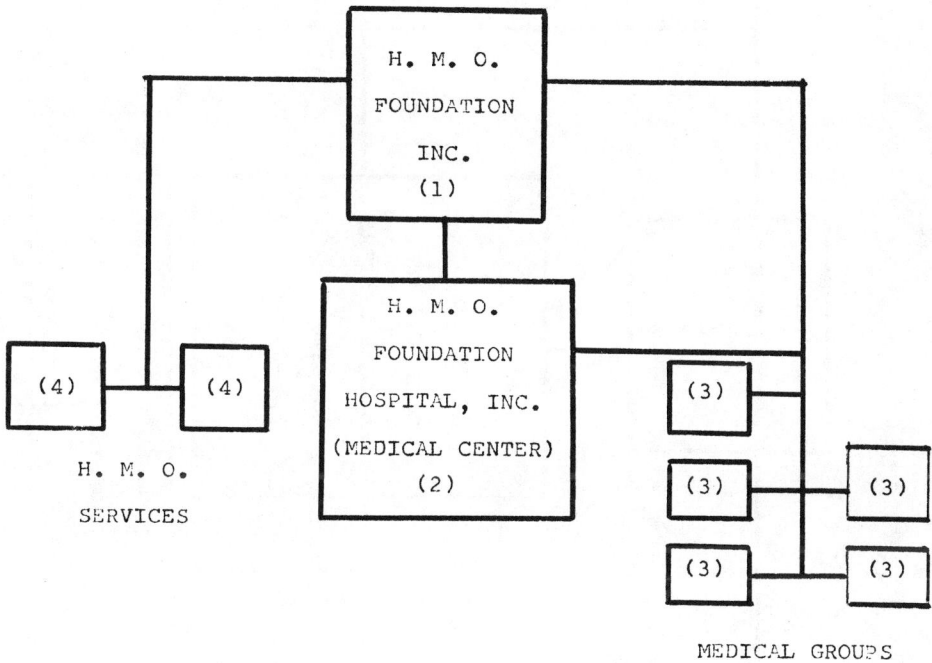

FIGURE II - 8

COMPONENTS OF AN HMO AT THE 500,000 MEMBER LEVEL

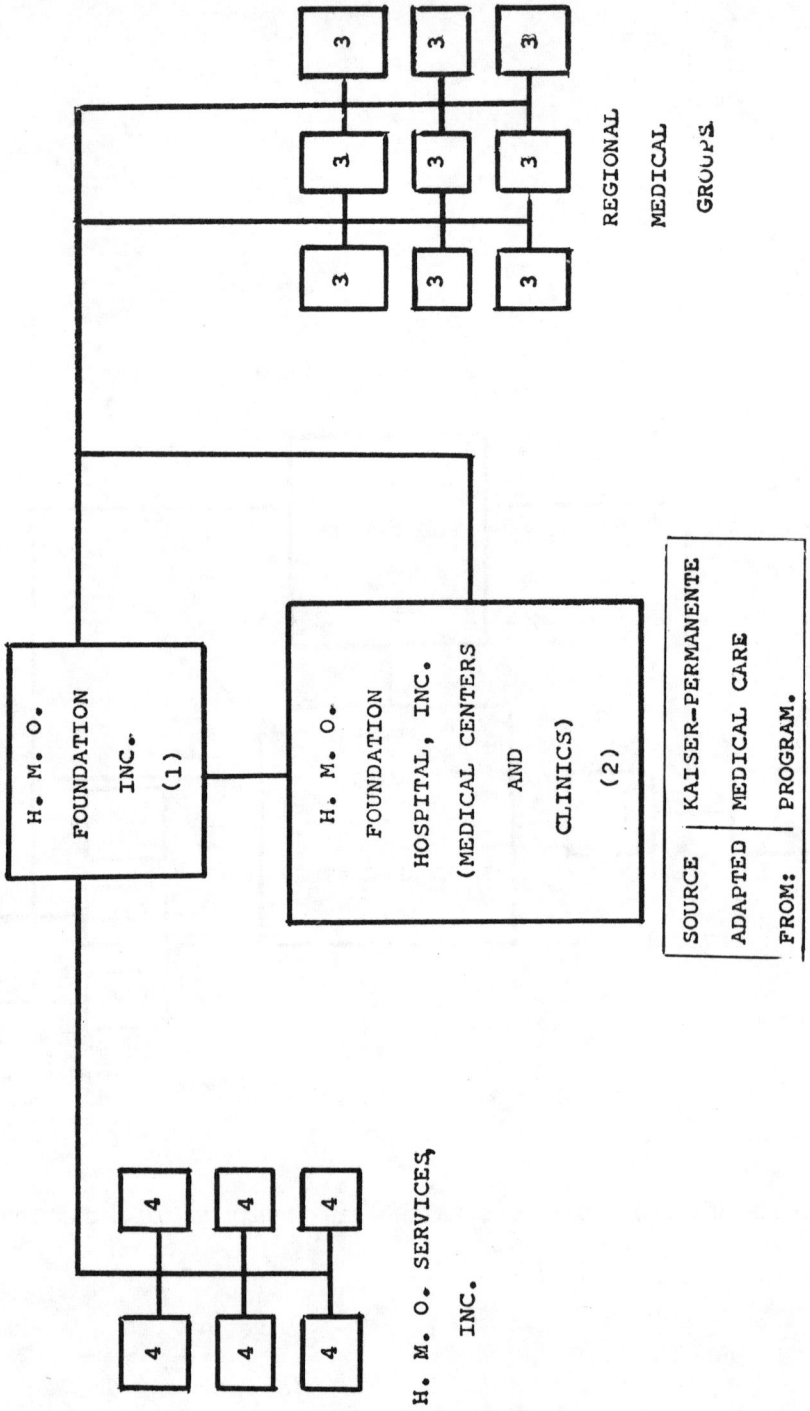

H. M. O.
FOUNDATION
INC.
(1)

H. M. O.
FOUNDATION
HOSPITAL, INC.
(MEDICAL CENTERS
AND
CLINICS)
(2)

REGIONAL
MEDICAL
GROUPS

H. M. O. SERVICES,
INC.

SOURCE	KAISER—PERMANENTE
ADAPTED	MEDICAL CARE
FROM:	PROGRAM.

CONCLUDING REMARKS

The organization plan which has been presented in this paper is offered as a solution to many of the difficulties in the present health care system.

Medical care stands at a critical point. One choice would be to adopt piecemeal legislation of the sort that in the past has seemed to depreciate the quality of care for both the sick and the well. The better choice is to create a rational, modern medical-care delivery system similar to the Health Maintenance Organization, which many believe would make it genuinely possible to achieve the principle of quality medical care as a right for all.

In conclusion, I would like to quote from the final report of the Committee on the Costs of Medical Care.

> Medical science has made marvelous advances
> during the last 50 years...We have the know-
> ledge, the techniques, the equipment, the
> institutions and the trained personnel to
> make even greater advances during the next
> 50 years. We know how to do many things
> which we fail to do or do in an incomplete
> and often most unsatisfactory manner. As
> a result of our failure to utilize fully the
> results of scientific research, the people
> are not getting the service which they need--
> first, because in many cases its cost is
> beyond their reach, and second, because in
> many parts of the country it is not available.
> Thousands of people are sick and dying daily
> in this country because the knowledge and
> facilities that we have are inadequately
> applied. We must promptly put this knowledge
> and these facilities to work.[92]

It is shocking to note that the foregoing statement was made in a 1932 report and yet its conclusion is strikingly similar to the one quoted in the introduction of this paper from the National Advisory Commission on Health Manpower (November 1967). Apparently progress in this field has been disappointingly slow.

---

[92] Medical Care for the American People, Committee on the Costs of Medical Care, (Chicago: University of Chicago Press, 1932), p.4.

BIBLIOGRAPHY

American Hospital Association. Journal of the American Hospital
    Association, (August 1, 1971).

Belsheim, Edmund O. Modern Legal Forms, Sections 2431-3160 Corporations,
    St. Paul, Minnesota: West Publishing Co., 1966.

_____. Modern Legal Forms, Sections 7501-8110 Release to Sale and
    Purchase of Land, St. Paul, Minnesota: West Publishing Co., 1966.

Bender, Matthew. Bender's Forms Consolidated Laws of New York Not-For-Profit
    Corporation 4C 101-1008. New York: Matthew Bender and Co., 1970.

Berg, Ronald H. "Who Can Afford to be Sick,?" Look Magazine, Vol. 32,
    No. 21, (October 15, 1968), pp. 38-43.

Blue Cross. Personal Interview with Ron Nick, Department of Associated
    Hospital Services, December 13, 1971.

"The Blue Sheet," Drug Research Reports, Vol.14, No. 41, (October 13, 1971),
    pp. 2 - 20.

Brigham, Eugene F., Fred, J. Managerial Finance, New York: Holt, Rinehard
    and Winston, 1969.

Bruner, Robert, Meyers, Donald, Rogatz, Peter. Organization and Quality of
    Health Services. Presented at Fairleigh Dickinson University,
    Teaneck, New Jersey, January 15, 1970.

California Medical Association. "Multiphasic Testing, 1971," Socio -
    Economic Report, Vol. XI, No. 1, (January 1971), pp. 1-15.

Collen, Morris F. "Implementation of a System," Journal of the American
    Hospital Association, Vol. 45, (March 1, 1971), pp. 48-49.

Committee on the Costs of Medical Care. Medical Care for the American
    People. Chicago, Ill.: University of Chicago Press, 1932.

Committee on Finance, United States Senate. Health Maintenance Organizations -
    Staff Questions With Responses of the Department of Health,
    Education, and Welfare. Washington, D.C.: U.S. Government
    Printing Office, 1971.

"Drugs and Health - Care Reform," The Christian Science Monitor, Vol. 63,
    No. 289, (November 6, 1971), p. 20.

Deutsch, Albert. "Group Medicine," Health and Medicine, (March 1957),
    pp. 135-138.

Egeberg, R., Finch, R. "Prepaid Group Practice," Harvard Law Review,
    Vol. 84, No. 4, (February 1971), pp. 884-955.

Fish, Hubert L., Holden, Paul E. and Smith, Hubert Z. Top-Management Organization and Control. New York: McGraw-Hill Book Co., 1951.

"Foundation Approach to Mass Health Care is Gaining," American Medical News, August 10, 1920.

"Foundations: Attack by Doctors of the Right and Left," New York Times, (January 2, 1972), p. 8.

Garfield, Sydney R. "The Delivery of Medical Care," Scientific American, Volume 222, Number 4, (April 1970), pp. 15-23.

H.E.W. Office of Research and Statistics. Health Insurance Plans Other Than Blue Cross or Blue Shield or Insurance Co., Research Report #5, Washington, D.C.: U.S. Government Printing Office, 1970.

Health Insurance Plan of Greater New York. Health Insurance Plan of Greater New York Report, New York, 1970.

Health Insurance Plan of Greater New York. Personal Interview with Julius Horwitz, Director of Public Relations, December 6, 1971.

Health Insurance Plan of Greater New York. Annual Report 1971 - "Tomorrow's Medical Care Today," Report of the President to the 24th annual meeting of the Health Insurance Plan of Greater New York, May 4, 1971.

"Increasing Dependence on Computer Seen," American Medical Association, (July 5, 1971).

Kaiser-Permanente. Kaiser Foundation Medical Care Program, Annual Reports, 1960-1970.

Kaiser-Permanente Health Plan. Letters From Mr. E. B. Bell, Director of Employee Relations, May 5, 1971; April 4, 1971.

Kaiser-Permanente Health Plan. Letters from Mr. Jack Chapman, Director of Public Relations, September 13, 1971; and October 15, 1971.

Kaiser Foundation Hospitals. Letters from William P. Davis, Facilities Planning, May 3, 1971.

Klarman, Herbert E. "Economic Aspects of Health Maintenance Organizations -- Their Impact on Hospitals," Presented at the annual meeting of Greater New York Hospital Association, April 28, 1971.

Kotler, Philip. Marketing Management, New Jersey: Prentice - Hall, Inc., 1967.

"Lid on the Fastest Riser,?" The Christian Science Monitor, Vol. 63, No. 263, (October 3, 1971), p. 12.

Long Island Jewish Hospital. Personal Interview with Barry Zeman on the Planning Council of the Long Island Jewish Hospital.

Macdonald, Larry K. "Computerized Test Measurements," <u>Journal of the American Hospital Association</u>, Vol. 45, (February 16, 1971), pp. 72-75.

MacEachern, Malcolm T. <u>Hospital Organization and Management</u>. Illinois: Physicians Record Co., 1962.

McFarland, Dalton E. <u>Management Principles and Practices</u>, London: The Macmillan Company, 1970.

Michael, Jerrold M., Spatafore, George and Williams, Edward R. "An Approach to Health Planning," <u>Public Health Reports</u>, Vol. 82 (December 1967), pp. 1063-1070.

Multiphasic Screening Guidelines Issued," <u>American Medical Association News</u>, (October 30, 1971).

Myers, Charles A., Pigors, Paul. <u>Personnel Administration</u>. New York: McGraw-Hill Book Company, 1969.

"New York's Approach to Prepaid Comprehensive Group Practice," <u>Newsletter - Medical Societies Reference Committee</u>, November 1970, pp. 2-4.

"The Non-Profit Medical Corporations Act," <u>Newsletter - Medical Societies Reference Committee</u>, November 1970, pp. 2-4.

Park East Hospital. Personal Interview with Eugene Burger, Hospital Administrator, August 25, 1971.

"Prepaid Medical Care: Nation's Biggest Private Plan," <u>Time Magazine</u>, LXXX; No. 11, (September 14, 1962).

"Review of A.M.H.T. Centers," <u>Journal of the American Hospital Association</u>, Vol. 45, (March 1, 1971), pp. 75-84.

Rhode Island Group Health Association. Personal Interview with Leo Pettitt, the Administrator and Director of Operations, November 5, 1971.

Rhode Island Group Health Association. Personal Interview with Dale Hover, Director of Enrollment, November 5, 1971.

Saward, Ernest W. "The Relevance of the Kaiser-Permanente Experience to the Health Services of the Eastern United States," <u>Bulletin, New York Academy of Medicine,</u> Vol. 46, No. 9, (September 1, 1970), pp. 707-716.

U.S. Department of Commerce/Bureau of the Census. <u>1970 Census of Population</u>. Advance Report prepared by the U.S. Department of Commerce/Bureau of the Census. Washington, D.C.: U.S. Department of Commerce, February 1971.

United States Employment Service. Job Descriptions and Organizational
        Analysis for Hospitals and Related Services, Washington, D.C.:
        United States Government Printing Office, 1952.

Weinerman, Richard E. "An Appraisal of Medical Care in Group Health Centers,"
        American Journal of Public Health, Vol. 46, (March 1956),
        pp. 300-309.

Williams, Greer. Kaiser-Permanente Health Plan - Why It Works. Oakland,
        California: The Henry J. Kaiser Foundation, 1971.

CHAPTER III

REACHING THE OPERATIONAL STAGE

Robert Brier

INTRODUCTION

Statement of Purpose and Approach

The Health Maintenance Organization is unique in that it represents
a relatively new and unexplored phenomenon. Because of this, it is most
important to emphasize material that has not yet appeared in print and would
be of some practical value to those working in the field.

Instead of discussing business planning fundamentals and then drawing links to the H.M.O. experience, I have chosen to attack the problem from
the opposite direction: to fully acquaint myself with the workings of the
H.M.O., and then, to bring in business useage if and when it is applicable.
As a result, the paper is not primarily made up of budgets and flow charts,
but instead, centers around some of the important variables with which the
H.M.O. planner must deal, such as: (a) the extent to which the government
will provide funds; (b) the economic potential of a plan; and (c) the pending
support legislation now in Congress.

These issues must be considered. It makes little sense to develop
complicated business plans that an H.M.O. might find useful after it has been
in existence five to ten years, when there is not enough seed money to start
operations.

Lack of Information on Long-Range Planning

It is difficult to apply conventional business ideas to H.M.O.
planning because the significant facts in certain key areas are not available.
The best example is the lack of information on the long-range planning process.
Few health plans (especially those in smaller communities) had gone beyond
developing a two-year operating budget when they first came into existence.[1]
The reasons are obvious. Funds presently available for starting H.M.O.'s are
very limited, and effective planning is simply too costly and time consuming
for a small H.M.O. planning council.

---

[1] Personal Interview - Jim Sleeth - H.I.P., November 19, 1971.

104

In addition, hospital accounting and financial techniques in the health field, while improving every day, have always been, and are still, imprecise. In the New York area, for example, a complicated Blue Cross reimbursement formula has forced hospitals into cost accounting procedures that have distorted the entire hospital accounting system.[2] With such a weak base, suddenly developing strong planning techniques to deal with H.M.O.'s is an incredibly difficult task.

Another problem in long-range planning arises from the fact that few H.M.O.'s have been in existence long enough to provide an experience base. The Kaiser-Permanente Plan and the Health Insurance Plan of Greater New York are the two long-established health care delivery plans. But one can hardly look to Kaiser or H.I.P. as a model for starting a small, under-capitalized plan with a completely different group of subscribers and geographic location. Kaiser, through its history, received sizable contributions from the family and estate of Henry Kaiser. This kind of generous support is not available to most H.M.O. organizers.[3]

Information Sources Used

While the Kaiser Plan may not be the ideal model for a small H.M.O. in the development stage, its organization has been so successful that we can hardly avoid using many of their techniques. Since the Kaiser people view themselves as the pioneers of successful H.M.O. operations in the U.S., they have wisely standardized operations data so that other H.M.O.'s can draw upon the Kaiser experience. A volume by Anne Somers entitled, "The Kaiser-Permanente Medical Care Program" offers, in some details, information on components of Kaiser's planning process.

Besides Kaiser, very few health plans have any documented data on planning. But bits and pieces from other health care delivery plans around the country are becoming available to the diligent and persistent researcher. Fragmentary data from the Columbia Plan (Maryland), the Harvard Plan, the New Haven Plan, Health, Inc. (Boston), the Community Health Foundation of Cleveland, Ohio, the Rhode Island Health Plan, the Rochester Plan, the Long Island Jewish Hospital-based plan, and Kaiser's new plan in Denver, Colorado have been assembled.

There is an enormous number of variations from one plan to the next; the most significant, for our purpose, is the source of funding. The Columbia Plan is almost completely financed by the Connecticut General Insurance Company;[4] the Cleveland Plan was originally financed partially by the Union

---

[2] Personal Interview, Barry Zeman, Planning Dept., Long Island Jewish Hospital, November 23, 1971.

[3] Author's assumptions.

[4] "The Columbia Plan and the East Baltimore Medical Plan," Robert M. Heyssel, M.D., Hospitals, (March 16, 1971), pp. 69-71.

Eye Care Center in Cleveland, and, in part, by Union Health and Welfare funds;[5] and, of course, the Kaiser Plan was given large sums for capital investment by the Kaiser family.[6]

Another major variable is the framework upon which the plan is based. For example, the Columbia Plan is a community-based plan, whereas, the Long Island Jewish Hospital Plan is centered around the hospital.

Chapter Summary

The planning process must take into account many important factors, some of which may seem peripheral at the outset. For that reason, data which may, at first glance, appear to be only tangentially relevant is necessary to proper development of H.M.O. plans. Some of these factors are: environmental consideration, start-up costs, sources of funds, Medicare and Medicaid programs, legislation and general business potential.

Environmental Considerations

In the planning process (especially long-range), all eventualities that may effect a health plan's viability must be accounted for. This is especially true for H.M.O.'s because the field is now so unstable that unexpected developments could have tremendous negative impact. One way to anticipate difficulties is to attempt to better comprehend those factors upon which the health plan's viability is founded. Such factors include: population characteristics, the economic conditions of the community in which the plan is located, and the community's attitude towards the prepaid group practice plans. The question as to whether an area has the resources and the desire to support an H.M.O. must be explored.

Start-up Costs

Good information on start-up costs can be found in texts by Somers, Yedidia, Bush and others (See Bibliography at end of Chapter). But much useful information has been obtained from various personal interviews. It is impossible to predict, in general, how much money an H.M.O. needs to get started and keep going, but a survey of different planning experiences may make it possible to arrive at an estimate.

Survey of Sources of Funds

This is a necessary part of the Chapter because it contains a survey of places from which organizers of a new H.M.O. may be able to secure funds for planning and initial operations. For example, the Department of H.E.W.

---

[5] Avram Yedidia, "Planning and Implementation of the Community Health Foundation of Cleveland, Ohio," (April 1968).

[6] Clifford H. Keene, M.D., "Financing A Total System of Medical Care - Case Study: The Kaiser Foundation Medical Care Program, pamphlet reprinted from: "Financial Implications of Hospitals in Comprehensive Health Care Planning," (Bloomington, Inc., Bureau of Business Research, 1969), p. 141.

represents one source. Others include insurance companies, Blue Cross-Blue Shield, G.H.A.A., unions, industry and various other government institutions.

Medicare and Medicaid

The Social Security Administration may be thought of as just another possible source of funds. However, the relationship between the H.M.O. and Medicare and Medicaid recipients might eventually determine whether a plan succeeds or fails. Besides surveying the current Medicare legislation (H.R. 1 and Senate Bill), interviews are used to elicit informed opinions on the future ties between H.M.O.'s and Medicare.

Legislation

Various pieces of legislation are discussed in the sections on Sources and Medicare, but in this Chapter, special emphasis is placed both on the "support" bills pending in the Congress and on informed opinions on how the Administration's proposed financial allocations may be compared and evaluated. Also, state "enabling" legislation, an essential environmental planning consideration, is discussed.

Business Potential

Since businessmen will not knowingly invest in a project that does not promise a favorable return on capital, answers to the question "Can and should an H.M.O. be run profitably?" are explored.

ENVIRONMENTAL CONSIDERATIONS

There are numerous factors involved in the formation of an H.M.O. which must be taken into account by those associated with the planning process. Some of these are broadly based and not limited to one particular H.M.O. They effect H.M.O. development as a whole and must be taken into account by all H.M.O. organizers. In this global category are (1) the current pending national health legislation; (2) economic factors which effect the health care consumer, such as the rate of inflation, disposable income trends and unemployment figures; and (3) medical industry trends.

However, there are also factors of a more predictable nature which differentiate one community from the next, and are important to the long-range planner because they will effect the plan's potential for membership growth (the major financial variable), the ability of potential enrollees to pay their monthly premiums, and the general financial health of an H.M.O. Of particular interest are:

(1) Population variables

(2) Economic consideration

(3) Community's social atmosphere

(4)   Medical facilities available

(5)   Setting of the health care delivery plan.

Population

Size and Location

The most important population variable is size. A community with
a population base of between 250,000 - 1,000,000 should be able to support an
H.M.O. Twenty to 25,000 enrollees are the minimum needed to make an H.M.O.
viable. According to H.E.W. studies, the population penetration averages 20
per cent.[7] In Kaiser's Northern California Region, the 1970 figures show
970,000 subscribers, about 17 per cent. There is a fairly wide variation.
In Sacramento and San Jose, the penetration is 13 - 15 per cent; in Berkeley,
25 - 30 per cent.[8]

Location is important. There must be good location for the H.M.O.
facility. Will it remain in one building, in one specific location, or will
it expand to several locations over a larger geographic area? If the latter,
both the population density of the overall target area and the specific towns
where centers are to be located must be known. A small, rural town with
8,000 population will not be populous enough for an H.M.O., unless it is a
close part of a large, more-densely populated region which could pick up the
slack.[9]

Age and Sex

Age and sex distribution have always been significant variables in
health care planning. The Kaiser people believe that age-sex distributions
are a major factor in determining utilization of facilities. Over the past
20 years, Kaiser's membership has a lower average age than the general
population. Again citing Northern California age statistics, 40 per cent of
the Kaiser members are under 20; and four per cent, over 65. This compares
to the general population of 37 per cent under 20 and nine per cent over 65.
Kaiser has a 50-50 distribution of males and females.

The age-utilization relationship is of particular importance in
determining the hospital-bed requirement of the subscribership. The number
of H.M.O. members that can be served by a 200-bed hospital varies with age
distribution. Age distribution is also important to the planner because it
is the basis for additional premium rates for Medicare people. Kaiser's data
for age-sex utilization are shown in Table IV - 1.[10]

---

[7]Personal Interview, Herman Schmidt, Field Director, G.H.A.A., Washington,
D.C., (February 25, 1972).

[8]Anne R. Somers, (Editor), The Kaiser-Permanente Medical Care Program, A
Symposium, "Characteristics of Health Plan Membership, Weissman & Richard
Anderson, (March 1971), pp. 33-43.

[9]Personal Interview, Leo Petit & Dale Hoover.

[10]Anne R. Somers, op. cit.

TABLE III - 1

KAISER'S HOSPITAL UTILIZATION RATES - BEFORE AND
AFTER AGE-SEX ADJUSTMENTS, 1969

	Per 1,000 Members Per Year	
Kaiser Utilization Rates:	Hospital Discharges	Hospital Days
A. Before Adjustment	78	488
B. After Adjustment to Northern California Population	87	605
C. After Adjustment - California Population	87	604
D. After Adjustment - U. S. Population	87	613

Source: Anne Somers, Kaiser-Permanente Medical Care Program, Symposium
March 1971, p. 41.

While the Kaiser people do place high emphasis on age and sex
distribution, most H.M.O. planners agree that this is not a major factor if
there is sufficient income in the community to pay for the H.M.O.[11] A judgment on this matter can be made by relating the level of health benefits
employers provide in the community to the age distribution. If the benefits
are not sufficient before establishment, an H.M.O. should probably not be
attempted.[12] The age and sex distribution are important for communities
where the distribution is significantly above or below the norm. In the
major eastern metropolitan areas where a majority of the new H.M.O.'s are
being formed, the age-sex differentials are negligible. However,new, rapidly
growing communities like Los Angeles after World War II, Phoenix and Columbia,
Maryland in 1972, represent areas that have a considerably younger population,
which fact must be taken into account by the H.M.O. planner. The Columbia
Plan, in spite of slow enrollment, benefitted by having an extremely low
hospital utilization rate.[13]

Competition

For each community, a key factor is the competition among the health
institutions.[14] For example, G.H.A.in Washington, D.C., competes with the

[11]Interview, Schmidt, op. cit.

[12]Ibid.

[13]Personal Interview, Lou Sacadelli, Director, G.H.A.

[14]Ibid.

other members of the government's Health Benefits Program. The population they attempt to enroll from the Washington area has the same age distribution and growth rate as the rest of the competition. The success of G.H.A. or any other H.M.O. in Washington is going to be determined by the quality and cost of care it provides, as compared to the other indemnity plans.

In all cases, a younger, faster growing town will be more attractive, because with new families constantly moving in, firm doctor-patient relationships have not yet been established,[15] and the H.M.O. will not meet this kind of competition.

Economic Considerations

Available Sources

Most of the newly-formed prepaid group plans have run into two major difficulties: slow enrollment and inadequate financial resources. Funds are needed for facilities, equipment, planning costs and for underwriting deficits that are inevitable, before the H.M.O. reaches breakeven. Funding may be provided by local sources such as a local bank or a labor union (this was done in Cleveland, New Haven and Rhode Island), but, in addition, the H.M.O. must obtain a strong external commitment from one or more of these: the government (H.E.W.), Blue Cross-Blue Shield, a private insurance carrier, or a charitable foundation. The amount of funds needed will depend very much upon whether a new medical center (including hospital) is built or whether existing hospital beds are initially available for the H.M.O.'s subscribers.[16]

Sufficient Funds to Pay Premium

Another key element in H.M.O. viability is the strength of the local economy. There must be enough money in the community to support the H.M.O. without a continuing demand for federal assistance. James Vohs of Kaiser estimates that about five to six per cent of regional, disposable income is needed to support an H.M.O.[17] Aside from the Medicaid and Medicare beneficiaries who have money for medical bills because of their entitlement by law, the working core of the community must be able to provide the bulk of the subscription income.[18]

One of the ways this potential can be estimated is by determining the level of benefits union groups have negotiated with their employers, and deciding whether or not health benefit money is sufficient to pay at least

[15] Personal Interview, Bruce Caputo, Inner City Fund.

[16] Anne R. Somers, Article by James Vohs, Exec. V.P. and Manager of Operations, Kaiser Foundation, "Considerations in Establishing New Program," pp. 155-58.

[17] Ibid.

[18] Interview, Schmidt, op. cit.

the usual $45 to $50 premium per family, per month. The enrollee (or his employer) must be able to pay this size premium because comprehensive health services cannot economically offer cut-down health care packages. Some health plans do have five, ten and 50 dollar packages, but an H.M.O. cannot avoid charging a fixed rate for its fixed comprehensive service. If the premium must be reduced, the services must also be cut down, and this negates the entire comprehensive care concept.[19]

Diversification

A useful measurement of the soundness of the local economy is the degree of diversification of industry. Diversification contributes to a stable labor market.

Government employees also make potential subscribers, as is the experience in New York (H.I.P.) and Washington (G.H.A.) reveals. It is important for the H.M.O. not to seek subscribers in one particular industry or from any one segment of the population. The H.M.O. must try to get members from a broad cross-section of industry to avoid being too closely tied to the vicissitudes of any one industry segment. For example, if the H.M.O. enrolled workers exclusively from a local steel plant, and the steel employment dropped, the H.M.O. might be in financial trouble, even if it had already reached its breakeven point.[20]

Community's Social Atmosphere

A community being considered for an H.M.O. should have some evidence of progressive leadership, a history of progress and a high level of community effectiveness in dealing with social problems. If a locality does not score well on these criteria, the H.M.O. organizers should hesitate entering that community. While these criteria are intangible, there are guidelines that can be used.

Labor Leadership

An important guideline is the community's labor leadership strength. In cities where this is a positive factor, for example, Cleveland and Detroit, the labor leadership has been able to raise the local unions' awareness of health care needs. If a community has a fragmented, loosely-knit, ineffective labor coalition, that fact is a negative element in determining H.M.O. potential.[21]

The connection between positive labor leadership and H.M.O. progress can be found in Cleveland, New Haven and Detroit. Cleveland's H.M.O. is a good example of this. Sam Pollack, business agent for the Meat Cutters

---

[19] Ibid.

[20] Interview - Petit and Hoover, op. cit.

[21] Interview - Schmidt, op. cit.

Union, gave the Cleveland Plan a tremendous lift from the start. Even before the H.M.O. was conceived, Pollack had helped develop a union eye-care program, so that the positive signs were present right at the beginning.[22]

The Rhode Island Plan is another example of a community plan with a strong union network. The state is small; in effect, is one large metropolitan area. Therefore, the various labor organizations have close contact with each other.

Organized labor is an important part of the power structure in State governments, and has tremendous prestige among State employees. These factors persuaded G.H.A.A. to set up a prepaid group plan in Providence. But there, the labor leadership did not offer the close support they had in Cleveland, and Providence has been slower in enrolling subscribers than hoped for at the beginning.[23]

Labor leadership's cooperation is particularly important because of their ability to mobilize and recruit their constituents. Organized labor has proven to be the most fertile source of subscribers for H.M.O.'s for two reasons: (1) the unions have negotiated good health benefits for their members, and (2) they have an organizational structure which can channel information and educational matter to their members.[24]

Management Leadership

Progressive business management is also important in some communities. In Winston-Salem, for instance, the initiative for establishing an H.M.O. came from the employers rather than the union.[25]

Rochester has proven to be an excellent place for an H.M.O., in spite of its reputation for conservatism, because the Xerox and Kodak managements decided in favor of a health care plan. Both corporations can draw upon their management personnel for qualified leadership to manage and promote the plan. Also, because 85 per cent of the Rochester population has some type of Blue Cross-Blue Shield coverage, key Blue Cross officials have been helpful in promoting the plan in the community.[26]

Leadership talent from industry can be valuable for an H.M.O. In some cases, people who have started plans have not had the proper managerial training to handle many of the everyday chores H.M.O. administrators face.[27] This certainly is less a problem in Rochester with Blue Cross, Xerox and Kodak providing a pool of trained managerial personnel.

---

[22]Ibid.

[23]Interview - Sacadelli, op. cit.

[24]Interview - Schmidt, op. cit.

[25]Ibid.

[26]Interview - Sacadelli, op. cit.

[27]Ibid.

State Laws

State laws which regulate the establishment of prepaid group
practice can serve as indicators of whether or not an area has the progressive
attitude necessary to start an H.M.O. There are still about 20 states which
prohibit a nonphysician from starting a health care or health insurance
program. These "Blue Laws" limit health care delivery organizations to those
which have a majority of physicians on the board and are open to any
physician in the state.[28] Many of the "Blue Laws" still on the books are
in the South. Connecticut is a northern state which had prohibiting legislation. There was a great deal of turmoil before the laws were changed, but
an amendment was enacted enabling only the Yale Corporation to organize a
prepaid group practice plan. The climate in the country is becoming more
hospitable to prepaid group practice.[29]

Medical Facilities Available

Hospitals

A vital factor in any H.M.O. feasibility study is whether the
area being considered has the facilities and physicians for a viable H.M.O.
The Kaiser people insist that proper efficiency and availability of beds
can only be assured if the H.M.O. has its own hospital.[30] But if there is
significant under-utilization of the hospital beds already available, the
H.M.O.'s founders might, instead, consider purchasing an existing facility.
Of course, if the H.M.O. is being organized by the hospital, as was the case
with the Long Island Jewish Hospital, then the following must be considered.[31]

1. Can it accommodate group-practice physicians?
2. Has it sufficient land and building space to
    support a new H.M.O. structure?
3. Is its financial position strong enough to
    absorb the start-up expenses?
4. Has it proven management capability?
5. Does its administrative board have a
    favorable attitude towards H.M.O.'s?
6. Are there large enough labor groups in
    the area for adequate enrollment?

Some recently-established H.M.O.'s have contractual arrangements
with existing hospitals in the community. Under this type of arrangement,
where hospitals are reimbursed just as they always have been by Blue Cross,
an H.M.O. should have no trouble finding willing hospitals with available
beds.[32]

---

[28]Ibid.

[29]Ibid.

[30]Somers, Article by James Vohs, op. cit., p. 157.

[31]Paper - Published by N.Y. Blue Cross - "Prepaid Group Practice and the
Health Maintenance Organization," Introduction - pp. 1 and 2.

[32]Interview - Schmidt, op. cit.

113

Personnel

The supply of medical and nonmedical personnel must also be considered. A minimum ratio of one doctor per 1,000 enrollees is required. A community must have a nucleus of competent physicians willing to change from individual practice to a prepaid, group practice. Since low enrollment in the early stages would not permit the H.M.O. to recruit specialists, the community must have specialists willing to accept referrals from the group, until adequate enrollment allows these doctors to be retained on a full-time basis.[33]

Where the community does not have an adequate supply of doctors to meet the H.M.O.'s requirements, recruitment from outlining areas becomes necessary. An important planning consideration is whether or not a community is attractive enough to draw this outside assistance.[34] This is a major problem in ghetto areas, where many doctors are neither willing to work nor live.[35]

Setting of Plan

H.M.O.'s are established in a variety of community settings. Each plan is unique in that it carries with it particular problems associated with its community. The early troubles of the Columbia Plan were very much related to the problems of establishing a new town between two large metropolitan communities - Baltimore and Washington.[36] The obstacles faced by H.I.P. in New York City, C.H.A. in Detroit and G.H.A. in Washington were, of course different, in that they are all in large population centers with extremely inefficient health care organizations.

H.M.O.'s born in a university setting (Harvard, New Haven and Columbia) have a totally original set of barriers.[37]

Advantages of University Setting

There are many advantages for an H.M.O. in affiliating with an academic institution. Harvard, Yale and Johns Hopkins, because of the prestige of their medical schools, are able to secure funds much more easily than nonuniversity plans.[38] Harvard, for example, received sizable loans from the Ford and Rockefeller Foundations.[39] The university plans also have

---

[33] Somers - James Vohs, op. cit.

[34] Ibid.

[35] Interview - Schmidt, op. cit.

[36] Ibid.

[37] Ibid.

[38] Interview - Leo Petit and Dale Hoover, op. cit.

[39] Personal Interview - Roger Birnbaum, Assistant Director, Harvard Community Health Plan, (March 5, 1972).

access to top medical personnel because they can use appointments to their medical school staffs as enticement to physicians to join.[40] To many doctors, an appointment to the Harvard Medical School is the most prestigious position possible.

Another advantage of the university setting is that individuals in an academic environment have more time for analysis and study, and for this reason, the most significant studies on H.M.O.'s have been conducted by university personnel, and time-consuming grant applications are always filled out to perfection.[41] Finally, a university setting is good for a new H.M.O. because a student health service may be run in conjunction with the community plan, and economies can be realized that can reduce the start-up losses.

If a university town does not have a large enough community popu-lation base to support an H.M.O., the student population may be used to expand that base. Burlington, Vermont, for instance, has a population of 40,000 inhabitants. Under ordinary circumstances, an H.M.O. could never succeed there unless it was started in conjunction with the medical school and the University of Vermont.[42]

Disadvantages

The university setting presents serious limitations. An H.M.O. must be concerned with securing the best possible competitive arrangements by having a hospital that is run efficiently and having doctors who devote themselves entirely to the enrollees. Both of these goals are best achieved outside the university setting. The Harvard Plan, for instance, is averaging about $150/day for hospital costs, because they use the university hospital. Fortunately, they have low hospital utilization. If they were using a community facility, their costs should be much lower.

An academic environment is generally oriented towards studying and planning, and when the transition must be made to move from planning to operations, there may be trouble. It took Yale ten years to make their program operational. While the Harvard Plan did not take as long, there was much friction before and after the transition period. Most large universities have the intellectual capacity to develop an H.M.O., but there are definite lags in the kind of decision-making that is required to get a plan opera-tional.[43]

---

[40]
Interview - Petit and Hoover, op. cit.

[41]
Interview - Schmidt, op. cit.

[42]
Interview - Petit and Hoover, op. cit.

[43]
Interview - Birnbaum, op. cit.

How Much for Initial Development Costs?

Initial development costs represent the money outlays required before the H.M.O. becomes operational.[44] The Roy Bill (H.R. 11728)provides for planning grants up to $250,000 for one year, and grants for initial development (for two years) up to $1 million.[45] Opinions vary as to how much money is actually needed for development costs. Lou Sacadelli, present Director of G.H.A. in Washington, estimates that the start-up money for an H.M.O. could range from $250,000 to $1 million, depending on how efficient the H.M.O. is in the early stages.[46] Ron Nick of Blue Cross identifies three kinds of costs:[47]

1. Planning Costs - reasonable estimates place this cost at between $50,000 - $100,000 over a one-to two-year period. The period is longer with a community-based H.M.O. because with greater non-professional involvement, the decision-making process takes more time.
2. Marketing Costs - generally considered hidden cost, these outlays should not be spared. If starting with zero subscribers, this could be a very significant element of cost.
3. Additional Cash Needs - Cost for equipment, down payments for construction, payments for renovation, and legal fees could run well over $1 million.

The New Haven Plan was on the drawing board at Yale for ten years before it began operations in 1971, and the federal government paid out almost $3 million to defray costs of the pre-operating period.[48] No community H.M.O. could afford such high preliminary costs, but if planning runs too far behind schedule, costs can mount to surprising levels.

Legal Fees

For early H.M.O.'s, the first preparatory expense may be the fee paid to legal counsel for helping change restrictive state legislation. Yale was faced with a very restrictive Connecticut statute which was eventually amended, but only after considerable expenditures of time and funds.[49] In Providence, a detailed feasibility study revealed that the existing laws

---

[44]Construction costs are dealt with in a separate section.

[45]Congressional Record - Thursday, November 11, 1971, H. R. 11728 - Bill sponsored by Hon. William Roy, "Health Maintenance Organization Act of 1971."

[46]Personal Interview - Lou Sacadelli, Present Director - G.H.A.

[47]Personal Interview, Ron Nick - Blue Cross.

[48]Interview - Sacadelli, op. cit.

[49]Ibid.

116

would not permit establishment of an H.M.O. Through the efforts of G.H.A.A. representatives and local union officials, a law was passed in the Rhode Island legislature on April 3, 1968, permitting the formation of a nonprofit plan.[50] Similar events took place in Cleveland in the early 1960's which led to the formation of Community Health Foundation.[51] The Group Health Association of America provides legal services to help gain favorable permissive legislation. The Rhode Island Plan, for example, was provided $50,000 worth of legal services by G.H.A.A.[52]

Other Personnel

Start-up costs are incurred for the services of personnel that make initial preparations for H.M.O. operation. These include architects, marketing people, and financial-resource advisors. The Cleveland Plan estimated an outlay of $55,000 for architectural fees, based on the schedule of the State Architectural Society.[53] Marketing and resource experts are needed during this initial period to:

1. define the population to be served
2. estimate the project's future enrollment potential
3. estimate the project's future utilization experience
4. negotiate contracts with third party, payors and providers of service
5. develop capital financing program for new facilities.[54]

Their services may be contracted for individually or they may be obtained as part of the services of a large sponsoring organization like Blue Cross or Connecticut General. Blue Cross is aiding a number of plans (i.e., the Long Island Jewish Hospital Plan[55] and the Rochester Plan[56]), and is providing a variety of preparatory services.

---

[50]"History and Rationale," Rhode Island Group Health Assoc. Inc., - paper published by plan.

[51]Avram Yedidia, "Planning & Implementing the Community Health Foundation of Cleveland, Ohio," Dept. of H.E.W., Public Health Service, (Washington,D.C.: U.S. Government Printing Office, April 1968).

[52]"History and Rationale," R.I.G.H.A., op. cit.

[53]Avram Yedidia, op. cit., p. 30.

[54]Paper Prepared by Leonard Cronkhite, Jr., M.D. "Operations and Cash Flow Projections of First Clinic for Initial and Second Fiscal Period," (Boston, Mass.: Health, Inc., August 7, 1970).

[55]Interview - Barry Zeman, Long Island Jewish Hospital, Planning Department, op. cit.

[56]Interview - Ron Nick, op. cit.

Other Start-up Costs

Other start-up costs often bunched together include such things as: purchase of supplies, equipment not capitalized because it has a small unit value and short useful life,[57] rent payments on facility (if such an agreement exists), and administrative expenses (telephone, secretary, etc.). Two new plans (Harvard, Columbia), have also made use of data systems analyses, making computer usage another pre-operating expense.

The pre-operational expenses (not capital expenditures) of the Community Health Foundation of Cleveland, Ohio, and the Columbia Plan, were as follows:

Cleveland[58] (Prior to opening January 1, 1964)

Architectural Fees	$ 55,000
Contingency	$ 50,000
Start-up Costs	$147,000
Interest Payments	$ 29,400

Columbia[59]

Feasibility Study (Hopkins)	$250,000	(June 1966-69)
Start-up Costs (Salaries, rent, telephone, etc.)	$ 78,000	(July 1969-Oct. 1969)
Research, Architectural Fees and Purchases	$173,000	(July 1969-71)
Data Processing	$ 75,000	

The Columbia Plan went through a much more extensive planning and development period than did the Cleveland Plan.

Capital Financing Considerations

Capital financing is tied to long-range planning because it involves funding an ambulatory facility, a hospital and the necessary equipment. These items will be of major financial concern for many years, and their costs must be balanced against annual projections of revenues and expenses. Capital financing of H.M.O.'s must be considered during both the start-up and the operational stages. The ambulatory facility and the equipment will have to be ready on Day One, so financial arrangements must be made beforehand. The considerations concerning the hospital are more complex. If the H.M.O. is to build its own hospital, construction costs must be estimated and the means for financing them must be obtained as early as possible. Cash down payments will be required before the construction begins. Also, if funds are borrowed from a conventional source, interest

---

[57]Avram Yedidia, op. cit.

[58]Ibid.

[59]Personal Interview - John Bayliff, Controller, (Columbia, Maryland: Columbia Plan, February 28, 1972).

payments become due almost immediately. So, while the facilities are generally thought of as long-term capital investments, their costs must be dealt
with before the H.M.O. begins operations.

Out-patient Facility

The Roy Bill has a provision for construction grants and construction loans. Grants up to $2,500,000 may be issued to various projects and
must not exceed 75 per cent of the cost of construction. Likewise, up to
$2,500,000 may be loaned for building the ambulatory facility and can not
exceed 90 per cent of the actual cost.[60] It is difficult to set any rule
of thumb for total construction costs of the facility because of the variation in costs from one area to the next, and the inflation in the health
care and construction industries. The Cleveland Health Plan spent $750,000
on its facility in 1964,[61] and the Rhode Island Ambulatory facility cost
$500,000 (not complete).

An H.M.O. must have a well-integrated system of health facilities,
both from a quality and a cost viewpoint. The planner must determine the
facilities needed to meet the needs of the potential subscriber population,
and at the same time, must keep in mind the total financial resources available. There are five options:

1. Construct new facilities.
2. Purchase existing facilities.
3. Lease (or rent) facilities.
4. Purchase facilities, sell them, and
    lease from buyer.
5. Contract for use of existing facility.

There are too many unpredictable variables, both financial and
otherwise, to develop a rule-of-thumb for providing facilities. The Rhode
Island Plan decided that they would build a smaller temporary structure, and
then, when enrollment reached a certain level, would move to a larger, more
efficient facility. An agreement was reached where R.I.G.H.A. would rent the
shell of the building (which the hospital built), and finish the interior
themselves. However, the $250,000 needed to renovate the interior could not
be financed because R.I.G.H.A. did not own the structure. As a result, by
1972 - years later - the interior still had not been completed.

In New Haven, the opposite approach was taken. The plan built
their own completed structure while enrollment was low, and used only a corner
of it. The H.M.O. must make the same mortgage payments, whether the enrollment is 1,000 or 30,000, and this makes for a very high initial fixed cost.[62]
One solution might be to lease out excess space to various business concerns

---

[60] Congressional Record - Roy Bill, op. cit.

[61] Yedidia, loc. cit.

[62] Interview - Petit & Hoover, op. cit.

119

until it is needed by the H.M.O.[63] The Harvard Plan leases the three bottom floors of a modern apartment building. They intend to continue this approach as the plan grows.[64] However, Harvard has the same renovation financing problems as Rhode Island because they, too, do not own the building.[65]

Equipment

Another important decision is the extent of investment in equipment. Typically, the investment in equipment for a new H.M.O. may run between $50,000 and $100,000.[66] R.I.G.H.A., for example, made an initial investment of $50,000,[67] while Health, Inc. of Boston spent $80,000.[68] The C.H.F. of Cleveland, with a greater financial base (in 1963) than most of the new pre-paid group practice plans, spent $150,000.[69] The equipment not purchased is borrowed from the H.M.O.-affiliated hospitals, for which they are charged as any outsider would be.

In Rhode Island, to save on capital investment, at first, x-ray equipment was not purchased, and arrangements were made with one of the local hospitals. If a small, portable x-ray machine had been purchased, the cost would have been considerably less than the $15/x-ray which the hospital was charging.

Hospital

The hospital is the focal point for all H.M.O. planning. To run efficiently, the H.M.O. should own and operate its own hospital. But this may not be feasible during the early stages of development. Even if capital funds for a new hospital were available from the outset, it certainly would not be wise to build a facility for 50,000 enrollees, when there are only 5,000 or 10,000 subscribers, unless the unused facilities can be otherwise employed. In Columbia, for instance, Connecticut General provided a $3.75 million loan for "the design and construction of permanent clinic facilities and a 60-bed acute general hospital in Columbia, as rapidly as the hospital deems it feasible and prudent to do so."[70] Up to 1972, however, the plan contracted for services with Johns Hopkins Hospital in Baltimore and others in the surrounding areas.[71]

---

[63]Interview - Barry Zeman, op. cit.

[64]Interview - Roger Birnbaum, op. cit.

[65]Interview - Petit & Hoover, op. cit.

[66]Interview - Ron Nick, op. cit.

[67]Interview - Petit & Hoover, op. cit.

[68]Cronkhite Paper, op. cit.

[69]Yedidia, loc. cit.

[70]Columbia Medical Plan Agreement, Section 4.1 - Provision of Hospital Care, January 8, 1971.

[71]Interview - Bayliff, op. cit.

Since hospitals are under-utilized in almost every city in the nation,[72] a more realistic approach might be to use facilities already in existence. One way for an H.M.O. to assure itself of adequate hospital space is to affiliate with a major medical school. This provides a certain degree of security but may increase operating costs, because the rates charged at most university teaching hospitals are among the highest in the country.[73] Another possiblity would be to organize an H.M.O. around an existing community-based hospital. This would reduce cost-reimbursement payments to the hospital (compared with university-based plans), and provide a broader base for enrollment.[74]

Other Costs

Land on which the medical center is to be constructed may be high-priced, depending upon location. The Cleveland Plan, for example, paid $135,000 for the ground on which it built its center.[75] Architectural and engineering fees are part of the basic construction costs and must be included.[76] There should be a contingency or reserve fund, so that if land acquisition and construction costs are underestimated, there will be funds available.[77] In many states, a reserve may be required by law.[78]

Long-Range Capital Considerations

The general instability (financial and otherwise) of all the newly-formed H.M.O.'s tends to make long-range planning extremely difficult. However, when the H.M.O. reaches its breakeven point, where enrollment, revenue and expenses can be predicted, five and ten-year plans become feasible. Kaiser,with its experience in expansion and growth, has developed the most effective long-range planning techniques in the field.

The Kaiser people say that a facility's plan must span a period of at least four to five years, to allow enough time for site determination, acquisition, planning, architecture, engineering and construction.[79] Kaiser uses standard ratios for hospital beds (1.8/1,000 members) and offices (one examining room suite/1,000), for aggregate planning. One of their prime concerns is properly estimating construction costs. If it takes three years

---

[72]Personal Interview - James Doherty, Director of Legal Department, (Washington, D.C.: G.H.A.A. February 25, 1972).

[73]Interview - Ron Nick, op. cit.

[74]Ibid.

[75]Yedidia, op. cit.

[76]Ibid.

[77]Ibid.

[78]Interview - Petit & Hoover, op. cit.

[79]Anne Somers, (editor), "Kaiser-Permanente Medical Care Program," A Symposium, Article by Walter Palmer, "Financing and Planning," (March 1971), pp. 75-80.

121

to build a major facility, costs can be expected to rise during that period. Over the past decade, Kaiser health facility costs have risen from $100,000/ 1,000 members to $235,000/1,000 members.[80]

Kaiser obtains up to 50 per cent of its needed capital financing from conventional lenders like insurance companies and banks, but it still must generate internal funds for:[81]

(1) the other 50 per cent of capital expansion;
(2) replacing worn or technically-obsolete
equipment;
(3) principal and interest payments on long-term
debt.

Working-capital requirements are less of a problem for an H.M.O. because subscriber premiums provide a steady and predictable cash inflow.[82]

Operating Expenses

General

The regular operating expenses of an H.M.O. can be divided into four categories:[83]

1. Cost of medical services.
2. Cost of hospital services.
3. Cost of prescription drugs and other appliances.
4. Property expenses.

The expenditures in each category depend on the enrollment level of the plan. But, there are some costs which are the same at the low enrollment levels as for high. An example is the OBS-Gynecologist requirements for a new group. At a 7,500 enrollment level, the equivalent of two Gynecologists would be required. At the 20,000 level, the number required is still two.[84]

The Roy Bill makes specific recommendations for initial operating grants and loans for H.M.O.'s, in medically-underserved areas. The grants or loans (or combinations) of this type, may be given for a period of not longer than three years. In the first year, the amount may not exceed $750,000 or 60 per cent of the costs; in the second year, $500,000 or 40 per cent of the costs; and in the third year, $250,000 or 25 per cent of the operating costs.[85]

---

[80]Anne Somers, op. cit., p. 77.

[81]Ibid.

[82]Ibid.

[83]Bush, op. cit., p.81.

[84]Interview - Barry Zeman, op. cit.

[85]Roy Bill, op. cit.

122

Whether these allotments are sufficient depends upon the initial enrollment level. The Cleveland Plan, by having 17,000 enrollees at the start, was able to avoid a deficit in their operating budget. They expected only 13,000 enrollees for the first half of 1964, which would have brought in $585,000 in dues, and caused $550,100 in expenses.[86] In Providence, the Plan was expected to open with 13,000 enrollees, but was forced to commence with only 1,300. This caused an initial operating deficit of $34,109.[87] Tables III - 2 and 3 show some of the cost data for the C.H.F. and R.I.G.H.A. health care plans.

Medical Staff Expenses

Doctors' salaries are the greatest single item of operating expense. For a new plan, physicians' costs may be divided into three categories:[88]

1. Those physicians who are regular members of the group and provide their full-time service, receive a salary or capitation payments. Full-time physicians provide services in medicine, pediatrics, obstetrics-gynecology, and general surgery.
2. Those physicians in specialties other than those above (orthopedist, urologist, radiologist, etc.). At the outset, they would not be regular members of the medical group and would be paid on a fee-for-service or other mutually-acceptable basis.
3. Physicians in other less-frequently-used specialties. Enrollees are referred by H.M.O. physicians and the H.M.O. would pay the specialist on a fee-for-service basis.

Method of Payment

Dr. Wilbur Reimers, Director of the Colorado-Permanente Medical, states that physicians may receive payment in one or more of the following ways: (1) salary; (2) hourly pay; (3) straight retainer; (4) retainers with membership adjustments; (5) per capital payments; (6) cost-related payments; and (7) fee for-service.[89] The three most common are fee-for-service, salary and capitation. The salary paid to the doctor reflects his training, position in the group, and experience. To provide an incentive factor, the capitation method is often used.[90]

There is no one method of payment that works well for all services because of the unique characteristics of each plan and each service. Trial and error experimentation is needed before a solid financial arrangement can be worked out. In Denver, for instance, because of high utilization rates,

---

[86]Yedidia, loc. cit.

[87]"History and Rationale," R.I.G.H.A., op. cit.

[88]Yedidia, loc. cit.

[89]Anne Somers, op. cit. Article by Wilbur L. Reimers, M.D., "The Denver Program: Development of a Kaiser-Permanente Program from Stratch."

[90]Bush, op. cit., p. 72.

TABLE III - 2

PROJECTION OF REVENUE AND EXPENSES

FIRST HALF - 1964

Cleveland Health Foundation

Membership	13,000 (Enrollees)
Number of Doctors (Full-time Equivalents)	12
Dues Revenue	$585,000
Expenses:	
Physicians	$102,000
Hospitalization	273,000
Clinic Personnel	85,800
Maintenance, Repairs	19,500
	$480,300
Excess before operating budget of C.H.F., and debt service and depreciation	$104,700
Operating Budget, C.H.F.	(39,000)
Debt Service	(30,800)
Total Expenses	$550,100

Source: Avram Yedidia, "Planning & Implementing, The Community Health Foundation of Cleveland, Ohio," H.E.W., Public Health Service, (Washington, D.C.: U.S. Government Printing Office, April 1968), p. 32.

124

TABLE III - 3

REVENUES AND EXPENSES - JUNE 1971

R.I.G.H.A.

Effective Membership	1,200 (Enrollees)

Receipts:

Subscribers	$14,000
Fee-for-Service	5,000
Pharmacy	400
Others	1,100
	$20,500

Disbursements:

Medical Staff	$17,600
Para-medical Staff	11,300
Administrative Staff	4,556
General Administration	10,806
Inpatient	5,580
Specialists	2,667
Outpatient	1,900
Out-of-Area	200
Reduction of Debt	-
Debt Service	-
Contingency Reserve	-
	$54,609
Balance (Deficit)	($34,109)

Source: Rhode Island Group Health Association, Inc., Operational
        Projections of Cash Flow, June 1971.

125

the payment of an outside urologist was changed from fee-for-service to per capita, so that a higher degree of cost predictability could be achieved.[91] Changes of this sort occur, from time to time, and are common in all H.M.O.'s.

Salaries

Salaries for doctors in the medical group are usually set by the medical marketplace. However, in under-capitalized operations, the physicians may not receive fully adequate compensation at the outset. The doctors, like other personnel in the group, may be asked to make financial sacrifices until the enrollment reaches an acceptable level.[92]

H.M.O. compensation schedules for the Kaiser Plan in Portland, Oregon are as follows:[93]

1. <u>Primary Care Physicians</u> - Average between $26,000-$36,000 (after ten years of practice). Also may receive $6,000-$12,000 in shares of the H.M.O.'s annual cost savings.
2. <u>Specialists</u> - Average between $30,000-$43,000 (after ten years) and also may receive $6,000-$12,000 in annual cost savings.

When the Cleveland Plan began in January 1964, the average pay for their 12 full-time physicians was $17,000 per year.[94] The plan was not affiliated with a major medical school[95] and was not able to use faculty appointments as offsetting compensation. The $17,000 appears low by today's standards. The Harvard Plan offers higher salaries and the prospect of teaching at the medical school. Table III - 4 gives further details on the Harvard Plan's starting salary schedules.

The Group Health Cooperative of Pudget Sound has a salary scale similar to Kaiser, but with a wider range. Salaries for the regular physicians in the group run from $23,000 to $45,000, with higher amounts for specialists. In H.I.P. new doctors start at $22,000 and $24,000 (slightly higher for specialists), with the possibility of advancing to between $50,000-$55,000.[96] Table III - 5 contains a comparison of physicians' salary ranges.

---

[91]Somers - Reimes, <u>op. cit.</u>

[92]Interview - Petit & Hoover, <u>op. cit.</u>

[93]Bush, <u>op. cit.</u>, p. 71.

[94]Yedidia, <u>loc. cit.</u>

[95]In early stages, broke relations with Western Reserve Medical School.

[96]"Prepaid Group Practice and Health Maintenance Organizations," paper prepared by Blue Cross, New York City, p. 3.

TABLE III - 4

HARVARD COMMUNITY HEALTH PLAN

STARTING SALARIES

Number of Years Experience & Training	Internal Medicine, Pediatrics, Allergy, Neurology, Hematology	General Surgery, Psychiatry, Obs.-Gyn.	Ophthalmology ENT. Orthopedics
Less than 5	$19,600	$22,540	$24,500
5-6	20,000	23,740	25,700
7-8	22,000	24,940	26,900
9-10	23,200	26,140	28,100
11-12	24,400	27,340	29,300
13-16	25,600	28,540	30,500
17-20	26,800	29,740	31,700

Source: "Group Practice: Planning and Implementing A Community-Wide Prepayment Plan," Ann S. Bush, New York State Health Planning Commission, (May 1971), p. 71.

TABLE III - 5

SALARY RANGE OF SELECT H.M.O.'s

Plan	Range	Average
Group Health Coop.	$23,000-$45,000	$33,000
Kaiser, Portland	$28,000-$38,000	$33,000
H.I.P.	$22,000-$55,000	$38,500
Harvard Community Health Plan	$19,600-$31,700	$25,650
Cleveland* (1964)		$17,000

* The 1964 figures cannot really be compared to
present-day figures, especially since Medicare
and Medicaid came about in 1965.

Source: "Prepaid Group Practice and Health Maintenance Organizations,"
paper prepared by Blue Cross, New York City, pp. 2 and 3.

Excess Payments

In the various Permanente Groups, it is usual for a doctor to become a junior partner in the group after two years service, and a full partner after three years. A full partnership entitles him to share equally in the profits of the group. In the Northern California Kaiser group, profits per physician averaged $9,000 per year.[97]

The East Nassau Medical Group has a similar arrangement. Physicians receive bonuses from H.I.P. in the form of additional capitation payments. Bonus payments are intended to encourage its participating groups to convert its doctors from part-time to full-time. A group presently receives a bonus of $12,000 for each full-time doctor. Extra evening hours also can lead to added bonuses.[98]

Fringe Benefits

Besides direct financial compensation, physicians also expect fringe benefits. Examples of fringe benefits are: life insurance, hospitalization and medical-surgical coverage, malpractice insurance, disability insurance, retirement benefits, and tax-deferred savings plans.[99] Addition of fringe benefits should be deferred until the H.M.O. achieves financial stability.

Para-medical and Nonprofessional Staffing Costs

The salaries of the para-medical staff in the clinics and the hospitals, and the medical group's administrative personnel, must be accounted for. The para-professionals that assist H.M.O. physicians include: nurses, medical and surgical assistants, laboratory and x-ray technicians, pharmacists, optometrists, physical therapists and others.[100] Table III - 6 contains a listing of annual rates of pay for 14 job categories.

Other Costs of Medical Service

Other important expenditures are out-of-area claims and expendable equipment and supplies for the clinic. Out-of-area costs vary from plan to plan. A large city plan, like H.I.P., incurs large out-of-area costs, while R.I.G.H.A. or Columbia do not. Rhode Island, in its first two months of operation, had approximately $140,000 in disbursements; only $350 of which were out-of-area costs.[101] The expendable supplies by the H.M.O. are similar in quantity and cost to the requirements of any other medical facility.

[97] Anne Somers, op. cit., Article by Wallace H. Cook, M.D., "Profile of the Permanente Physician," p. 105.

[98] Personal Interview - Marvin Leeds, Director of East Nassau Medical Group, December 28, 1971.

[99] Bush, op. cit., p. 73.

[100] Bush, op. cit., p. 70.

[101] Rhode Island Group Health Assoc. Inc., Cash Flow Statement - June 1971, May 1972.

TABLE III - 6

SALARIES OF NON-PHYSICIAN PERSONNEL
OF HEALTH, INC.

Position	Annual Rate of Pay
Regular Nurses	$ 9,000
Lic. Pract. Nurses	$ 7,000
Lab. Technicians	$ 7,000
X-Ray Technicians	$ 7,000
Medical Record Technicians	$ 7,000
Ass't. Med. Record Technician	$ 6,000
Secretary/Receptionist	$ 6,500
Admitting Receptionist	$ 8,200
Billing Clerk	$ 6,200
Payroll/Purchase Clerk	$ 6,200
Clinic Manager	$15,000
Sec. to Clinic Manager	$ 7,300
Pharmacy Assistant	$ 6,500
Social Service Worker	$ 9,000

Source: Paper prepared by Dr. Leonard Cronkhite, Jr., M.D. Health, Inc.
Boston, Mass. "Operations and Cash Flow Projections of First
Clinic for Initial and Second Fiscal Period, August 7, 1970.

Costs of Hospital Services

The hospital expenditures would include: (1) salaries and fringe benefits of hospital-based physicians, para-medical health personnel, administrative staff and other hospital personnel; (2) the costs of food and other goods and services; and (3) expendable equipment and supplies.[102] It must be remembered that to the extent that an H.M.O. successfully maintains the health of its enrollees, hospital utilization, and thus, hospital costs, will be reduced. In Columbia, for instance, much larger start-up deficits would have been incurred if the hospital utilization rates had not been so low.[103]

Prescription Drugs and Appliances

Costs incurred in this category are:[104]

1. Drugs
2. Glasses
3. Hearing Aids
4. Various orthopedic devices

H.M.O.'s have different coverages with regard to items (2) through (4).

Property Expenses

These costs include:[105]

(1) depreciation and replacement of facilities and equipment;
(2) maintenance and repair;
(3) rental fees and contractual payments;
(4) taxes;
(5) insurance and interest payments.[106]

SOURCES OF FUNDS

It is easy to list all the financial sources an H.M.O. might tap for funds, but getting money from those sources is something else again. While Washington seems to favor the H.M.O. concept, large funds were not yet made available by early 1972. The research and interviews upon which this Chapter is based indicates that every H.M.O. started in the

---

[102]Ann S. Bush, op. cit.

[103]Interview - John Bayliff, op. cit.

[104]Ann S. Bush, op. cit., p. 81.

[105]Ibid.

[106]For further details in any of these cost categories, individual planning experiences must be consulted - i.e., the Cleveland Plan (Yedidia), Columbia, Harvard, etc.

last five years has had serious financial difficulties at the outset, unless some large, wealthy, sponsoring organization came in and assumed the initial financial burden. An example is the Harvard Plan. One might think a plan sponsored by the Harvard Medical School, in the heart of the Boston area, would certainly be able to raise all the necessary funds for initial development, either through government or private sources. Dale Hoover, formerly affiliated with the Harvard Plan and now with the Rhode Island Group Health Assoc. reports that when the Harvard Plan was in its initial stages, those in administration often did not know from where money for the next payroll was coming.[107] Two years after the Harvard doors were opened, the Plan still faced financial stringency,[108] and uncertainty.

The Rhode Island Plan, serving the Providence area and outlying suburbs, also faced financial starvation at the outset.[109] Costs in the initial stage were partially covered by $250,000 raised locally from union members, $50,000 in services received from the Group Health Association of America, and a grant of $157,700 from H.E.W.;[110] but this was not nearly enough.

According to Marie Henderson of the Federal Employees Health Benefits Program, an H.M.O. needs enough financial backing at its inception for five years of operation, if the organization is to function properly.[111] Unless adequate funds can be obtained, the fledgling H.M.O. will run into trouble.[112]

Hill-Burton

Perhaps the savior of all pioneering H.M.O.'s is the health legislation now in Congress. While funds for planning an H.M.O. have always been small and difficult to come by,[113] government funds for new H.M.O. facilities and redevelopment of old facilities are even more difficult to obtain.[114] Titles VI and XI of the Public Health Service Act provide some capital funds.[115] Title VI, or Hill-Burton, has been the main government source for

---

[107] Interview - Petit and Hoover, op. cit.

[108] Ibid.

[109] Ibid.

[110] "History and Rationale," op. cit.

[111] Interview - Petit and Hoover, op. cit.

[112] Ibid.

[113] Biggest Government Planning Source is G.H.A.A.

[114] Harvard Law Review, op. cit., p. 983.

[115] Ibid.

loans and grants to hospitals and health facilities since its creation in
1946.[116]   But because of administrative obstacles, Hill-Burton has not yet
been widely utilized by group plans.[117]   One difficulty is that funds through
Hill-Burton have been apportioned solely for full-scale hospital construction.

During the past two decades, 3,500 communities have benefited from
these funds.   More than 8,800 projects have been approved, representing a
total cost of $8.8 billion in construction money.   Hill-Burton funds totaled
more than $2.7 billion, and were matched by $6.1 billion from state and local
funds.[118]

According to Mr. Leo Petit at the Rhode Island Plan, administrators
of Hill-Burton money are beginning to place new emphasis on ambulatory care
facilities.   However, where Hill-Burton Funds are appropriated is often
determined by how much a state is entitled to, and how much has already been
committed.   State allocations already parceled out cannot be changed.[119]
Therefore, in spite of the added emphasis by the Nixon Administration on the
H.M.O. concept, current Hill-Burton funds cannot be an immediately significant source because of prior commitments to hospital construction.[120]

Group Practice Facilities Act

Title XI of the P.H.S. Act was authorized by Congress in 1966 as
a program of the Federal Housing Administration, to provide mortgage insurance to group practice facilities.   The purpose of the program was "to assure
the availability of credit on reasonable terms to units or organizations
engaged in the group practice of medicine, optometry or dentistry, particularly those in smaller communities and those sponsored by cooperative or
other nonprofit organizations, to assist in financing the construction and
equipment of group practice facilities."

The F.H.A.-insured mortgage may be used to build, rehabilitate,
equip, and furnish structures for group practice.[121]   Each application must
be presented by a sponsor and mortgagor.   The sponsor is an organization
that organizes and promotes the plan.   It may be sponsored by a nonprofit

---

[116]"Hospital Capital Funds: Changing Needs and Sources," Hospitals,
   Robert M. Sigmond, (August 16, 1965), p. 52.

[117]Harvard Law Review, op. cit., p. 984.

[118]"Many Federal Programs Finance Hospital Construction," Hospitals,
   Harold M. Graning, M.D. (April 1968), p. 43.

[119]Interview - Petit and Hoover, op. cit.

[120]My own observation.

[121]"H.U.D.-F.H.A. Program for Group Practice Facilities," Pamphlet,
   H.U.D.-146-F, (August 1970).

group that will lease the facility to a group of doctors, or by a group of health care specialists who will create a separate nonprofit entity to qualify as mortgagor and owner of the facility.

The mortgagor is the entity which owns the property secured by the F.H.A. mortgage. The mortgagor must also be organized on a nonprofit basis, and none of its earnings may go to any private stockholder or individual.[122]

Those who participate in the plan must be part of a group intending to provide ambulatory care to the community with a comprehensive program. Patients can pay the plan on a prepayment basis or fee-for-service. The medical group must consist of five or more full-time doctors, with at least one on general practice or internal medicine. In sparsely-populated communities, as few as three doctors are allowed.

Unfortunately, Title XI funding for group practice appears to be even more remote than Hill-Burton financing. Applicants to the program must prove that they were not able to obtain a mortgage loan of similar terms from any other source, without F.H.A. assistance. In addition, H.E.W. must approve the proposed facility before H.U.D. or F.H.A. can act. While some money has been distributed, the time factor and the excessive red tape have proven to be deterrents.[123]

O.E.O.

The basic concept of the O.E.O. Community Neighborhood Health Service Program is to establish new ambulatory care centers in areas where there are insufficient facilities for the poor, and to staff these centers with some form of medical group practice.[124] Six basic guidelines were set down to govern each prospective O.E.O. applicant:

(1) high quality comprehensive, outpatient health services - both acceptable and accessible to the people being served must be available;
(2) representatives of the population being served should be included in the planning and administration of the plan;
(3) there must be provisions calling for continuous, personalized relationship between the health service providers and the patients;

---

[122] Ibid.

[123] Harvard Law Review, op. cit., p. 984.

[124] "Integration of an O.E.O. Health Program into A Prepaid Comprehensive Group Practice Plan," Theodore Columbo, Ernest Saward, M.D., Merwyn Greenlick, Journal of Public Health, (Jan.-June), p. 641.

(4) there must be training and employment of
neighborhood residents for the project;
(5) plans must be coordinated with other
anti-poverty programs;
(6) services must be provided in a way that
may be easily analyzed and observed.

These points are consistent with the basic principles of the Kaiser
Foundation, and because of this, the Oregon region, which was firmly committed
to the Kaiser concept, submitted a proposal in 1965 for a project to be
funded under O.E.O.'s Research and Development Program.[125] Thus, the Kaiser
Foundation in Portland, Oregon became the first prepaid group practice plan
to receive an O.E.O. grant for planning of comprehensive services. Since
that time, O.E.O. has funded the planning of N.H.C.'s in about a dozen
cities.[126]

Initial Mistakes

The Portland Plan was not actually funded by O.E.O. until late
1966, when specific monies became available under the Community Neighborhood
Health Service Amendment.[127] Two erroneous assumptions made by O.E.O.
officials in 1965 retarded all C.N.H.S. development. One error was the
belief that Title 18 and 19 funds would finance 50 to 75 per cent of the
costs of running the centers. Experience has shown that only ten to 20 per
cent of the cost of care is reimbursable through third-party government
funds.[128] The second wrong projection was that funds would be available
through Hill-Burton. Hill-Burton funds were committed years in advance, and
until just recently (June 1971), they had not committed any funds to N.H.C.
development. All construction funds have come through Title XI mortgage
loans.[129]

Recent O.E.O. Activity

In 1972, the O.E.O. was seeking to develop wide-range programs
through the H.M.O. concept. The agency was looking for six communities where
broad-based plans may be set up to service populations of 100,000 to 200,000.
Planning grants of two to three million dollars was to be awarded to each
organization. In 1971, two O.E.O. planning grants were given to the South
Philadelphia Health Action Corporation, and an organization servicing Orange
and Chatham Counties in North Carolina.[130] Tufts University's Community

---

[125]Ibid.

[126]"O.E.O. Officials: Clinics Could Become H.M.O.'s," Modern Hospital,
(September 1970), p. 34 (no author).

[127]"Integration of an O.E.O......." op, cit.

[128]"O.E.O. Officials:........" op. cit.

[129]Ibid.

[130]Ibid.

Health Action Program had earlier received O.E.O. research and demonstration grant in 1967, which helped launch their Columbia Point Health Plan in a Boston ghetto.[131] The East Baltimore Medical Plan, opened in April 1971, is at least partially being financed by O.E.O. funds. It is patterned after the Columbia Plan (Columbia, Maryland), except that it services a low-income population and has drawn most of its funds from government sources. The program is being financed both with Title 19 funds and Section 314 of P189-49 and the O.E.O. The O.E.O. funds have gone mainly to covering those individuals (approximately 30 per cent) in the area not covered by the other government programs. The major funding problem of the East Baltimore Plan was that medical programs available to the population are "categorical;" that is, an individual may be eligible one day and not the next. Thus, many people cannot fit into one particular category and may not participate in the plan. The O.E.O. program has been providing funds to support these excluded people.[132]

Smaller Sources

Other government agencies that have in the past participated in health care funding and may be tapable as supplementary sources for H.M.O. financing are: Small Business Administration, Model Cities Program (H.U.D.), Regional Medical Programs, Public Health Service, Medicare and Medicaid, Bureau of Health Manpower, Internal Revenue Service and Civil Service Commission. Since 1956, the Small Business Association has been making loans for hospital construction, nursing homes, and other health facilities that are operated for profit and qualify as a small business. Loans are made for construction, equipment and working capital.[133] A nonprofit-oriented H.M.O. will find that this source is not presently available.

The Model Cities Program of H.U.D. is involved with the F.H.A. Mortgage Insurance Program. Other than that, its contributions are very limited.

H.U.D., the F.H.A. and H.E.W. are all connected when it comes to funding health facilities, but quite often, grant applicants have difficulties in dealing with the multiplicity of governmental agencies involved. Doctors Robert Blenton and Clifton Gaus, affiliated with the East Baltimore Plan, claimed that the Johns Hopkins Medical School had to deal with three levels of government and 12 separate agencies. Each had its own definitions, guidelines, administrative processes and funding cycles.[134]

---

[131]"The Tufts Comprehensive Community Health Action Program," William F. Maloney, M.D., _Journal of American Medical Association_, (October 30, 1967), Volume 202, No. 5, p. 110.

[132]"The Columbia Medical Plan and the East Baltimore Medical Plan," Robert M. Heyssel, M.D., _Hospitals_, (March 16, 1971), Volume 45, pp. 69-71.

[133]Harold M. Graning, M.D., _op. cit._

[134]"Drug Research Report," - "The Blue Sheet," (July 7, 1971), Volume 14, No. 27, pp. 12-13.

H.E.W.

        The Department of Health, Education and Welfare is the central government agency for dealing with H.M.O. planning and development. Unfortunately, federal resources today "are scattered in categorical, earmarked pigeon-holes"[135] instead of properly being gathered in one common package."[136] The Nixon Administration is attempting to develop "a single point of access in the Government with a single instrument for the combination of resources needed to achieve the purposes."[137] H.E.W. would be responsible for creating this instrument.

        President Nixon's new health plan (other bills also) proposes financial assistance to those H.M.O.'s already in operating stages. While little money will be available until some new health legislation is padded by Congress, H.E.W. has stated that there are some funds already appropriated which may be used by newly-formed H.M.O.'s, mostly for planning purposes.[138]

Situation as of 1972

        Section 314(e) of the Public Health Service Act is being used as the mechanism for financial and by H.E.W.[139] Section 314(e) authorizes two types of grant programs: (1) "Projects to provide health services (included related training) to meet health needs of limited geographic scope or of specialized regional or national significance; and (2) projects to develop and support new program of health services."[140] Grants may be made to cover a part of the cost of the project, and applicants must prove that they can provide the remainder of the cost. The extent of coverage by 314(e) will depend on the type of grant awarded, depending on whether the request for funds is an "initial" request, a request for "additional" funds or for "supplemental" funds.[141]

Grant Cycle

        Specific grant cycles, as set down by H.E.W., are another important consideration.[142] These cycles must be anticipated because there are three deadline dates per year, and "....there is a rather involved review process

---

[135]"Towards A Comprehensive Health Policy for the 1970's," A White Paper, Dept. of H.E.W., (May 1971), p. 37.

[136]Ibid.

[137]Ibid.

[138]"Health Maintenance Organizations," The Concept and The Structure, Dept. of H.E.W. and H.S.M.H.A., Rockville, Md., (no date), 6 pages, p. 3.

[139]Letter (form), from Regional Office of H.E.W., Region II (N.Y.) to Glenn E. Hastings, Project Director, Nassau-Suffolk Comprehensive Health Planning Council, Centereach, N.Y. (April 8, 1971).

[140]"Instructions for Preparation and Submission of Application for Health Services Development Project Grant," (Rockville, Md.: H.E.W. and H.S.M.H.A.), p. 1.

[141]Letter from Regional Office of H.E.W., op. cit.

[142]Personal Interview with Dr. Lawrence Clare of H.S.M.H.A.-H.E.W., Regional Office #2, (Feb. 8, 1972).

that involves both the regional and headquarters offices of the H.M.O. effort."
The first deadline for the 1972 fiscal year was October 15th. The second was
originally scheduled for January 15th, but the government made a change a
week before the applications were due, changing the mechanism from grants to
contracts and giving applicants another month to receive contract materials
and make revisions. Approximately 3½ million dollars in grants will be distributed in this second cycle. The final cycle will have an April 15th
deadline.[143]

Grants and Contracts

The grant-contract relationship is somewhat complicated. Changing
from grants to contracts and back is a technique devised by H.E.W. to make
more funds available. "A grant is an award of money to carry out a program
purpose, that purpose having been intended to be carried out by a nongovern-
mental effort." While the government may set down some guidelines and give
some assistance, the final product, in a sense, is the undertaking, and
ultimately, the property of the grantee.

Contracts are supposed to be a much more tightly controlled
bidding on a rather specific product. The product becomes the responsibility
of the government to provide, and the contractor, in effect, becomes an extension of the government. Anything the contractor produces becomes the government property and is more tightly controlled by the government. In the
present funding cycle (#2), the contract mechanism is being used with a great
purpose because it is the way to get at available money.[144] This administrative revision and others, along with the constantly changing deadlines
and quantity of appropriated funds, adds to the uncertainty that presently
exists, and will continue to exist in H.E.W. until some H.M.O. legislation
is passed.

Application

The main ingredient in applying for any H.E.W. grant or contract
is the submission of a detailed, line-by-line budget in which all costs and
revenues are included. The projections should be made on an annual basis,
up to three years in advance. Each individual cost category must be identified, and utilization rates must be projected. Annual revenue will be a
key factor, with the dues' rate structure being the most significant
variable.[145] Based on revenue and cost projections, the financial statements
and supporting documentation that should be prepared for the government, as
well as for any other prospective lender, include:

(1) Cash flow chart, by month, for the first year, and
by six-month intervals for the next two years.

---

[143]Ibid.

[144]Ibid.

[145]"H.M.O. Development Checklist," paper received from H.E.W. - no date or
author.

(2) Statement of Sources and Uses of Funds for
    each six-month period - for first three years
    of operation.
(3) Statement of income and expenses for each
    quarter of the first year and each half of
    the second and third years.
(4) A projection of cash flow breakeven and total
    operational breakeven in terms of time and
    money.
(5) A statement of the amount of money to be
    borrowed, and a description of the uses to
    which the funds will be put.
(6) A general description of the H.M.O. and
    the activities it will be conducting.
(7) A short biographical sketch of key officers
    in the H.M.O.[146]

314(e) grant applications are sent to the regional H.E.W. office, where they
are evaluated and sent on to the central office in Washington.[147]

Filling out government grant applications is a lengthy, but
important procedure. When an H.M.O. is first being organized, grants
management becomes one of the more important responsibilities. Most large
hospitals employ a well-trained specialist to deal with grant applications.[148]

Recent Funding

H.M.O.'s received $6.5 million in planning funds from H.E.W. during
fiscal year ending June 1971. Secretary Elliot L. Richardson stated that 66
grants were given to: physician groups, medical schools, neighborhood health
centers, community hospitals, existing H.M.O.-like organizations, medical
society foundation plans, private corporations, and state and local health
departments, to develop H.M.O.'s.[149]

Grants and contracts were awarded to the two agencies directly
involved in the H.M.O. development program in H.E.W. - the Health Services
and Mental Health Administration (H.S.M.H.A.) and the Medical Services
Administration (M.S.A.) of the Social and Rehabilitation service. H.S.M.H.A.
made 35 planning grants and 16 grants for feasibility studies. These 51
awards totaled $5,391,924. M.S.A. funded 15 research and demonstration
projects at a total of $1,100,000. M.S.A. projects are primarily concerned
with developing H.M.O. options for Medicaid recipients.[150] Of the 51 grants

[146]Ibid., pp. 19-20.

[147]Letter from Regional Office of H.E.W. op. cit.

[148]Interview - Petit and Hoover, op. cit.

[149]"H.E.W. News," Office of Public Affairs, H.E.W., (July 20, 1971).

[150]Ibid., p. 2.

139

and contracts distributed by H.S.M.H.A., 18 were over $100,000 and seven
were $200,000 or more. The Department of Public Health in Philadelphia
received the largest sum ($525,000). There were two R & D grants (M.S.A.)
over $100,000. One was given to Temple University ($130,954) and the
other to the Department of Social Services and Housing in Honolulu ($144,511).
(See Table IV - 7).[151]

Short-Range Funding Prospects

As of 1972, the most accurate figure on funds available through
H.E.W. to H.M.O.'s is "less than 27 million dollars."[152] The H.E.W. budget
has authorized approximately 57 million dollars for the 1972 fiscal year, but
that would depend on the passage, by Congress, of the H.M.O. Assistance Act.
The Act may not be passed until the end of 1972, and if this occurs, certainly
H.E.W. would not be able to distribute an additional 20 million dollars right
at the end (i.e., last month), and so much of the appropriated funds for 1972
would go unused. If the Act is passed within a reasonable time limit, the
Administration expects to spend about 57 million dollars in 1972 and 60
million in 1973.

Meantime, H.E.W. is borrowing money from other programs (314e).
So far, all that has been spent in 1972 is about 9¼ million dollars, so that
hopefully, an additional 20 million dollars will be spent in 1973. It will
be spent on further initial developmental and planning grants, as well as
"second stage grants," to plans which were awarded funds in May and June of
1971.

This, of course, does not imply that H.E.W. will simply go to the
grantee and give them funds for another year. The department expects "not
only success in terms of moving forward, but an ability to carry success to
a further stage next year," and what this probably means is that some of the
grantees of last June will probably be able to secure much larger grants, as
they develop their plan to an advanced stage, while others may simply be
turned down.[153]

Local (New York and New Jersey)

On the local level, Donald Logsdon, the H.M.O. coordinator for
the Region II office of H.E.W.,[154] said in June of 1971 that he had received
22 applications for general development grants, running from $50,000-$500,000.
Development expenses covered: staff recruitment, marketing costs, study of
physician and community attitudes, determination of legal issues and barriers,

---

[151]Ibid., pp. 3-7.

[152]Interview - Clare, op. cit.

[153]Ibid.

[154]Speech made at the Institute, sponsored by the Hospital Association of
New York State, One-Day Institute on Prepaid Group Practice, Non-Profit
Medical Corporation and Health Maintenance Organization, held on June 15,
1971 in Albany.

TABLE III - 7

GRANTS - H.S.M.H.A. - 1971

Recipient	City & State	Amount of Grant	Recipient	City & State	Amount of Grant
Matthew Thornton Health Plan, Inc.	Hollis, N.H.	$ 21,000	American Assoc. of Medical Colleges	Washington, D.C.	$127,688
Harvard Community Health, Inc.	Boston, Mass.	98,795	Florida Health Care Plan	Daytona Beach, Fla.	75,000
Health, Inc.	Boston, Mass.	121,858	State of Franklin Health Council	Cullouhee, N.C.	40,000
Blue Shield of Rhode Island	Providence, R.I.	23,250	Abraham Lincoln Memorial Hospital	Lincoln, Ill.	56,000
Martin Luther King, Jr.	Bronx, N.Y.	52,850	Consumer Cooperative Group Health Plan	St. Paul, Minn.	99,875
Hunterdon Medical Center	Flemington, N.J.	99,682	Lovelace-Bataan Medical Centr. & Presbyterian Medical Services	Albuquerque, N.M.	79,681
Mt. Sinai Hospital	New York, N.Y.	53,029	Bexar County Medical Foundation	San Antonio, Tex.	63,820
New York City Health & Hospital Corps.	New York, N.Y.	100,000	Hillcrest Medical Center	Tulsa, Okla.	72,151
GHAA-Blue Cross/Blue Shield	Rochester, N.Y.	212,540	Dodge City Medical Center	Dodge City, Kans.	122,270
Nassau Medical Services Foundation	Garden City, N.Y.	64,000	Rocky Mountain-Grand Junction County Medical Society	Grand Junction, Colo.	13,000

141

TABLE III - 7 (continued)

Recipient	City & State	Amount of Grant	Recipient	City & State	Amount of Grant
Georgetown University	Washington, D.C.	$130,892	Metropolitan Denver Foundation for Medical Care	Englewood, Colo.	$ 52,550
Missoula Comprehensive Health Planning Council	Missoula, Mont.	55,985	Cuyahoga County Hospital	Cleveland, Ohio	80,075
Alamosa Community Hospital	Alamosa, Colo.	35,385	Detroit Health Facility, Inc.	Detroit Mich.	79,650
Denver Health and Hospitals	Denver, Colo.	80,228	Carbondale Health Plan	Carbondale, Ill.	77,085
Health Services Alliance of San Jose, Inc.	San Jose, Calif.	77,000	Health Facilities Research, Inc.	Port Charlotte, Florida	55,000
Lutheran Hospital of Southern California	Los Angeles, Calif.	100,000	Tennessee Group Health Foundation, Inc.	Nashville, Tenn.	230,105
Foundations for Medical Care of Sonoma County	Santa Rosa, Calif.	102,750	Univ. of Ky. Research Foundation	Lexington, Ky.	51,250
Medical Care Foundation of Sacramento	Sacramento, Calif.	101,266	Group Health Cooperative of Puget Sound(Olympia)	Seattle, Wash.	90,500
Consumer Cooperative - Puget Sound	Seattle, Wash.	99,000			

Source: H.E.W. News, Office of Public Affairs, H.E.W., July 20, 1971, pp. 3-7.

142

TABLE III - 7 (continued)

CONTRACTS - H.S.M.H.A.

Recipient	City & State	Amount of Grant	Recipient	City & State	Amount of Grant
Community Health Center Foundation	Salt Lake City, Utah	$ 77,000	Boise State College	Boise, Idaho	$110,000
Genesee Region Health Planning Council	Rochester, N.Y.	250,000	East Los Angeles Health Task Force	Los Angeles, Calif.	250,000
Penobscot Bay Medical Center	Rockport, Maine	107,000	N.Y.-Pennsylvania Health Planning Council	Binghamton, N.Y.	65,000
Maryland Health Maintenance Committee, Inc.	Baltimore, Md.	250,000	Health Planning Council, Inc.	Tucson, Arizona	250,000
American Assoc. of Medical Clinics	Alexandria, Va.	199,796	Dept. of Public Health	Philadelphia, Pa.	525,000
Texas Instruments	Dallas Texas	99,963	Mon Valley Community Health Center	Monessen, Pa.	4,000
Bionetics Research Labs., Div. of Litton Industries	Bethesda, Md.	40,000 (approx.)			
Family Health Care, Inc.	Washington, D.C.	68,955			

143

TABLE III - 7 (continued)

RESEARCH AND DEMONSTRATION GRANTS - M.S.A.

Recipient	City & State	Amount of Grant	Recipient	City & State	Amount of Grant
Survey Research Center, University of California at Los Angeles	Los Angeles, Calif.	$ 86,484	Harvard Community Health Plan, Inc.	Boston, Mass.	$ 33,557
Jefferson County Department of Health	Birmingham, Alabama	69,786	Department of Public Welfare	Columbus, Ohio	74,219
Mesa County Medical Society	Grand Junction, Colo.	36,195	Department of Public Welfare	Boston, Mass.	72,388
The Atchison, Topeka and Santa Fe Memorial Hospitals, Inc.	Topeka, Kansas	55,800	Institute of Health Services Research, Tulane University	New Orleans, La.	81,707
Penobscot Bay Medical Center, Inc.	Rockport, Maine	54,240	Temple University	Philadelphia, Pa.	130,954
Greater Woodlawn Assistance Corporation	Chicago, Ill.	45,000	The Regents of the University of Michigan	Ann Arbor, Michigan	58,560
South Philadelphia Health Action	Philadelphia, Pa.	62,530	Department of Human Resources	District of Columbia	94,069
Department of Social Services and Housing	Honolulu, Hawaii	144,511			

consultant costs and others. Applicants were asked (according to the readiness of their organizations) to request for funds in one of these, or any other area they felt important. Of the 32 applications, 17 were considered appropriate, and from those, four were approved. The four chosen were affiliated with (1) a neighborhood center; (2) a medical school; (3) a public hospital; and (4) a hospital in New Jersey. These four awarded grants were to be of a "demonstrative" nature, and would last for a total period not to exceed over one year, with the option of extending that grant for an additional year, if the funds are available.[155]

Long-Range Prospects

Based on pending health legislation in Congress, H.E.W. has estimated its own potential H.M.O. development program through 1976. Their estimates are based on 50 million additional subscribers by the end of the decade.[156] H.M.O. "units" are used to project H.E.W. grants for planning, development and operating support. Each H.M.O. unit would average 30,000 members.[157] Table III - 8 contains a summary of the number of H.M.O.'s in development.

According to pending legislation, H.E.W. will provide $23 million in planning grants through 1976. They will average $250,000 and range between 50 and 500 thousand dollars. In operating support, H.E.W. (under the proposed H.M.O. Assistance Act and Health Manpower Bill) would have three individual programs. First, H.E.W. would provide $22 million of initial operating grants, contracts or loans to H.M.O.'s that serve predominantly poor, underserved areas. New H.M.O.'s serving a cross-section of the population, could receive working capital loans in the first three years or operation, and grants for ambulatory facilities and equipment approximating $300 million.

H.E.W. will also provide up to 75 additional dollars for each Medicare-Medicaid beneficiary enrolled in the schools' H.M.O. plan.[158] In total, H.E.W. estimates it would spend $813 million on developing H.M.O.'s up to 1976 (see Table III - 9). However, in the Senate Health Subcommittee hearing on July 20, 1971, H.E.W. Assistant Secretary DuVal, cut the figure to $598 million.[159] Senator Kennedy, who was conducting the health

---

[155] Memorandum - Long Island Jewish Medical Center, "One Day Institute on Prepaid Group Practice, Non-Profit Medical Corp., and H.M.O.," Held on June 15, 1971, Albany, June 22nd (date of Memorandum), pp. 5-6.

[156] Long Island Jewish Medical Center - Legislative Bulletin #5, August 5, 1971, Released by Joseph Levi, p. 1.

[157] A 30,000 subscriber unit may be an individual H.M.O., or it could be a large H.M.O. which has expanded from 30 to 60 thousand.

[158] L.I.J.M.C. - Legislative Bulletin, op. cit., pp. 2-5.

[159] Drug Research Report, Volume 14, No. 29, (July 21, 1971), "Kennedy Attacks Ambiguity of Administration's Planning of H.M.O.'s; Javits Sees H.M.O.'s Needed Under Any Proposed National Financing Scheme," pp. 19-21.

TABLE III - 8

HEALTH MAINTENANCE ORGANIZATIONS DEVELOPMENT PROGRAM

(Units = 30,000 enrollees)

	Fiscal Year					
	1972	1973	1974	1975	1976	1972-6
H.M.O.'s in Planning	92	236	272	200	200	1000
H.M.O.'s Operating:						
With H.E.W. Support	122	230	314	392	442	1500
Without	6	17	59	68	50	200
Total	128	247	373	460	492	1700
Cumulative	128	375	748	1208	1700	1700
Enrollment (millions)						
Potential.	3.78	11.25	22.46	36.30	51.00	
Actual	1.26	5.03	12.52	23.37	36.66	
Budget Authority (millions)	$ 49	$131	$186	$205	$241	

Source: "Legislative Bulletin #5," Long Island Jewish Hospital, August 5, 1971, Page 2.

TABLE III - 9

H.E.W. PROGRAM - H.M.O. DEVELOPMENT

(Dollars in Millions)

	Fiscal Year '72		Fiscal Year '73		Fiscal Year '74	
	Units	Amounts	Units	Amounts	Units	Amounts
Planning	92	$ 23	236	$ 59	272	$ 68
Operating Grants	36	$ 18	70	$ 35	100	$ 50
Loans	1	$ 4	6	$ 24	9	$ 36
Medical School Grants	10	$ 4	24	$ 13	50	$ 32
Total Budgetary Authority		...$49		...$131		...$186

	Fiscal Year '75		Fiscal Year '76		Fiscal Year '72-76	
	Units	Amounts	Units	Amounts	Units	Amounts
Planning	200	$ 50	200	$ 50	1,000	$250
Operating Grants	94	$ 47	90	$ 45	160	$195
Loans	12	$ 48	12	$ 48	40	$160
Medical School Grants	75	$ 60	100	$ 98	100	$207
Total Budgetary Authority		...$205		...$241		...$812

Source: "Legislative Bulletin #5," Long Island Jewish Hospital, August 5, 1971, Page 5.

Subcommittee hearings, claimed that H.E.W. and the Administration were purposely making their proposals on H.M.O. financing vague so that no commitments would actually be made until President Nixon's health legislation is passed.[160] Also, in the July 20th hearing, it was noted that H.E.W. grants and contracts. Dr. DuVal said they were for exploration and R & D, so that cost-control regulations could be instituted.[161]

G.H.A.A.

Group Health Association of America is a nonprofit organization devoted to the development of prepaid group practice plans around the nation. While G.H.A.A. does not give planning funds, it may be classified as an indirect source because it helps in making feasibility studies and the avail- ability of consultation with H.M.O.'s.[162] If a plan is not yet developed and the climate appears right for establishing an H.M.O., "Group Health" will send in a field respresentative to help organize the community.[163] While G.H.A.A. offers a limited amount of technical assistance themselves, they often arrange for consultants from the various member plans like Kaiser, H.I.P. and Group Coop. of Puget Sound, to assist a new plan in a more thorough manner.

G.H.A.A. was organized in 1959 through an H.E.W. grant. As stated in its Articles of Incorporation, the organization's basic purpose is to "promote the health and well-being of the people of North America, especially through application in health care programs of the principles of:

1. Prepayment of the cost of health care;
2. Group practice of medicine;
3. Comprehensive health care of high quality
    under the direction of qualified professional personnel;
4. Direction of policy and administrative functions
    be in the interest of consumers of health
    services."[164]

It has received various additional grants from H.E.W. One recent grant was used to set up the Education and Training Department, of which Mr. Jeffrey Prussin is the Director. G.H.A.A. also relies on income from

[160]Ibid., p. 19.

[161]Ibid., p. 20.

[162]Harvard Law Review, op. cit., p. 953.

[163]Personal Interview with Jeffrey A. Prussin, Director of Dept. of Education and Training, (Washington, D.C.: Group Health Association of America, January 31, 1972).

[164]This is G.H.A.A., (pamphlet), Prepared by Group Health Association of America, Inc.

dues paid by its member plans.[165] However, because H.E.W. grants provide most of the financial backing, G.H.A.A. must abide by grant stipulations, which state that the organization may take only a limited part in an H.M.O.'s formation.[166]

Aside from the assistance that is given new plans, G.H.A.A. also does lobbying, educational training, and distributes various pamphlets and folders on the H.M.O. concept. There is a prepaid group practice school which has a series of workshops on group practice, hosted by various member plans and which gives an in-depth look at the several member plans. G.H.A.A. is also developing a series of special interest workshops on subjects on legal matters and industry enrollment. They work with labor groups and can help in H.M.O. enrollment on a local level.

G.H.A.A. is not simply a public relations organization for H.M.O.'s. It is more a "how-to-do-it" type of situation where professionals are given basic training in overcoming obstacles to H.M.O. formation. It has materials of interest to management, labor, doctors, and the general public.[167]

Blue Cross-Blue Shield

If the H.M.O. is to become a dominant force in the health industry, Blue Cross must aid its development. But the fundamental concept of "the Blues" is inconsistent with a prepaid group practice. Blue Cross has a financial role as an insurance company which pays the cost of hospitalization. This may change, and signs of change are appearing. Blue Cross seems to be interested in setting up H.M.O.'s because of their leadership in the health insurance industry, and the prospect of creating a more efficient mechanism of their own.[168]

Blue Cross has played a variety of roles in relation to H.M.O.'s. In some nonhospital-based plans like H.I.P., subscribers carry Blue Cross or other hospitalization insurance. Thus, there is a close tie between the two, with H.I.P. providing the ambulatory care, and Blue Cross, the financing for hospitalization.[169]

This relationship, or one of a similar nature, is mutually advantageous because none of the newly-formed H.M.O.'s are able to set up their own hospital facilities, and as a result, cannot insure hospitalization coverage without outside assistance. While the New Haven Plan was partially

---

[165]"Prepaid Group Practice," (folder), A workshop series on fundamentals of prepaid group practice, sponsored by G.H.A.A., Inc.

[166]Interview - Prussin, op. cit.

[167]Ibid.

[168]Harvard Law Review, op. cit., p. 905. Also, interview with Barry Zeman at Long Island Jewish Hospital.

[169]Ibid., p. 912.

self-financed and did its own underwriting, Blue Cross is still used as a financial agent for reimbursing the hospital.[170] The Harvard Plan has used a variety of private insurance companies, including Blue Cross, to underwrite and assist in marketing the plan.[171]

Blue Cross is particularly interested in H.M.O.'s developed within a hospital setting, because if they encourage an efficient hospital-based H.M.O., they may reap the benefits.[172] The Long Island Jewish Hospital H.M.O. will be a test of the relationship between the hospital-based plans and the Blues, because New York Blue Cross is providing L.I.J. with planning funds and its marketing organization.[173]

Reasons for Present Lack of Support

Blue Cross states that it "is capable of offering to emerging group practice plans the means of obtaining a sound financial base, marketing, benefit structure, financing and reimbursement, computer capacity and systems skills, and physician and hospital relationships.[174] Also, Blue Cross can best handle the problem of out-of-area coverage, with which all H.M.O.'s are faced.

While it readily admits that it favors the H.M.O. concept, for many reasons it has so far been limiting its support. One reason is Blue Cross' relationship with Blue Shield in each state. Dr. Joseph Dorsey, the Harvard Plan's Medical Planning Director, told a Senate Subcommittee on October 6, 1971 that once the Harvard Plan had proven itself, Blue Cross had guaranteed H.C.H.P. 11,000 new members within one year, or it would pay "the fixed costs of providing ambulatory care, to the extent the enrollment falls short of the commitment.[175] In contrast, Massachusetts Blue Shield declined to participate. This conflict may be complicated in an area where Blue Shield is more powerful. In Providence, Blue Shield has large cash reserves, while Blue Cross does not. Thus, the immediate prospects of an H.M.O. obtaining capital from a physician-controlled Blue Shield organization is not good.

In both Rhode Island and Boston (Harvard), Blue Cross continued to support the H.M.O.'s, albeit with a small capital investment. After an H.M.O. proves that it can function effectively, the Blue Cross may increase their participation.[176]

---

[170]Ibid., p. 916.

[171]Ibid.

[172]"Prepaid Group Practice and H.M.O.'s," paper printed by New York Blue Cross, Introduction, pp. 1-2 (no author or date).

[173]Interview - Barry Zeman, op. cit.

[174]Blue Cross Paper, op. cit.

[175]Interview - Petit and Hoover, op. cit.

[176]Ibid.

H.M.O.'s Effect on "Blues" Present Position

The competitive force which H.M.O.'s present to Blue Cross has had a number of effects. Wherever an H.M.O. springs up, Blue Cross rearranges the benefit packages. As soon as the Rhode Island H.M.O. opened, Blue Cross adjusted their state and local employee program so that it included diagnostics, outpatient services, and other benefits not originally offered. So, even though Rhode Island did not get the number of enrollees it had anticipated, in effect, it caused upgrading of Blue Cross coverage for the entire community. This has also occurred with the various Kaiser plans in the west.[177]

"Blues" Present and Future H.M.O. Development

This line of reasoning has led to an increase in the number of Blue Cross Service plans actively engaged in the formation and organization of H.M.O.'s. In March 1970, the 74 members of Blue Cross were polled on their relationships with prepaid group plans in their area. Five Blue Cross members stated that they were actively involved in H.M.O. development (N.Y., L.A., Wash., D.C., St. Louis, and Boston). Eight others were presently exploring the possibility of involvement, and an additional eight expressed interest, or had studies concerning H.M.O.'s under way.[178]

The "Blues" have recently been involved with the Marshfield Clinic in Wisconsin, Medi-Groups in New Jersey, and various plans in the South, all of which are H.M.O.'s.[179] A major effort to set up a successful H.M.O. has been made by the "Blues" in Rochester, where Dr. Ernest Saward now presides as acting Chief Administrator of the plan. Because of Dr. Seward's excellent reputation and other favorable factors concerning the Rochester Community, Blue Cross has made it one of its largest H.M.O. investments in funds and services. A "new town," similar to Columbia, Maryland, is being built close by, which will increase the subscription potential for the Rochester Plan.[180]

Each of the 74 Blue Cross-Blue Shield plans is in a different state of development with respect to its attitude towards the H.M.O. concept. In California, the attitude of any health insurance organization towards the H.M.O. is positive, while in the South, where no established H.M.O.'s have yet proven themselves, the relationship is still unformed. Blue Cross is a non-profit organization responsible to the various state insurance departments, and therefore, cannot use its monies to support questionable experimental programs. Some Blue Cross-Blue Shield plans do not have the surplus resources to devote additional staff time, research time, and fund support to a new H.M.O. plan.[181]

---

[177]Ibid.

[178]"Group Practice: Planning and Implementing A Community-Wide Prepayment Plan," Ann S. Bush, New York State Health Planning Commission, (May 1971), p. 35.

[179]Interview - Marvin Leeds, op. cit.

[180]Interview - Petit and Hoover, op. cit.

[181]Interview - Ron Nick, op. cit.

151

Opinion of H.M.O. Leadership

There appears to be division within the various Blue Cross-Blue Shield organizations as to whether or not an H.M.O. is a worthwhile investment. There is also division among H.M.O. administrators concerning the desirability of a strong H.M.O.-Blue Cross relationship. Some believe that the real future of prepaid group practice is intimately connected with the Blue Cross, because the "Blues" have the real power in the health field with their tie-ins with county medical societies and close relationship with the hospitals in each state.[182] Leo Petit of R.I.G.H.A. believes that the "Blues" might become a significant force in H.M.O. development, but he also believes that there were certain areas, like marketing, where their effectiveness could be improved.[183]

Insurance Companies

As was the case with Blue Cross-Blue Shield, the commercial insurance carrier, because of its experience, is a natural ally of an H.M.O. Insurance companies are "trustees of their insured," with the responsibility of looking after their best interest, and must constantly re-evaluate their product so that they keep pace with advances in technology and the organization of health care.[184] So, it would be logical for them to play an active role in experimentation with the H.M.O. concept.

History

The first real step in establishing a relationship between prepaid group practice and the commercial insurance came in September of 1967, when H.E.W. Secretary Gardner told the National Conference on Private Health Insurance that insurers should become actively concerned with making coverages available for group practice care, on a dual-choice basis.

This was followed by additional conferences throughout 1967 and 1968 which helped develop, in a more concrete fashion, the relationship between the carrier and the H.M.O.[185] In 1967 and 1968, another major development occurred when the Harvard Plan, the New Haven Plan and the Rhode Island Group Association all began exploring the possibilities of having major insurance carriers participate in their development. Harvard appointed a committee to give consideration to the possible relationship. The committee established sub-groups to consider legal, administrative, actuarial, and marketing considerations.[186]

---

[182] Interview - Marvin Leeds, op. cit.

[183] Interview - Petit and Hoover, op. cit.

[184] J.F. Follmann, "Insurance Companies and Group Practice," Health Insurance Association of America, 1968, (Paper).

[185] It must be remembered that the term H.M.O. was not yet developed in 1967 and 1968. Here, H.M.O. meant prepaid group practice.

[186] J.F. Follmann, op. cit.

Other events occurred in 1968 which further expanded the possibilities. H.I.P. worked out an arrangement with two insurance carriers,
Metropolitan Life and Continental Assurance, whereby H.I.P. would provide
medical services, and they provide the hospital insurance and marketing
effort. The insurance companies agreed to make possible the choice of major
medical or H.I.P. in certain of its insured groups. In May of 1968,
Metropolitan Life Insurance made a $100,000 demonstration grant for an
ambulatory medical care program at Washington University, with the prospect
of similar-sized donations over the next four years. Funds provided by those
grants went to pay salaries of professional and nonprofessional personnel, to
buy office equipment and supplies and to pay for data-processing equipment.[187]

Despite the many encouraging signs throughout 1967 and 1968, there
are only a few situations where insurance companies have a major financial
stake in an H.M.O., because of the uncertainty that surrounds most H.M.O.'s.
There is no proof, aside from the Kaiser-Permanente Plan, that a prepaid group
practice can generate its own funds and provide a reasonable rate of return
on investments. Unlike Blue Cross and Blue Shield, commercial carriers are
profit-oriented organizations and do not make investments unless they can be
assured of a favorable return. In the beginning, some carriers said that
"since this is a brand new situation, let's get our feet wet and maybe everybody will benefit." As the newness faded away, the major commitments have
also.[188] Connecticut General's venture into Columbia, Maryland is one exception. Also, Equitable Life has invested $3.5 million in a program sponsored
by the National Medical Association in Washington, D.C., and has loaned $1.5
million to the New Haven Health Plan. The Harvard Plan has contracts with
ten different insurance companies who are offering the program as a dual-
choice option to 170 employer groups.[189]

The Columbia Experience

Connecticut General's Relationship to the Plan

There are three basic components in the Columbia Plan's organizational framework: the Columbia Hospital and Clinic Foundation, Inc., with a board
of directors consisting of a Joint Committee of Trustees of Johns Hopkins
University and Hospitals; the Columbia Medical Group, consisting of a limited
partnership with the Dean and Associate Deans of Johns Hopkins Medical School;
and Connecticut General, which serves as the lead carrier in the development
process.[190] Connecticut General has provided the mortgage financing for
building a new hospital and ambulatory care facilities through a $3.75 million
loan.

---

[187]Ibid.

[188]Interview - Clare, op. cit.

[189]Bush, op. cit., p. 34.

[190]"The Columbia Medical Plan," speech presented by Harold R. Thalheimer,
   Medical Programs Department, Connecticut General Life Insurance Company,
   before the American Association of Hospital Planning and the Association
   of Hospital Consultants, (August 16, 1969).

There are also significant development costs, and this is being treated by Connecticut General and the other carriers involved as a typical insurance risk. Many of the losses will eventually be paid back to the insurance company; first, in the form of a 25 per cent retention factor added to the monthly premium, and second, through an agreement which stipulates that if and when the Columbia Plan starts making profits and accumulates cash in excess of one-month's operating expenses, then that money will go to reducing the deficit.[191]

Reasons for Connecticut General's Involvement

With the large potential risk in the Columbia Plan, the question arises as to why Connecticut General would get involved as deeply as they have. One reason is that C.G. had about $50 million invested in the real estate development of Columbia, even before the health plan was started, and they got involved with the health plan because it made good real estate investment sense. Certainly, when a person is considering moving to a new town, the quality of the health facilities available are an important incentive.[192]

Secondly, Connecticut General is one of the largest writers of health insurance each year of any commercial carrier, and consequently, they are making a sound business decision in order to protect an investment already made. They are looking for ways to keep themselves from getting hurt in their health insurance business, which seems to be the present trend for all carriers.

Columbia represents C.G.'s experiment with the H.M.O. concept as a possible mechanism of increased cost control. The $20 million investment is not necessarily an overwhelming sum, if considered an investment which may lead to a reduction of C.G.'s other health losses.[193]

Aside from the financial investment, C.G., along with all large carriers, believes that they have a definite responsiblity to their insured, and if they help develop a modality which improves the cost and quality of the present health delivery system, that responsibility would be met.[194]

---

[191] Personal interview with Ira Shimp, Assistant Director of Columbia Medical Plan, and John Bayliff, Controller of Columbia Plan, February 28, 1972.

[192] Personal Interview with Bruce Caputo, Director - Inner City Fund, New York and Washington, February 18, 1972. The Johns Hopkins Hospital, according to my interview at the Columbia Plan, is not the closest, nor is it the only hospital used by Columbia. Hopkins is used for routine admissions but emergency admissions go to St. Agnes Hospital, or Montgomery County General Hospital. Other scattered places are also used for orthopedic services and the like.

[193] Interview - Shimp and Bayliff, op. cit.

[194] Thalheimer Speech, op. cit.

Unions and Private Industry

Unions

Since organized labor is the second largest purchaser of health care in the United States, it is reasonable that they would have a real interest in H.M.O. development. The Griffith and Kennedy National Health Insurance Legislation is the result of increasing disenchantment by the A.F.L.-C.I.O. with the quality and cost of health care provided to their members. In California, the California Council for Health Plan Alternatives (C.C.H.P.A.), an organization which includes representatives from 14 of the largest unions in the state, has been formed to change the state's tradition-al fee-for-service practices into community-wide prepaid group practice plans.[195] Strong union backing has been responsible for the creation of other plans around the country.

In Detroit, the Community Health Association, with over 70,000 enrollees, was created in 1956 by the United Auto Workers. The Community Health Foundation of Cleveland is one of the few prepaid group plans which immediately started "in the black" because Sam Pollock, President of the Meat Cutters Union, promised and delivered 10,000 meat cutters as members of the plan in its very early stages.[196] While union enrollment has not been nearly as swift with the Rhode Island Plan, organized labor's unhappi-ness with the limitation of Blue Cross and Physician Service Plans ignited the initial spark more than 15 years ago.[197]

In Cleveland, various union concerns participated in funding the Foundation in its early planning stages. The Retail Clerks' Health and Welfare Fund passed a resolution to lend the C.H.F. $300,000 for construct-ing and developing the center. The Union Eye Care Center, which was interes-ted in new types of health services for its members, started the project in 1961 with a $25,000 grant. The center, between 1961 and 1963, continued to finance the cost of exploring the feasibility of a prepaid group plan in Cleveland, and up to June 1963, they had contributed a total of $51,500. The Meat Cutters Union also voted to loan C.H.F. $300,000. In addition, during the Fall of 1962 and 1963, a campaign was initiated, within all sponsoring unions, to raise capital for the building fund. Of the $1,401,500 raised by C.H.F. prior to 1964 (scheduled opening), union efforts provided more than half.[198]

In Providence, eight different A.F.L.-C.I.O. Unions, plus the Teamsters, participated in the start-up program for R.I.G.H.A., and a total of $250,000 was accumulated. So, while unions play a significant role in almost every H.M.O. development program, their financial resources may often be limited.[199]

---

[195]Ann S. Bush, op. cit., p. 36.

[196]Interview - Lou Sacadelli, op. cit.

[197]Edwin C. Brown, "How We Did It and Are Doing It - Providence (Hospital Model)," from Public Health Service - Labor Seminar on Consumer Health Services, Washington, D.C., (January 22-23, 1968).

[198]Avram Yedidia, op. cit., p. 30.

[199]Interview - Lou Sacadelli, op. cit.

Industry

While Kaiser has set an excellent precedent for industry participation in developing prepaid group practice plans, no other large corporation has duplicated the Kaiser situation, although there seems to be a reasonable cause for a large corporation getting involved. North American Rockwell, for instance, spends in the neighborhood of $35 million annually on health benefits for its employees, and a more efficient system would be most welcome.[200] Texas Instrument, with its 10,000 employees in Dallas, is looking for an alternative health organization. They have received a large planning grant from H.E.W., jointly with the University of Texas Medical School, and they have been trying to write a benefits plan, estimate its cost, and figure out how doctors and hospitals will be tied in under a non-profit organization in a similar pattern to the Kaiser Plan.[201]

Since it is likely that by the end of the 1970's there will be many more H.M.O.'s, the question as to what part the large corporation will play in this development becomes important. While some corporations probably will have satellite H.M.O.'s, the larger pattern will probably be groups of 20 to 25 doctors that service employee groups without being explicitly related to one. The Kaiser Plan is almost that way now, with Kaiser Industries' employees representing only about five per cent of the patient load.[202]

MEDICARE AND MEDICAID
(SOCIAL SECURITY ADMINISTRATION)

The term Health Maintenance Organization was first created by the House Ways and Means Committee in preparing the Social Security Amendment of 1970.[203] This amendment states that individuals eligible for coverage under Parts A and B of Medicare would be able to choose a new Part C, where their care would be provided by an H.M.O. The Social Security Administration would then reimburse the H.M.O. on a capitation basis.[204] Today, Medicare provides protection for more than 95 per cent of the elderly, the Medicaid provides some protection for 15 million of the aged poor, the blind, the disabled and families with children.[205]

---

[200]Ann S. Bush, op. cit., p. 35.

[201]Interview - Bruce Caputo, op. cit.

[202]Ibid.

[203]"Legislation and Prepayment for Group Practice," Bulletin N.Y. Academy of Medicine, Louis L. Feldman, M.B.A., Vol. 47, No. 4, (April 1971), p. 418.

[204]Ibid., p. 419.

[205]"Towards A Comprehensive Health Policy for the 70's," p. 13.

History

Prepaid group practice was originally tied to the S.S.A. through the 1965 Social Security Amendments which provided for Medicare and Medicaid. After the amendments were drawn, a phrase was added to Section 1833 of Title 18 (Medicare) calling for the participation of prepayment organizations on a basis other than fee-for-service. The Social Security Administration interpreted this as meaning an organization with three or more full-time physicians (or the equivalent) and a prepayment system where the people who are members pay, or have payments made for them, in advance.[206] In spite of the provision made for prepaid group practice, the S.S.A. was totally oriented towards reimbursing costs on an item-by-item basis. Because H.M.O.'s do not determine the costs for each particular service, the total costs of services made to Medicare and Medicaid patients had to be roughly estimated, and a portion of that cost allocated to the S.S.A. Also, the $50 annual deductible and 20 per cent co-insurance requirements of Medicare, had to be changed to an equivalent monthly premium rate which Medicare subscribers would pay.[207]

These and other Administration complications have caused much confusion for the individual plan and for the government. However, the larger, established H.M.O.'s have been quite successful in enrolling Medicare recipients.[208] H.I.P. for example, has 55,000 Medicare enrollees in its plan, and approximately four per cent of Kaiser's enrollees are 65 years or more.[209]

Cost Savings

Whether the Social Security Administration is a financial source of H.M.O.'s is a matter of interpretation; health plan officials will argue that it is the plans that are providing additional funds for the S.S.A. by sizably reducing the reimbursement figures. According to 1968 figures, the Group Health Cooperative of Puget Sound saved the S.S.A. $206.96 per Medicare enrollee[210] (See Table III - 10). Figures compiled by the U.S. Civil Service Commission indicate that in Portland, Kaiser Plan Medicare patients used 1,700 hospital days per year, as compared to the national average of over 2,700 days.[211] In the 65-and-over category, Group Health Association of Washington, D.C. (according to 1966 figures) had 1,617 hospital days per 1,000 people per year, while the Blue Cross figures in the same area were 2,914 hospital days per 1,000. The annual admissions (over 65) for the G.H.A.

---

[206]Louis L. Feldman, op. cit., pp. 415-416.

[207]"Drug Research Report," op. cit.

[208]Harvard Law Review, op. cit., p. 990.

[209]Somers, Appendix Table #8, op. cit., p. 202.

[210]Harvard Law Review, op. cit., p. 990.

[211]"The Relevance of Prepaid Group Practice to the Effective Delivery of Health Services," Ernest W. Saward, M.D., Speech presented at 10th Annual Group Health Institute, Ontario, Canada, June 18, 1969, Reprinted by H.E.W., O.H.E.W. Pub. No. 72-6302, p. 14.

TABLE III - 10

COMPARISON: NATIONWIDE MEDICARE COSTS AND
GROUP HEALTH COOPERATIVE MEDICARE COSTS

	Part A Hospital Insurance		Savings	Part B Supplementary Medical Insurance	
	S.S.A. (A)	G.H.C.(B)		S.S.A.(A)	G.H.C.(B)
Admissions	10.6 mil.	2,159			
Cost	$6.3 bil.	$836,424			
Cost/Admission	$594.34	$387.41	446,762		
Med. Insur.					
Enrollees				35.8 mil.	10,144
Cost				$2.1 bil.	$656,956
Per Enrollee Year			($61,878)	$58.66	$64.76
Net Savings			$384,884		

Source: (Article) "Impact of Medicare on Group Practice Prepayment
Plans," Harold F. Newman, Journal of Public Health,
(Jan.-June, 1969), p. 633.

plan were 126 per 1,000 persons, while the Blue Cross average was 232 admissions per 1,000 persons.[212]

A good deal of the success Kaiser and others have had with Medicare enrollment can be attributed to efficient formulas worked out for integrating Medicare patients into the mainstream of the plan's services. Kaiser, in 1966, developed a new type of coverage, "M", by taking the most comprehensive group coverage they had to offer and adding in certain Medicare benefits the Kaiser plan did not ordinarily offer. A monthly dues rate was then established by dividing the health plan into two separate ratings and eliminating those parts of the plan not covered by Medicare reimbursements.[213] Health Insurance Plan of New York also has a separate Medicare classification called H.I.P. Care, where Medicare eligibles pay a small supplemental premium ($3 or $5 per month) and get comprehensive care. In addition, Medicare enrollees are the only H.I.P. members allowed to enter the plan on an individual basis.[214]

Reimbursement

The most significant point concerning the present and future relationship between the prepaid group practice plan and Medicare is the reimbursement mechanism used. G.H.A. of Washington, D.C., which has a clinic-based plan, does not deal with the S.S.A. directly. Instead, they work through regional fiscal intermediaries on a fee-for-service basis.[215] Kaiser and H.I.P. deal directly with the S.S.A. and are considered the fiscal intermediaries. Part A (hospital-based benefits) are reimbursed to the plan on a reasonable cost basis; and Part B (medical services) are reimbursed by a monthly per-capita payment for each Part B beneficiary who belongs to the particular plan. The G.H.C. of Puget Sound eliminates the intermediary concept completely and deals directly with the S.S.A.[216]

Regardless of which relationship between the plan and the government is maintained, the method of reimbursement is extremely cumbersome, especially when it comes to determining capitation payments under Part B. While the H.M.O.'s are not necessarily under-reimbursed by the S.S.A., there are higher administrative costs involved in the entire procedure, and a general lack of incentive to provide Medicare services in the most efficient manner. The way in which the 1965 Social Security Amendment presently operates is that after a $50 deductible, 80 per cent of either the "reasonable cost, or the "reasonable charges" for a particular service are

[212]"The Federal Employees Health Benefits Program," Enrollment and Utilization of Health Services 1961-8, Prepared by George S. Perrott, Office of Group Practice and Development, H.E.W., p. 15.

[213]"Towards A Comprehensive Health Policy," op. cit., pp. 53-54.

[214]Interview - Marvin Leeds, op. cit.

[215]Harvard Law Review, op. cit., p. 990.

[216]"The Impact of Medicare on Group Practice Prepayment Plans," Harold F. Newman, M.D., M.P.H., Journal of Public Health, (January-June 1969),p.629.

reimbursed by the S.S.A. to the H.M.O.[217] The 1965 Amendment was not specifically designed for group practice plans, and even the present legislation in Congress states that the H.M.O. may reimburse physicians any way they desire, including fee-for-service.[218] Thus, physicians can still be paid for the services they render, providing their fees meet rather loose standards.[219]

Prepaid groups that provide comprehensive, efficient care at lower costs do not gain by providing it; if they cut their costs 20 per cent, the amount they are reimbursed also drops 20 per cent. The same is also true with hospitals. One way to rectify this disincentive problem is to reward plans that provide care at below average costs and penalize those who do not save on costs.[220] Incentive reimbursement experiments are incorporated in the current Medicare legislation now in Congress.[221]

Medicare Legislation

H.R. I

As of 1972, both the Senate and the House had legislation before them directly dealing with the H.M.O. concept as it applies to Medicare. The House Bill (H.R. I - was passed in 1971) appears to be less precise than the Senate's. It provides that any organization that offers a subscription-type arrangement and can prove to H.E.W. that it has the capacity to provide comprehensive, quality health care, may participate in the Medicare program.[222]

The House Bill does not provide an incentive formula and merely states that an H.M.O. may collect up to 95 per cent of their costs. It would be up to the Secretary of H.E.W. to determine an appropriate reimbursement formula for those plans providing the same services well below the 95 per cent level.[223]

The House version is also lacking in that it does not include any incentive for the Medicare recipient to join an H.M.O. There are no additional funds appropriated to the H.M.O. that will help it provide those services covered by Medicare, plus additional services.

---

[217] Harvard Law Review, op. cit., p. 989.

[218] Ibid., p. 991.

[219] "Health Care in the 70's: Dollars and Delivery-The Latest Dichotomy in Public Health," Beverlee A. Myers, M.P.H., Speech presented at Opening Session of 1971 Meeting of Western Branch; American Public Health Assoc. June 15, 1971, in Los Angeles, California, p. 9.

[220] Ibid., p. 11.

[221] Ibid.

[222] Harvard Law Review, op. cit., p. 992.

[223] Ibid., p. 993

Thus, a Medicare recipient who joins an H.M.O. may not receive all the benefits he is entitled to under the Medicare program. To make matters worse, if he joins the plan, he becomes ineligible to receive any benefits from the S.S.A. that are not covered in his individual plan.[224]

According to the Administration's present health strategy, President Nixon wishes to "restructure the delivery system around that segment of the population that already has some form of health coverage.[225] Included in this group would have to be Medicare and Medicaid beneficiaries, and in that case, the lack of resolution of the "95 per cent payment" question may hurt the President's cause.[226] The question repeatedly asked at the legislative hearings held last year concerning the Bill was: "Will the legislation state that the provider will be reimbursed on a capitation basis; i.e., a flat 95 per cent of the average Medicare payment for the area, or will it be up to 95 per cent?" If the "up to 95 per cent" interpretation prevails, the H.M.O. and Medicare cannot favorably unite.[227]

Senate Bill

The Senate Finance Committee has recommended a more effective bill. It requires a greater amount of efficiency within the H.M.O.'s that participate in the Medicare program, by providing for annual meetings between the H.E.W. Secretary and the health organization, where the contract between the two may be cancelled if the quality of care and the plan's economic efficiency falter.[228] The brightest part of the Senate's plan is that it provides an incentive-oriented reimbursement formula. The amount reimbursed is based on the rate charged to "under 65" members of the plan, with certain adjustments that take into account Medicare patients' increased utilization of facilities and added cost to the plan.[229] In spite of the positive points, the Senate, like the House, has created a piece of legislation with too much generality and imprecision.[230]

Impact of Legislation

There are those who feel that the general concept of H.R. I (House Bill) is not as significant as many H.M.O. advocates would have us believe,

[224]Ibid., pp. 993-995.

[225]Reprint from Hospitals, Journal of American Hospital Association, Volume 45, (March 16, 1971), "Health Maintenance Organizations," (no page numbers), first page of "Conference Analysis."

[226]"Health Care in the 70's," Second page of "Guidelines of Implementation," op. cit.

[227]Ibid.

[228]Harvard Law Review, op. cit., p. 992.

[229]Ibid., pp. 993-994.

[230]Ibid.

basically because it has no effect on the middle class, nontitle 18 and 19
beneficiaries. Many people have the mistaken belief that through it, the
Federal government will be able to set up the rules and regulations and
approve some H.M.O.'s and reject others. Actually, the approval of medical
facilities and systems is entirely a state function, and there has been a
lot of wishful thinking in which people hope that with the passage of H.R. I,
the Federal government would be able to override state manpower laws and
restrictive acts which make illegal a nonphysician-sponsored prepaid group
practice.[231]

      Dr. Clare of H.E.W. states that "even if H.R. I were passed, the
restrictive state laws would remain in litigation for years, making the
process a very gradual state-by-state thing. Decisions made in one Supreme
Court will not effect the decision made in the next state." So, in one
sense, all that H.R. I really does is give Social Security "the authority
they felt they didn't have to pay prepaid group practices for the work that
they do on a capitation basis."

Importance of H.R. I

      According to Dr. Clare, the passage of H.R. I will have an impor-
tant, more subtle effect on H.M.O.'s if the full 95 per cent reimbursement
of costs is made. Kaiser claims that they can cover Medicare services for
about 85 per cent of the prevailing costs, and if the S.S.A. reimburses 95
per cent of the costs, it is feared that some "fly-by-night, fast-buck
operators" who would be out to make some extra money on the ten per cent
differential, could try to take advantage of the situation.

      As a result, it has been suggested that strong regulations be
made so that the difference between the 85 and 95 per cent be returned to
the beneficiary through more services. This implies that the additional
premium paid by Medicare recipients in an H.M.O. plan would be knocked down.
Presently, the Social Security Administration does have a complicated Group
Practice Prepayment Plan (G.P.P.P.),[232] which does pay prepaid group practice
on a capitation basis, "more or less." It is really a cost reimbursement
for covered services, and noncovered services, which are preventive (Medicare
does not cover preventive medicine), would have to be paid for by an additional premium to the prepaid group practice by the Medicare eligibles. This
means that a premium ranging between six and 12 dollars has to be paid by
the over-65 member, in addition to the capitation payment made by the Social
Security Administration. Only with this additional payment would the
Medicare patient be eligible for all the additional covered services like
annual physicals, refractions, etc. With the passage of H.R. I, the present
premium could be lowered to between two and five dollars per month, and this
would be the real benefit of H.R. I to Title 18 beneficiaries.[233]

---

[231] Interview - Dr. Clare, op. cit.

[232] The G.P.P.P. is the provision made in the 1965 amendment providing
for the $50 deductible and the 80 per cent reimbursement of reasonable
cost.

[233] Interview - Dr. Clare, op. cit.

Extended Coverage

Another hazy area which eventually must be clarified is the extent
to which H.M.O.'s under H.R. I would be required to provide broader "health
maintenance" services not included in Sections A and B. This includes
"periodic examinations, complete immunization programs, surveillance of
dietary, personal and social situations which can detract from health,
tuberculosis care and other special programs." These additional services,
if provided, could have a significant effect on the costs of the H.M.O. and
the premium charged Medicare enrollees. According to H.E.W. sources involved in the creation of H.R. I, "the Medicare package of hospital and
medical services would continue to receive major emphasis, with additonal
services being included to the extent that they are covered under the
program."[234]

It was further stated that while an annual physical examination
and other thorough medical screening procedures will hopefully be offered to
the older beneficiary as an inducement to enroll in the H.M.O., the government "cannot require that an H.M.O. offer such services, since the current
Medicare program does not cover routine physical examinations. However,
since H.M.O's emphasize preventive care, it is believed that many will, as
a matter of policy, offer such services without charge to Medicare beneficiaries."[235] While this statement may be valid, certain plans have recently
been debating whether or not to totally discontinue their annual physicals,
due to the large financial burden they produce.[236]

Medicaid

Most authorities believe that there is tremendous potential for a
relationship between the H.M.O.and Medicaid eligibles. Marvin Leeds, the
Director of the East Nassau Medical Group,[237] believes that while it was
important for an H.M.O. to "avoid the stigma of being considered a poor
people's plan," the potential of recruiting Medicaid recipients would make
it possible to develop a nucleus around which an entire H.M.O. may be built.
East Nassau provides care to 2,500 Medicaid eligibles on a capitation basis,
with O.E.O. paying the capitation. Others expressed similar viewpoints.
Jeffrey Prussin of G.H.A.A. states that Medicaid recipients would have to be
part of an integrated H.M.O. network, in order for the plan to succeed.
Obviously, an H.M.O. must be organized in an area where the population base
can afford to pay a premium of 40-60 dollars a month, whether it be the

---

[234]Committee Print - Health Maintenance Organizations; Staff questions with
responses of the Department of Health, Education and Welfare,
Committee on Finance, U. S. Senate, (Washington, D.C.: U. S. Government
Printing Office, September 27, 1971), p. 16.

[235]Ibid.

[236]Personal Interview with Dan Sullivan, Public Relations Director,
(Washington, D.C.: G.H.A., January 31, 1972).

[237]Interview - Marvin Leeds, op. cit.

employer who pays it, the employee, or the government, through Medicare or Medicaid. The H.M.O. concept is presently geared for the working and middle-class population, and as a result, O.E.O. does not know exactly what to do with it, although the potential is there.[238]

Recruitment

One of the keys to developing an H.M.O. in low-income areas is determining a fair method of recruitment. Dr. Paul Ellwood, in the January, 1972 edition of The American Journal of Public Health,[239] notes that an H.M.O. might be tempted to enroll low-risk groups and throw off high-risk and sick populations to the system-at-large. This would occur because the system-at-large does not require enrollment, whereas H.M.O.'s do, and as a result, would go after young families instead of older couples and enrolled Medicaid populations, instead of unenrolled. This problem is found in cities where there is a fairly large Medicaid population and also a large population which is not eligible for Medicaid, but is still not able to pay for its own health care. In these cities, there are voluntary hospitals which practice on a regular fee-for-service system and also have a money-losing, "charity," out-patient load. If an H.M.O. went after the Medicaid-enrolled population and left the non-Medicaid enrollees for the voluntary hospital, the hospital would be in worse shape than it was previously, because they would be taking care of the medically-indigent population, but they would receive no reimbursement at all.[240]

Since Medicaid is administered through various state social service agencies, the Administration, through H.R. I, has attempted to increase the state's incentives to set up various H.M.O.'s. Presently, there is a rather strong resistance on the part of state agencies and a tendency to delay and be cautious about getting involved with an enrollment capitation situation. One reason for this is that they don't really know what the capitation amount should be and they don't want to overpay.[241]

What H.R. I proposes is that the federal matching for Title 19 services delivered under an H.M.O. will be increased 25 percentage points. Federal matching in New York and New Jersey is presently 50 per cent, so if services were delivered under an H.M.O., the matching would go up to 75 per cent. This obviously means that a state which wants to maximize its federal dollar and minimize its state spending in medical care will have a very strong incentive to have care provided under an H.M.O.[242]

Eligibility

Another area not yet clear in H.R. I is the Medicaid eligibility question. The H.M.O. premium is based upon a pre-determined group of

---

[238]Interview - Jeffrey Prussin, op. cit.

[239]Dr. Paul Ellwood, "Implications of Recent Health Legislation," American Journal of Public Health, (January 1972), pp. 20-23.

[240]Ibid., Also, Interview with Dr. Clare.

[241]Interview - Dr. Clare.

[242]Ibid.

subscribers. Welfare Departments question how the medically-indigent are to be identified in advance, when they are constantly going in and out of eligibility. Certainly, it would make their capitation payments very difficult to determine. In response to this issue at the Senate hearings, an H.E.W. representative replied that "the medically needy would /be chosen/ on the basis of income level. If not identified in advance and at a time coincident with an open enrollment period of the H.M.O., except possibly on a one-time, fee-for-service basis.[243] While state welfare departments place major emphasis on the eligibility issue, H.E.W. is not quite as worried. They claim that the majority of the public assistance population does not move back and forth between eligibility, and the welfare departments are unnecessarily concerned.[244]

ADDITIONAL LEGISLATION

Introduction

The Nixon Administration is sponsoring H.R. I in the House and the Javits Bill in the Senate (actually H.R. I is being discussed in the Senate). Both cover broad areas of health reform with specific sections dealing with H.M.O. funding, the H.M.O.'s relationship to the Medicare and Medicaid programs, and definitions of the characteristics an H.M.O. must possess to be classified as such. The Javits Bill has within it the H.M.O. Assistance Act, which deals with funding H.M.O.'s over the next four years.

Aside from the Administration's bills, there is other H.M.O.-oriented legislation. The Kennedy Bill (S3) and the Griffith Bill in the House are the major proponents of National Health Insurance concept which many feel must be passed in some form, in order for the H.M.O. to succeed. The Harvard Law Review concludes that: "A national health insurance program can thus create continuing incentives for providers to move toward comprehensive health service organizations that follow the principles of prepaid group practice.[245] The Griffith Bill calls for grants to be distributed to organizations which provide a full range of services. The Kennedy Bill authorizes that the Secretary of H.E.W., upon the recommendation of a 13-member Health Maintenance Organization Review Council, will make grants to academic health centers to assist in planning or studying the feasibility of developing H.M.O.'s. The bill also provides for developmental and construction grants and a loan program for operating the H.M.O. in its beginning stages.[246] The Kennedy and Griffith Bills, along with the Javits (Administration) Bill, all provide for the government to bear a certain percentage of the nonconstruction start-up costs of H.M.O.'s. The Javits Bill provides that

---

[243] Committee Print - Health Maintenance Organizations, op. cit.

[244] Interview - Dr. Clare, op. cit.

[245] Harvard Law Review, op. cit., p. 1001.

[246] "H.M.O.'s" - Fact Sheet on five Senate bills pending before the Committee on Labor and Public Welfare concerning Health Maintenance Organizations (received from H.E.W., but no actual source given).

percentage should be "up to 80 per cent; the Griffith Bill, up to 75 per cent; and the Kennedy Bill, up to 90 per cent for new organizations, and up to 80 per cent for enlarging existing plans.[247] The Kennedy Bill covers construction costs with grants and loans matching up to 90 per cent of non-federal funds used.[248]

Other Recent Bills (Pell and Javits)

Two other Senate Bills proposed in 1971, dealing with H.M.O.'s are the "Minimum Health Benefits and Health Services Distribution and Education Act of 1971," proposed by Senator Pell of Rhode Island, and the "Local Comprehensive Health Services Systems Act of 1971," proposed by Senator Javits of New York.[249] The Pell Bill is unique in that it creates Community Health and Education Corporation, which will be a profit institution, and as far as practicable, provide the benefits of a prepaid group practice. It is hoped that the corporation can become a self-sufficient, economic entity without need of federal assistance, after 20 years of operation. It will be financed, in part, through the issuance of common and pre-ferred stock.[250]

The Javits Bill authorizes the Secretary of H.E.W. to make loans and grants, and to provide technical assistance to help develop Comprehensive Health Care programs.[251] The Secretary may make grants to and contract with: any public or nonprofit hospital, and medical school or other institution of higher learning, any insurance carrier or nonprofit prepayment plan providing health coverage, and any nonprofit community organization providing health coverage in a geographically defined, primary service area, and representing a broad range of income and social groups. H.E.W. could agree to pay up to 80 per cent of the costs of planning and developing the "Comprehensive Health Service System."[252] This Javits' Bill is actually his own National Health Insurance Bill, and, in effect, it states that Medicare should be applied to the under-65 population.

While both the Administration and the Kennedy Bills attempt to promote the H.M.O. concept, there is wide variation in the method each uses. The Kennedy Bill aspires to get into all aspects of health reform, including training, manpower education, form of delivery services, organization and everything else. The Administration prefers to break these things up and tackle one thing at a time under its own authority.[253] However, most health authorities agree that most of the legislation mentioned thus far, including

---

[247] Harvard Law Review, op. cit., p. 987.

[248] Ibid.

[249] Not to be confused with the other Javits' Bill, which is the Administration's health strategy.

[250] H.M.O. - Fact Sheet, (#2), op. cit., pp. 1-3.

[251] The definition of Comprehensive Health Care Systems coincides with the definition of Health Maintenance Organization.

[252] H.M.O. - Fact Sheet, (#6). op. cit.
[253] Interview - Dr. Clare, op. cit.

166

the Administration's, does not deal adequately with the development of
H.M.O.'s. Because of this, there has recently been a new wave of more-direct
health bills dealing specifically with financial support of H.M.O.'s. These
"support bills" include the Roy Bill and the Stagger Bill, with a new Kennedy
support bill soon to follow.

"Regulators" and "Reformers"

Dr. Paul Ellwood, in the January edition of The American Journal
of Public Health,[254] divides all health legislators and planners into two
broad categories: "regulators" and "reformers." The "regulators" are those
who feel that centralized planning and stricter regulations are the only way
to deal with the current health crisis. They are dealing with the "here-and-
now," and aim their policy at controlling health care costs through more
stringent utilization procedures, price controls, increasing the controls of
planning agencies over the construction of hospital beds, and establishing
an inspector general for health.

The "reformers" want to bring about changes in the health industry
which would increase internal regulation, and thereby reduce the need for
external restrictions. They would do this "through the creation of competition among providers, the use of cost-effective incentives, and the promotion
of health services delivery by organizations which would be responsible for
defined populations."

Most of the health legislation before Congress, including H.R. I,
brings together the viewpoints of both these groups. While these two opposing groups do exist, Dr. Ellwood states that one cannot necessarily separate
the two along party lines. The Administration forces do not go along with
the National Health Insurance Bills as proposed by the liberal Democrats
(Kennedy), but they definitely are in favor of the H.M.O. concept, which is
the foundation of the "reformer" philosophy. In fact, every serious National
Health proposal, with the exception of the A.M.A. Bill and the Aetna Bill,
advocate the formation of H.M.O. delivery units.[255] So there appears to be
a narrowing of the gap of opinions within the Congress, and this may result
in more adequate legislation.

Current Support Bills

The Bill introduced in the House by Congressman William Roy, on
November 11, 1971, while lacking in certain areas, is still considered by
many to be the most constructive support legislation produced in either
house. The Administration has major support bills in both the House
(Staggers Bill) and Senate (Javits-H.M.O. Assistance Act), which appropriates
$45 million in direct money for H.M.O.'s, $23 million of which goes to capital
construction in underserved areas, and $22 million of which goes to general
H.M.O. planning in 1972.[256] Congressman Roy, in creating this Bill, felt that

---

[254]Dr. Paul Ellwood, "Implications of Recent Health Care Legislation,"
American Journal of Public Health, (January 1972), pp. 20-23.

[255]Ibid.

[256]See Section on H.E.W. - Chart of projected Administration Figures 1972-76.

the Administration's legislation does not go far enough in terms of the Administration's goals of setting up 1,700 H.M.O.'s by 1976, and giving 90 per cent of the U.S. population the opportunity of having H.M.O. care available to them by the end of the decade.[257] So he restructured the Administration's goals by selling for 1,600 H.M.O.'s by 1981, and appropriating approximately 1½ billion dollars over that time in grants and loans, so that each H.M.O. gets about $5 million.

The Roy Bill also makes planning and feasibility for an H.M.O. much easier, with $25 million being allotted in the first year for these two purposes. With 100 H.M.O.'s planned for the first year, that would be $250,000 per H.M.O. In underserved areas (facilities are not available), the Roy Bill provides for direct loans, loan guarantees, federal grants and interest subsidies. In established areas, the Roy Bill provides for interest subsidies and loan guarantees on the theory that a lot of facilities are already available in nonunderserved areas. The Roy Bill is different from the Administration Bill in that it operates under the realistic assumption that an H.M.O. once established, may lose money. To compensate for this, it provides for a 60 per cent federal subsidy the first year, 40 per cent the second year, and 20 per cent the third, so that the initial cost is not so high.[258] (See Table IV - 11).

State Legislation

Funding

On the state level, "enabling" legislation is of far more significance than "funding" legislation. In New York State, there are only two possible sources available to H.M.O.'s through state regulations. First, there is the New York State Health and Mental Hygiene Facilities Improvement Corporation, which authorizes loans at low interest rates for the construction of municipally-owned health facilities. The New York State Housing Finance Agency floats the bonds which are requested for each project by the corporation.[259] Second, there is the "hospital mortgage loan construction law" (Article 28-B). The purpose of the law is to encourage the "construction and modernization, including the equipment, of hospitals and other health facilities with mortgage loan participation by the New York State Housing Finance Agency." The Article authorizes mortgage loans with conventional financing of up to 90 per cent for modernization.[260]

Enabling Legislation

In 1969, the Aspen Systems Corporation was given a grant to analyze the various state laws which affect the group practice of medicine.[261]

---

[257]"Towards a Comprehensive Health Policy for the 1970's," op. cit.

[258]Personal Interview with James F. Doherty, Legislative Representative of G.H.A.A.,and Steve Lewis, of the Legal Department of G.H.A.A., Washington, D.C., February 25,1972.

[259]Ann S. Bush, op. cit., p. 35.

[260]Summary of Article 28-B, Provisions 2871-2874.

[261]Ann S. Bush, op. cit., p.52.

168

TABLE III - 11

COMPARISON OF SUPPORT BILLS

Administration	1,700 H.M.O.'s	812 million
(Stagger-House)	by	dollars
(Javits-Senate)	1976	through
		1976
Roy Bill	1,600 H.M.O.'s	1.5 billion
(House)	by	dollars
	1981	through
		1981
		(Grand Total)
Kennedy Bill	?	?
(Senate)		

Source: From figures stated in this section.

It was concluded from the study that in less than half of the 50 states, the legal environment is such that a voluntary prepaid group practice may be organized. New York is considered one of those with an open, permissive, enabling legislation. The Non-Profit Medical Corporations Act (5704-A), or the Lombardi Law, signed by Governor Rockefeller in July 1971, allows groups of doctors to form prototype H.M.O.'s. Health Service Corporations would also be encouraged to use their assets to organize prepaid, comprehensive medical care groups.[262] These Medical Corporations could enter into contracts to provide professional medical service and hospital service, with health service corporations and medical expense indemnity corporations, municipal hospitals, and hospital corporations, as organized under state regulations. Medical corporations may also enter into contracts with the New York State Housing Finance Agency for mortgage loans, receive assistance from any Federal, State, municipal government, or any person, firm or corporation by

---

[262]"The Non-Profit Medical Corporation Act," Article from Newsletter - Medical Societies' Reference Committee, (no date) - (received at L. I. Jewish Hospital). Also, Non-Profit Medical Corporation's, Article 44, Public Health Law, New York's Approach to Prepaid Comprehensive Group Practice - Considerations for Applicants, New York State Dept. of Health, Hollis S. Ingraham, M.D., Commissioner, July 1971.

contracts or otherwise. Among other advantages, the Medical Corporation is offered preferred federal and state tax status, eligibility for low interest, 90 per cent mortgage loans, and exemption from real property taxes.[263]

Restrictive state laws for H.M.O. development can be classified in one of two broad categories: incorporation and regulation. Some states, especially in the South, have common laws that prohibit the corporation from joining with any medical practice. These laws were passed because it was common belief that a "corporation" lacked the educational and ethical qualifications to be associated with the practice of medicine. Originally, the laws were created to protect the uninformed layman from inefficient, profit-motivated health care. However, as is the case with the New York State Law, a nonprofit health service corporation is certainly no longer a menace to health care, if it is properly organized.[264]

Blue Laws

The Blue Shield laws are the regulating statutes that impede H.M.O. growth. Most of them were created by medical societies in the 1930's in order to keep health insurance practices under the control of local physicians. These laws provide a barrier on consumer and community-oriented plans, because they prohibit a health service from forming until it is run by physicians. In many states with Blue Laws, the only way a prepaid group practice can be formed is by allowing itself to be classified as an insurance company, and thereby be subject to the authority of the State Insurance Commission.[265] While H.I.P. in New York went along with this classification for many years, Kaiser fought hard against this principle and is regulated by the State Attorney General's office instead.[266]

BUSINESS POTENTIAL

The conventional funding institutions that make up the capital markets today are interested in reasonable return on their investment. Investing in an H.M.O. would not ordinarily excite the financial community for one simple reason: they are classified as nonprofit institutions, and if they earn sizable surpluses, they jeopardize their income tax exemption.[267] With a disincentive to earn profits, most H.M.O.'s have not made obvious financial changes that would dramatically increase profit, and the result has been little investment interest from the capital markets.

---

[263]Ibid.

[264]Group Health and Welfare News, published by G.H.A.A., 1717 Massachusetts Ave., Washington, D.C., Vol. XIII, No. 2, (February 1972).

[265]Ibid.

[266]Interview - Lou Sacadelli, op. cit.

[267]Dr. Paul Ellwood, "Health Maintenance Organization Patterns," (Paper), also prepared by staff of American Foundation, Minneapolis, Minnesota, April 1971, pp. 10-12.

Profit-Oriented H.M.O.

The proprietary or for profit H.M.O. is potentially important, but its nonuse further widens the gap between the H.M.O.'s and the investment community. Of the prepaid group practice plans, almost without exception, they are all organized on a nonprofit basis. The only exceptions are those organized by physicians. The best-known of these is the Ross-Loos Clinic in Los Angeles, where 85-90 per cent of the work is on a prepaid basis, and the doctors are extremely cost- and profit-oriented. Among other things, they own and run their cafeteria and parking lots for a profit. However, profit is not really labeled as such by the group. Instead, it turns up in the distribution to the partners on an income basis, over and above a drawing account, and is lumped in with other things like savings on hospitals. There's another such group called the Western Clinic in Tacoma, Washington, which is much smaller (about 30,000 enrollees - about one-half are in pre-payment). This particular group is unique in that the doctors underwrite hospitalization.[268]

Upjohn Plan

Other more-venturesome profit plans have sprung up in California. One of the best publicized is the Upjohn Clinic. Harold Upjohn has made an agreement to take over the Southern Pacific Railroad Hospital Association, which has the responsibility of caring for the employees of the Southern Pacific Railroad, between San Francisco, Los Angeles and Tucson. Within the Association, there is an 80-year-old, 400-bed hospital in San Francisco, and a renovated, converted train depot in Tucson, which has been made into a 45-bed hospital. The railroad workers must get their hospital care in one of these railroad hospitals, and their outpatient care in various locations between these three major points. The railroads pay a premium to the Association, and Upjohn has agreed not to increase the rate for more than three years. He thus has the right to use the facilities and the medical staff, and has borrowed about three million dollars to develop a separate outpatient facility and a nursing home.[269]

Omnicare

Omnicare, another proposed profit-making plan, in California, has had legal troubles with the State Attorney General. Victor Stein, the President, proposes to motivate the doctors by selling them stock in Omnicare Corporation. The Attorney General questions whether by owning stock in the corporation, the doctors would be more induced to provide less care than they should in exchange for increasing their profits.[270] The plan's mechanism would be similar to Kaiser, with the major difference being that sale of stock would make funds easier to obtain. Capital gain, as opposed to dividend yield, would provide the main incentive to invest.[271]

---

[268]Interview - Lou Sacadelli, op. cit.

[269]Ibid.

[270]Ibid.

[271]Harvard Law Review, op. cit., p. 918.

Judging from the profit plans mentioned, the profit-making H.M.O. is a phenomena of the West Coast, where prepayment is well-established. For example, Ross-Loos might well have gone to fee-for-service, had it not been for the strong influence of Kaiser in the Los Angeles area. The same is true of the Western Clinic, which is very close to the Group Cooperative of Puget Sound. In addition, the Kaiser Plan also provides a clue that within a non-profit plan, a profit could be made. The clue is that Kaiser includes within its premium something between four and five per cent for what is called expansion, and this finances Kaiser growth. Presumably, a businessman would call this profit. General Motors, for instance, finances its expansion out of profit by planning on 20 per cent (of capital) as profit. Out of that, they give a small per cent back to the stockholders, and the rest is used for capital expansion.[272]

For-Profit Opposition

In spite of the progress made on the West Coast, there are definite reasons why the profit-oriented H.M.O. has not quickly caught on. There is an historical, legal precedent in many states opposing profit plans. For instance, Omnicare, as previously mentioned, must secure legal approval from the State Attorney General.[273] New York State has the Non-Profit Medical Corporation Act which opens the doors for H.M.O.'s in the State, but only those organized on non-profit basis.[274] H.R. I includes a specific provision designed to guard against retention of excessive profits or funds collected for Medicare beneficiaries. It says that the Secretary of H.E.W. will require, following each accounting period, a certified public statement from each H.M.O., of the funds collected and the rate of retention with respect to Medicare enrollees and others.[275] While H.R. I does not eliminate the possibility of having profit H.M.O.'s along with government-supported, non-profit ones, it does indirectly create an unfavorable air for their development.

Ellwood's Views

There are many individuals in the health field who are strongly in favor of proprietary H.M.O.'s. Dr. Paul Ellwood states that "planners should recognize that H.M.O.'s sponsored by profit-making corporations are not necessarily bad, although for-profit organizations whose primary objective is to maximize profits, could pose problems. In addition, for-profit H.M.O.'s should be sponsored by Corporations with a reputation to uphold, that have demonstrated locally that they are responsible organizations, and that they have the capacity to invest substantial capital with the prospect that they will have to wait for a return on their investment.[276]

---

[272]Interview - Lou Sacadelli, op. cit.

[273]Harvard Law Review, op. cit., p. 918.

[274](Non-Profit Medical Corp. Act)., op. cit.

[275]Questions and Answers - Senate Hearing, op. cit.

[276]Dr. Paul Ellwood, "Implications of Recent Health Care Legislation," op.cit.

Ellwood, who is strongly in favor of integrating the for-profit and nonprofit H.M.O. into one coordinated health system, has made various proposals for improving the business potential of the present H.M.O. Increased leverage is the key component. The typical nonprofit H.M.O. has low percentage return on net worth and return on equity, simply because it does not wish to increase profitability, and thereby, jeopardize its tax position. The H.M.O. in certain aspects can be likened to a public uility, in that it has stable earnings that are highly predictable. The big differ- ence between the two is the debt-to-equity ratio which is well above 2:1 for utilities, and less than 1:1 for H.M.O.'s. If the ratio was raised to 2:1 for H.M.O.'s, it would not hurt their tax situation and still increase their return on equity.[277] Table III - 12 shows the differece.

The return on equity may be further expanded for a profit-oriented H.M.O. by leasing, instead of owning, land and real estate investments in clinics and hospitals. This reduces the initial investment in an H.M.O., but increases the routine operating expenses. The move would increase profit- ability because H.M.O. operations are significantly more profitable than real estate management for the health plan.[278] Table IV - 13 shws the difference in return on equity. It must be remembered that the figures used to determine increased return on equity are taken from plans that have always been non- profit entities. If figures were available for a profit-oriented H.M.O., the return would be even higher.[279]

Some people are opposed to the for-profit H.M.O. because in an attempt to maximize profit, they fear it might very well sacrifice quality care and increase premiums. Dr. Ellwood disagrees and states that the proprietary H.M.O., with more efficiency-oriented management, would have more incentive to use:

1. Para-professionals
2. Computer-based health records
3. Multi-phasic testing
4. Preventive health procedures

Management in a for-profit plan would be less likely to buy unnecessary, sophisticated medical equipment or to hire physicians or other skills that could be bought more economically on a fee-for-service basis.[280]

Other Favorable Points

Bruce Caputo of the Inner City Fund, a consulting firm that works with H.E.W., conducted a systematic study as to whether proprietary, for- profit health institutions were less efficient than those organized on a nonprofit basis. After a rigorous investigation of hospitals, nursing homes,

---

[277] Dr. Paul Ellwood, "H.M.O. Patterns," op. cit.

[278] Ibid.

[279] Ibid.

[280] Ibid.

173

TABLE III - 12

RETURN ON EQUITY - H.M.O.'s

	Present Return on Equity	Return on Equity Assuming 2:1 debt to Equity ratio & 10% Interest Rate
Kaiser Health Plan	10.0%	11%
G.H.A. - Washington	5.9%	7%
Group Health Cooperative	5.0%	6%

Source: Paper by Dr. Paul Ellwood, "Health Maintenance Organization Patterns," (Minneapolis, Minnesota: American Rehabilitation Foundation, April 1971), p. 11.

TABLE IV - 13

RETURN ON EQUITY -
WITH AND WITHOUT LEASING

(For Group Health Cooperative of Puget Sound)

	With Present Debt/Equity Ratio	With Debt/Equity Ratio of Two
Own Fixed Assets	5.0	6.0
Lease Fixed Assets	15.3	22.8

Source: Paper by Dr. Paul Ellwood, "Health Maintenance Organization Patterns," (Minneapolis, Minnesota: American Rehabilitation Foundation, April 1971), p. 11.

physicians, etc., it was concluded that "there is no statistically discernable difference in quality, by the profit/nonprofit distinction." Since there is really no way to measure whether one group provided better quality than the next, quality was not measured by results, but rather by inputs, like the width of the corridor in the hospital, the number of nurses per bed, and even the presence or absence of television sets in hospital rooms.

These input studies were inconclusive. Some found that the proprietary organizations were superior, while others found that the reverse was true. If there was any significant statistical distinction, it was that the larger organization - whether profit or nonprofit - provided lower costs and better inputs. So that if the government is interested in regulating health care providers or favoring a particular class with subsidies or loan guarantees, they're much better off discriminating on the basis of size than on the basis of ownership.[281]

Another significant point is that it is so easy to juggle classifications, that it is foolish to discriminate on the basis of ownership. An example would be a group in Southern California called the California Medical Group, which is a nonprofit, prepaid organization that contracts with a proprietary physicians group. They also contract with a for-profit hospital chain, a voluntary hospital, and the public city hospitals. That group has involved itself in all three modes - government, nonprofit and for-profit - and could legally be classified under any one. Obviously, any single classification would be misleading.[282]

Another common, for-profit misconception had to do with the management of a profit-oriented organization. Many would say that there would be a much greater tendency to have extortionary practices in a for-profit plan than in a nonprofit one. However, those who are going to abuse the system and make unconscionable profits from it are more likely to get into a non-profit mode, because from a public relations viewpoint, the for-profit organization is infinitely more vulnerable.[283]

Taxes

Since taxes provide the primary financial disincentive for the establishment of profit-oriented H.M.O.'s, their various classifications must be further explored. A for-profit H.M.O. does not ordinarily wish to increase return on investment or else it could lose its exemption under 501C3 (federal income tax). Aside from the federal income tax, however, an H.M.O. has a certain liability for local property tax. The amount they must pay depends on whether they get 501C3 or 501C4 treatment under the code. The latter is exempt from the local property tax, but to be the latter, an H.M.O. would have to prove that it is a charitable organization, not one that merely serves local social interests. An example of a 501C4 is the Red Cross.

---

[281] Interview - Bruce Caputo, op. cit.

[282] Ibid.

[283] Ibid.

175

The Kaiser Plan, in spite of numerous attempts to be classified 501C4, is still considered 501C3, because they don't really have the "color" of a totally-charitable institution because too many people make their living off of it.[284]

Of course, even if a particular health institution is classified as a charitable organization, that does not mean that if it receives non-related income from outside activities, that this income is also tax-exempt. This principle may have an important effect on the setting up of a hospital-based H.M.O. An example would be a charitable hospital that plans to develop an H.M.O. They decide that a medical center for ambulatory care must immediately be purchased, and to maximize return until the H.M.O. is ready to utilize the center, they will lease out the space to local businesses. Ordinarily, under the Federal and State Tax on Unrelated Business Income, the income the hospital receives from business lease tenants is taxable. However, if the hospital can prove that it will use the facility within the next ten years for exempt purposes, income earned will be nontaxable.[285] Voluntary hospitals may also be able to issue tax-free bonds for added long-term financing. Whether or not they are eligible depends upon an Internal Revenue Service ruling issued in 1963, and how the hospital is classified under it.[286]

CONCLUSION AND RECOMMENDATIONS

The present time (1972) is critical because Congress has before it various bills which could make the Health Maintenance Organization an integral part of a restructured health system in this country. This proposed legislation can provide the sorely-needed funds which each new plan must have. While Blue Cross-Blue Shield and the private insurance company may eventually also help financially, the government must lead the way and provide the bulk of the investment. If the legislation fails or is not substantial enough, many new plans will falter, because people simply have not yet been convinced that the H.M.O. route is the best way.

Because of the general lack of uniformity in the H.M.O. area, no two people view the plans exactly alike. For that reason, an attempt was made in this Chapter to bring together a variety of viewpoints on various aspects of H.M.O. financial development. The result of this collection of data and opinions is difficult to assess. If anything definite can be stated about the past and present H.M.O. planning experiences, it is that in almost every instance, financial needs were underestimated. This is certainly to be expected because the area is simply too new and too unpredictable to set

---

[284] Interview - Bruce Caputo, op. cit.

[285] Interview - Barry Zeman, op. cit.

[286] Gerald Sears, "How Hospitals Could Use Tax-Free Bonds," The Modern Hospital, Vol. 107, No. 5, (November 1966), pp. 129-133, 182-183.

universal standards. That is why the Kaiser Plan, as large and successful as it is, cannot be used as an exclusive blueprint for an H.M.O. in Boston or Texas. There are just too many special conditions in each location that will effect the plan's financial success.

Interviews with those administrators closely tied to the planning and operations of newly-formed H.M.O.'s can be most informative, if they help to define the special problems each plan faces and those actions employed to rectify the problems. Essentially, this paper has revealed the financial difficulties associated with three important H.M.O.'s.

The Rhode Island Plan is a good example of an H.M.O. with a strong population base and a solid administrative foundation (small, but solid), that was not initially able to raise sufficient funds for operations.

The Harvard Plan is quite different from Rhode Island. It is sponsored by one of the most prestigeous medical schools in the entire country; it is located in a city where high enrollment is almost assured; and it has received substantial planning grants from a number of foundations. Still, money problems haunted them constantly through the early years, and have not yet subsided.

The Columbia Plan is unique because of its location in the "new town" of Columbia, Maryland, and its relationship with Connecticut General Life Insurance Company. Its problems center around enrollment and its relationship with Connecticut General.

These three plans are experiencing difficulties common in any new, unexplored area. Hopefully, by studying the obstacles they encountered and their mistakes, others will be able to apply the H.M.O. mechanism with greater efficiency and confidence in the future.

Bibliography - Personal Interviews (By Date)

Jim Sleeth, Vice-President for Administrative Management of H.I.P.,
November 19, 1971.

Barry Zeman, Planning Department, Long Island Jewish Hospital,
November 23, 1971.

Joseph Levi, Administrator at Long Island Jewish Hospital,
November 24, 1971.

Leo Petit, Head Administrator, and Dale Hoover, Marketing and Enrollment
Director, Rhode Island Group Health Association, Inc.,
Providence, R.I., December 7, 1971.

Marvin Leeds, Director of East Nassau Medical Group, December 28, 1971.

Dan Sullivan, Public Relations Director, G.H.A., Washington, D.C.,
January 31, 1972.

Jeffrey Prussin, Education and Training Director, G.H.A.A.,
January 31, 1972.

Ron Nick, New York Blue Cross Administrator, February 4, 1972.

Dr. Lawrence Clare of H.S.M.S.A. - H.E.W., Regional Office Two,
February 8, 1972.

Bruce Caputo, Director of Inner City Fund, New York and Washington,
February 18, 1972.

Lou Sacadelli, Executive Director of G.H.A. of Washington, D.C.,
former Associated Executive Director of G.H.A.A.,
February 25, 1972.

James F. Doherty, Legislative Representative of G.H.A.A., and Steve Lewis,
of the Legal Department of G.H.A.A., Washington, D.C.,
February 25, 1972.

Herman Schmidt, Field Director, G.H.A.A., Washington, D.C., February 25,
1972.

Ira Shimp, Assistant Director of Columbia Medical Plan, and John Bayliff,
Controller of Columbia Plan, February 28, 1972.

Roger Birnbaum, Assistant Director, Harvard Community Health Plan,
March 5, 1972.

(Telephone Interview) - Fran Brissette, Medical Programs Department,
Connecticut General Life Insurance Company, March 12, 1972.

BIBLIOGRAPHY

Brown, Fred R.   "Government Financial Support for Health and Medical
          Services in the U.S." (Dissertation - Political Science),
          University of Pennsylvania, 1959.

Bush, Ann S.   "Group Practice: Planning and Implementing A Community-Wide
          Prepayment Plan, New York State Health Planning Commission,
          May 1971.

"Capital Financing: Methods, Sources, discussed at Duke Forum," Hospital
          Topics, August 1967, pp. 48-9.

Cash Flow Statements - June 1971-May 1972, Rhode Island Group Health
          Association, Inc.

Colombo, Theodore, Saward, Ernest, M.D. & Greenlick, Merwyn, "Integration
          of an O.E.O. Health Program Into A Prepaid Comprehensive Group
          Practice Plan," Journal of Public Health, Jan.-June, p. 641.

"Columbia Medical Plan" (3-page publicity paper), October 1971.

Columbia Medical Plan Agreement - Connecticut General, Johns Hopkins
          Medical School and Columbia Medical Plan, Sept. 22, 1969.

Committee Print - Health Maintenance Organizations; Staff Questions with
          Responses of the Department of Health, Education and Welfare,
          Committee on Finance, U. S. Senate, Washington, D.C.: U. S.
          Government Printing Office, Sept. 27, 1971.

"Community Health Service," Publications Catalog, U. S. Dept. of H.E.W.,
          1969 Edition.

"COMP," Columbia Medical Plan, (News Release), Volume 1, Number 3,
          July 1971.

Congressional Record, Thursday, Nov. 11, 1971, H. R. 11728 - Bill Sponsored
          by William Roy, "Health Maintenance Organization Act of 1971."

Cronkhite, Dr. Leonard, Jr. "Operations and Cash Flow Projections of First
          Clinic for Initial and Second Fiscal Period," Boston, Mass.:
          Health, Inc. August 7, 1970.

Dearing, W.P. M.D., "Developments and Accomplishments of Comprehensive Group
          Practice Prepayment Programs," Washington, D.C.: Group Health
          Association of America, Inc. Revised Edition, January 1, 1970.

Drug Research Report, Volume 14, No. 29, 7/21/71, "Kennedy Attacks Ambiguity
          of Administration's Planning of H.M.O.'s; Javits Sees H.M.O.'s
          Needed Under Any Proposed National Financing Scheme," pp. 19-21.

Ellwood, Dr. Paul M. Jr. & Staff of the American Rehabilitation Foundation,
          "Health Maintenance Organization Pattern," Minneapolis, Minn.
          April 1971.

Ellwood, Dr. Paul, "Implications of Recent Health Legislation," <u>American Journal of Public Health</u>, Jan. 1972, pp. 20-23.

Esselstyn, Caldwell B., M.D., "The Outlook for Group Practice Payment, Direct Service Plans During the Next Twenty Years," reprinted from <u>Michigan Medicine</u>, Volume 66, July 1967, pp. 829-45.

"Facts for Bargaining,"Part Two of "What's New In Collective Bargaining Negotiations and Contracts," Washington, D.C.: The Bureau of National Affairs, Inc. Major Health Proposals, Copyright 1971.

"The Federal Employees Health Benefit Program," Enrollment and Utilization of Health Services 1961-8, prepared by George S. Perrott, Office of Group Practice and Development, H.E.W., p. 15.

Feldman, Louis L. "Legislation and Prepayment for Group Practice," <u>Bulletin N.Y. Academy of Medicine</u>, Vol. 47, No. 4, April 1971, p. 418.

Follman, J. F., "Insurance Companies and Group Practice," Health Insurance Assoc. of America, 1968.

<u>G.H.A.News</u>, published for the members of Group Health Association, Inc. Vol. XXXIV, No. 2, June 1971.

Graning, Harold M. "Many Federal Programs Finance Hospital Construction," <u>Hospitals</u>, April 1968.

Greenberg, Ira G. & Rodburg, Michael L. "The Role of Prepaid Group Practice in Relieving the Medical Care Crisis, <u>Harvard Law Review</u>, Vol. 84, No. 4, Feb. 1971.

<u>Group Health and Welfare News</u>, published by G.H.A.A., 1717 Mass. Ave., Washington, D.C. Vol. XIII, No. 2, Feb. 1972.

"Harvard Community Health Plan," publicity folder.

<u>Health Maintenance Organizations</u> - <u>The Concept and the Structure</u>. Rockville, Md.: Dept. of H.E.W. & H.S.M.H.A. pp. 3-9.

<u>H.E.W. News</u>. Office of Public Affairs, H.E.W., July 20, 1971.

"H.M.O. Development Checklist," paper received from H.E.W. (no date).

<u>H.M.O.'s</u> - Fact Sheet on Five Senate Bills Pending Before the Committee on Labor and Public Welfare - Concerning Health Maintenance Organizations.

<u>H.M.O.'s</u> (paper) Summary of Five Senate Bills concerned with H.M.O.'s, sent to me by Association of American Medical Colleges, Washington, D.C.

Heyssel, Robert M. M.D., "The Columbia Medical Plan & The East Baltimore Medical Plan, <u>Hospitals</u>, March 16, 1971, pp. 69-71.

H.R. 5614, in the House of Rep. - March 4, 1971, sponsored by Staggers, Health Manpower Assistance Act of 1971.

H.R. 11728, in the House of Representatives - Nov. 11, 1971, sponsored by Roy, Health Maintenance Organization Act.

"H.U.D. - F.H.A. Program for Group Practice Facilities," (Pamphlet) H.U.D. - 146-F, August 1970.

"Instructions for Preparation and Submission of Application for Health Services Development Project Grant," Rockville, Md.: H.E.W. and H.S.M.H.A.

Johnson, Richard I. "Money Shortage Tightens Noose Around Traditional Capital Financing Sources," Modern Hospital, Vol. 107, Number 5, November 1966.

Kaiser Foundation Medical Care Program 1969, Annual Report.

The Kaiser Permanente Medical Care Program, A Symposium, Edited by Anne R. Somers, New York: Commonwealth Fund, 1971.

Keene, Clifford H. M.D., "Financing A Total System of Medical Care - A Case Study: The Kaiser Foundation Medical Care Program" - reprinted from Financial Implications of Hospitals in Comprehensive Health Care Planning, Bloomington, Ind.: Bureau of Business Research, 1969.

Klarman, Herbert E. Economic Aspects of Health Maintenance Organizations - Their Impact on Hospitals, New York University, presented at Annual Meeting of Greater N.Y. Hospital Association, April 28, 1971.

Leeds, Marvin M. Testimony Before Committee on Health, Assembly, State of New York, September 18, 1969, State University of New York at Stonybrook.

Logsdon, Donald. Speech Made at One-day Institute on Prepaid Group Group Practice, Non-Profit Medical Corporation and Health Maintenance Organization, held on June 15, 1971 in Albany.

"Long Island Jewish Medical Center, Legislative Bulletin," August 5, 1971, Bulletin #5, Subject: H.M.O., Hill Burton.

Long Island Jewish Medical Center - Memorandum, "One Day Institute on Prepaid Group Practice," June 15, 1971, pp. 5 & 6.

Lopik,William Van. "Financial Management," Hospital, Vol. 42, April 1, 1968, pp. 53-8.

Lucas, Patricia. "The Aurora Plan: Joint Effort Makes Health Care a Community Affair," Hospital Topics, August 1967, pp. 53-8.

Magraw, Dr. Richard M. "Patterns for the Future," Group Practice, August 1968, pp. 26-31.

Maloney, William F. M.D., "The Tufts Comprehensive Community Health Action
        Program," Journal of American Medical Association, Volume 202,
        No. 5, Oct. 30, 1967, p. 110.

Message from the President of the U. S. - Relative to Building a National
        Health Strategy, Washington, D.C.: U.S. Government Printing
        Office, February 18, 1971.

Myers, Beverlee A. M.P.H., Health Care in the 70's: Dollars and Delivery -
        The Latest Dichotomy in Public Health, Speech presented at
        opening session of 1971 meeting of Western Branch, Los Angeles,
        Calif: American Public Health Association, June 15, 1971.

_____. "Health Maintenance Organizations: Objectives and Issues,"
        based on speech at annual conference of State Comprehensive
        Health Planning Agencies on April 7, 1971 in Washington, D.C.

Newman, Harold F. M.D., "Impact of Medicare on Group Practice Prepayment
        Plans," Journal of Public Health, Jan.-June 1969, p. 629.

"Non-Profit Medical Corporations Act," Article 44, Public Health Law,
        New York's Approach to Prepaid Comprehensive Group Practice -
        Considerations for Applicants, N.Y. State Dept. of Health,
        Hollis S. Ingraham, M.D., Commissioner, July 1971.

"The Non-Profit Medical Corporation Act," Article from Newsletter -
        Medical Societies Reference Committee (Received at L. I. Jewish
        Hospital).

"O.E.O." Officials: Clinics Could Become H.M.O.'s," (no author),
        Modern Hospital, Sept. 1970, p. 34.

"Planned Surplus Gives Doctors Incentives - Keeps Facilities Up to Date,"
        Modern Hospital, February 1971, pp. 91-2.

"Prepaid Health Care: The Way It Works, What's Being Planned," U. S. News
        & World Report, March 29, 1971, pp. 76-7.

"Prepaid Group Practice," (folder), A Workshop Series on Fundamentals of
        Prepaid Group Practice, Sponsored by G.H.A.A., Inc.

"Prepaid Group Practice and H.M.O.'s," paper printed by New York Blue Cross.

"Promoting the Group Practice of Medicine," Report on the National
        Conference on Group Practice, October 19-21, 1967. U. S. Dept.
        of H.E.W., P.H.S. Pub. No. 1750.

Prussin, Jeffrey A. Director, Dept. of Education and Training - G.H.A.A.,
        "This is Prepaid Group Practice Medical Care," Speech before
        Group Health Care Symposium, Newtown, Pennsylvania, January 15,
        1972.

"Publications of the Health Services and Mental Health Administration,"
        PHS Publication No. 2156, January 1971.

"Public Health Services - Labor Seminar on Consumer Health Services,"
Washington, D.C.: U. S. Dept. of H.E.W. Public Health
Services Publication No. 1845, January 22-23, 1968.

Reed, Louis S. "Health Insurance Plans Other Than Blue Cross or Blue Shield
Plans or Insurance Companies, 1970 Survey," U. S. Dept. of
H.E.W. Office of Research And Statistics, Research Report No. 35.

Regional Office of H.E.W. (Letter), Region 11 (N.Y. & N.J.) to Glenn E.
Hastings, Project Director, Nassau-Suffolk Comprehensive Health
Planning Council, Centereach, N.Y. April 18, 1971.

Renthal, Dr. Gerald, "A Community Hospital," Medical Care Administration -
Case #6, U. S. Dept. of H.E.W., May 1968.

_____. "Medical Care Planning in a Small Urban Area," Medical Care
Administration - Case #1, Part 11, Dept. of H. E. W. January
1967.

Rhode Island Group Health Association, Pamphlet, "History & Rationale."

Saward, Ernest W. M.D., "The Relevance of Prepaid Group Practice to the
Effective Delivery of Health Services," Speech presented at
10th Annual Group Health Institute, Ontario, Canada, June 18,
1969, Reprinted by H.E.W., Pub. #72-6302.

Saward, Dr. Ernest, Blank, Janet D. and Greenlick, Merwyn R. "Documentation
of Twenty Years of Operation and Growth of a Prepaid Group
Practice Plan," Medical Care, Vol. 6, p. 215, 1968.

Sears, Gerald P. "How Hospitals Could Use Tax Free Bonds," Modern Hospital,
Dec. 1966, pp. 129-32.

Selected Notated Bibliography on Health Maintenance Organizations, Dept. of
H.E.W., H.S.M.H.A., Community Health Service May 1971,
reprinted July 1971.

Selected References on Group Practice, U. S. Dept. of H.E.W., Public Health
Service, 1969.

Sigmund, Robert M. "Hospital Capital Funds: Changing Needs and Sources,"
Hospitals, August 16, 1965, p. 52.

"Source Book of Health Insurance Data," 1969, Health Insurance Institute,
277 Park Avenue, New York.

A Study of National Health Insurance Proposals - Introduced in the 92nd
Congress, A Supplementary Report to the Congress, Department
of Health, Education and Welfare, Elliot L. Richardson,
Secretary, July 1971.

Thalheimer, Harold R. (Speech), "The Columbia Medical Plan," Secretary,
Medical Programs Dept. Connecticut General Life Insurance
Company, given before American Association of Hospital Planning,
(no date given).

"This is G.H.A.A." (Pamphlet) Washington, D.C.: Group Health Association
          of America, Inc,

"Toward A Comprehensive Health Policy for the 1970's" - A White Paper,
          U. S. Dept. of H.E.W., May 1971.

Walters, Frank C. "Group Health Association, Inc. of Washington, D.C."
          reprinted from Group Practice, Volume 10 - No. 9, September 1961,
          Copyright by American Association of Medical Clinics.

"Wanted: Comprehensive Medical Care at a Reasonable Cost," (folder)
          prepared by G.H.A.A., Washington, D. C.

West, Howard, "Group Practice Plans in Governmental Medical Care Programs,
          American Journal of Public Health, Vol. 59, No. 4, pp. 624-9.

Yedidia, Avram, "Planning and Implementing of the Community Health
          Foundation of Cleveland, Ohio," Public Health Service
          Publication No. 1664-3, Washington, D.C.: U. S. Government
          Printing Office, April 1968.

CHAPTER IV

A PLAN FOR MARKETING H.M.O. SERVICES

Alan J. Gartner

INTRODUCTION

Purpose

This chapter presents a marketing plan for attracting subscribers to the H.M.O. The plan is designed to obtain at least 50,000 subscribers from a local population of about 500,000 persons. Experts in the field suggest that at least a ten per cent enrollment from a population is necessary for the success of a prepaid health maintenance organization in any locality.*

Organization

As in many commercial organizations, the marketing function of the H.M.O. will have a director of marketing who reports to the chief executive officer. The director will have jurisdiction over the following functional areas: marketing planning, service management, advertising management, marketing research, personal selling, and public relations (see Figure IV - 1). Although the functions in Figure IV - 1 are shown as being discrete, it is quite possible in a small H.M.O. or in the early stage of growth, that two or more of these functions can be entrusted to one person. The boxes depict functions and not necessarily positions.

Director. The major responsibility of the marketing executive is to formulate and carry out the marketing plan in a manner consistent with H.M.O. objectives.[1] In accomplishing these ends he will require the co-ordinated assistance of all his subordinate functions, especially that of planning.

---

*Background letter from Kaiser-Permanente marketing staff, Oakland, California, March 17, 1971.

[1] Mark E. Stern, Marketing Planning: A Systems Approach, (New York: McGraw-Hill Book Company, 1966), p. 6.

FIGURE IV - 1[a]

THE MARKETING ORGANIZATION OF THE H.M.O.

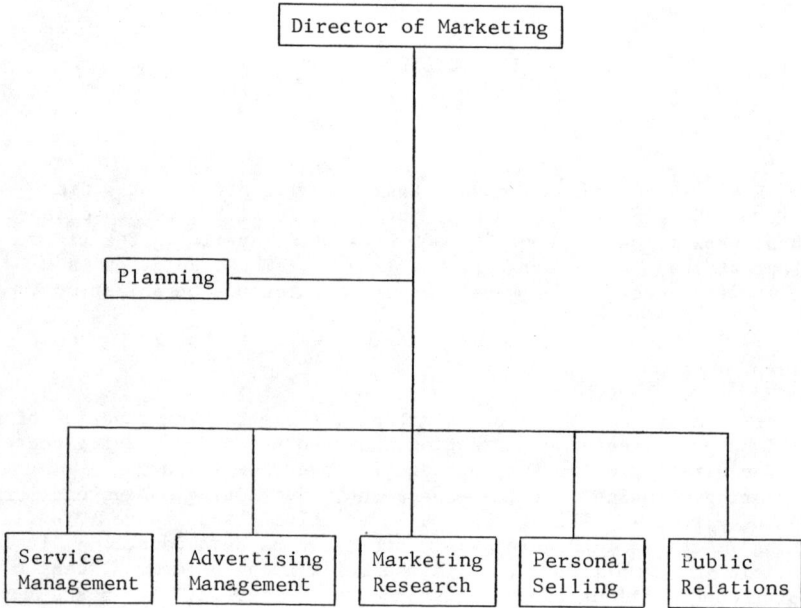

```
                    ┌──────────────────────┐
                    │ Director of Marketing │
                    └──────────────────────┘
                                │
┌──────────┐                    │
│ Planning │────────────────────┤
└──────────┘                    │
        ┌───────────┬───────────┼───────────┬───────────┐
┌───────────┐ ┌───────────┐ ┌───────────┐ ┌──────────┐ ┌──────────┐
│ Service   │ │Advertising│ │ Marketing │ │ Personal │ │ Public   │
│Management │ │Management │ │ Research  │ │ Selling  │ │Relations │
└───────────┘ └───────────┘ └───────────┘ └──────────┘ └──────────┘
```

[a]Adapted from Mark E. Stern, op. cit., p. 17.

186

Planning. The planning area is responsible for the forward thrust of the company's marketing effort. Information collected by the line personnel is molded into a cohesive plan and this is directed toward the achievement of the organization's marketing objectives.[2,3]

Service Management. The responsibility of service management is to develop that part of the marketing plan geared to the basic health needs of the subscriber primarily through subscriber education.[4] Service management must study the market carefully so as to identify significant trends that could affect the outlook for subscriber activity. The department is responsible for the preparation of catalogs, bulletins, and other service-selling aids. It must be sure of the quality and appeal of these instruments since they will figure predominantly in the advertising program.[5]

Advertising Management. The intangible nature of the H.M.O.'s service makes it extremely difficult to promote.[6] Therefore, advertising management's role in marketing is to illustrate the advantages of the service to the population of potential subscribers. The main task of selling a service such as the H.M.O., is to make the intangible seem real and tangible. Imaginative advertising is required in order to paint a picture that will clearly portray to the prospective customer the merits of what he is being asked to buy. It is also vital that advertising management, in its campaigns, relates the advantages of the H.M.O. to the health needs of the subscriber.[7]

Subscriber satisfaction must also be aided by advertising management. This can be done by creating an image of high quality and efficiency. The image must have a real basis and reflect the true character of the H.M.O. because it can exert an important influence on the selection process of individual subscribers and upon subscription renewals.[8]

The advertising mission is accomplished through advertising copy and proper media selection. Advertising management must determine the copy theme which must be executed effectively and forcefully. Those advantages

[2] Ernest C. Miller, Marketing Planning: Approaches of Selected Companies, (American Management Association, 1967), p. 10.

[3] Handbook of Modern Marketing, ed. by Victor P. Buell, (New York: McGraw-Hill Book Company, 1970), pp. 8, 62.

[4] Ibid.,p. 8-22

[5] Ibid., p. 8-23.

[6] Eugene M. Johnson, An Introduction to the Problems of Service Marketing Management, (Wilmington, Delaware: University of Delaware, 1964), p. 17.

[7] Ibid., p. 18.

[8] Albert J. Wood, "New Dimensions in Marketing Research for Banks," Banking, LI, (April 1959), p. 56.

and qualities of the H.M.O. in which subscribers have the greatest interest must be emphasized.[9]

One the basic theme of copy has been determined by management, the actual writing of copy follows. In the case of the H.M.O., the services of an independent advertising agency will probably be utilized. Advertising agencies are qualified in the tactical aspects of copywriting and can create campaigns given certain financial bounds to work within.[10]

The concomitant task of advertising management is that of media selection. The advertiser and his audience are separated by a gap of time and space. It is the function of media to bridge this gap by economically carrying the message to the audience.[11]

Marketing Research. The collection and interpretation of facts that help the marketing organization to get its service more efficiently to the consumer are the missions of the marketing research department.[12]

Two categories of marketing research applications are explored in this chapter. The first is environmental research and the second actionable research. Environmental research involves the collection of data about the nature of things as they are.[13] An example is a study of consumer satisfaction with prepaid group practices in selected areas. This kind of study can be used by the H.M.O. marketing research department to evaluate existing prepayment plans.

Actionable studies represent those studies aimed specifically at a particular management decision. These types of studies are intended to reduce risks and to provide direction.[14] A pertinent example is a concept test of the probable consumer appeal of the H.M.O.

Personal Selling. The relationship between the production and consumption of the H.M.O. service results in a close personal relationship between buyers and sellers quite different from that in the marketing of most commodities. We call this indirect personal selling. The H.M.O. may be modern and efficient with highly trained personnel, but the impression a subscriber gets from employees is a major factor in determining his attitude toward the service enterprise. Furthermore, the attitudes and actions of the personnel may negate promotional efforts which had previously led to the

---

[9]Buell, op. cit., p. 13-19.

[10]Ibid., pp. 13-20

[11]Ibid.

[12]A. B. Blankenship and J.B. Doyle, Marketing Research Management, (American Management Association, 1967), p. 1.

[13]Buell, op. cit., pp. 6-42.

[14]Ibid.

customer's patronage. Therefore, the successful operation of a service organization is related directly to the quality of the indirect personal selling performed.[15]

A survey conducted by a trade magazine showed that approximately 91 per cent of those who dropped out as customers of service organizations, did so because of dissatisfaction. Proper consideration, courteous treatment, better handling of complaints, and recognition of the importance of satisfied customers probably would have retained these drop-outs.[16]

Since the H.M.O. will probably receive a large portion of its subscription income from unions and corporations, direct personal selling also is necessary. Individual subscriptions can be obtained through indirect and promotional methods, but group recruitment calls for a more concentrated sales effort.

The H.M.O. will require a trained salesman who is thoroughly familiar with the health maintenance organization - its uses, limitations and superiority over existing prepaid group plans. He also must have a detailed knowledge of the prospective group subscriber. He must have studied their problems, their policies, and the individuals who have influence on the ultimate subscription decision. A salesman, so equipped, can sell corporations and/or unions more effectively than can any other promotional method.[17]

Public Relations. Public relations is unpaid advertising and for the purpose of convincing people that they should adopt a certain attitude or pursue a certain course of action.[18] In the case of the H.M.O., the initial task of the public relations function, in conjunction with a P.R. agency, is to present the organization and its services in a favorable light.

An effective way to promote an organization like the H.M.O. is to make it meaningful to the self-interest of each group or individual involved. The assumption is that enlightened self-interest will cause people to respond favorably.[19]

Once the organization is in operation, public relations must shift emphasis to another area. News of efficient service and cordial reception

---

[15] Johnson, op. cit., p. 63.

[16] "The Diminishing Service Dollar," NADA Magazine, XXVIII, No. 10, 1956, p. 16.

[17] David D. Seltz, Successful Industrial Selling, (Englewood Cliffs, N.J.: Prentice Hall Inc., 1958), pp. 2-3.

[18] Howard Stephenson ed., Handbook of Public Relations, (New York: McGraw-Hill Book Company, 1971), p. 8.

[19] William S. McNary, "PR and the Health Industry," Public Relations Journal, X, No. 9 (1954), p. 12.

will become promotional vehicles. But, always it is necessary that good
service precede the news of it.[20]

Another task of the public relations department is to neutralize the
effects of negative reactions toward the H.M.O. Opinions from self-styled
experts or subscribers which are harmful to the organization must be countered
carefully. This is done to prevent dissatisfaction among actual and potential
members who may look to such adverse opinions.

Marketing Planning

Peter Drucker[21] defines planning as the continuous process of
making present entrepreneurial decisions systematically and with the best
possible knowledge of futurity. The efforts needed to carry out these
decisions must be organized so that results can be measured against expecta-
tions through organized systematic feedback. In a similar manner, Lyndell
Urwick[22] describes planning as an intellectual process and a mental disposition to do things in a orderly way, to think before acting and to act
in the light of facts, rather than guesses.

Thus, it can be seen that there is an important common point in
these definitions that characterize all planning. That is, the purpose to
manipulate the present systematically to make preparation for the future.
This is also the basis for marketing planning and the marketing planning
process.[23]

Marketing planning is an extension of planning in general. It is
a set of activities and processes involved in establishing marketing goals,
assessing market opportunities, generating possible strategies through which
to achieve these objectives, designing detailed marketing programs, integrating the individual programs into a marketing plan, and adjusting the plan to
changes in the environment.[24]

The marketing planning process can be viewed as a systematic step-
by-step flow routine.[25] As shown in Figure IV - 2, the process flows from
the basic marketing objective through systematic stages until the optimal
plan is realized. Mark Stern briefly discusses the highlights of the
planning process as follows:[26]

---

[20]Scott M. Cutlip and Allen H. Center, Effective Public Relations, (Englewood,
Cliffs, N.J.: Prentice-Hall, Inc., 1965), p. 362.

[21]Peter F. Drucker, "Long Range Planning: Challenge to Management Science,"
Management Science, V, No. 3 (1959).

[22]Lyndell Urwick, The Elements of Administration, (New York: Harper and Row
Publishers, Incorporated, 1944), p. 33.

[23]Stern, op. cit., p. 411.

[24]Ibid., p. 9.

[25]Ibid., p. 12.

[26]Stern, op. cit. pp. 12-16.

190

FIGURE IV - 2

THE MARKETING PLAN PROCESS FOR THE H.M.O.[a]

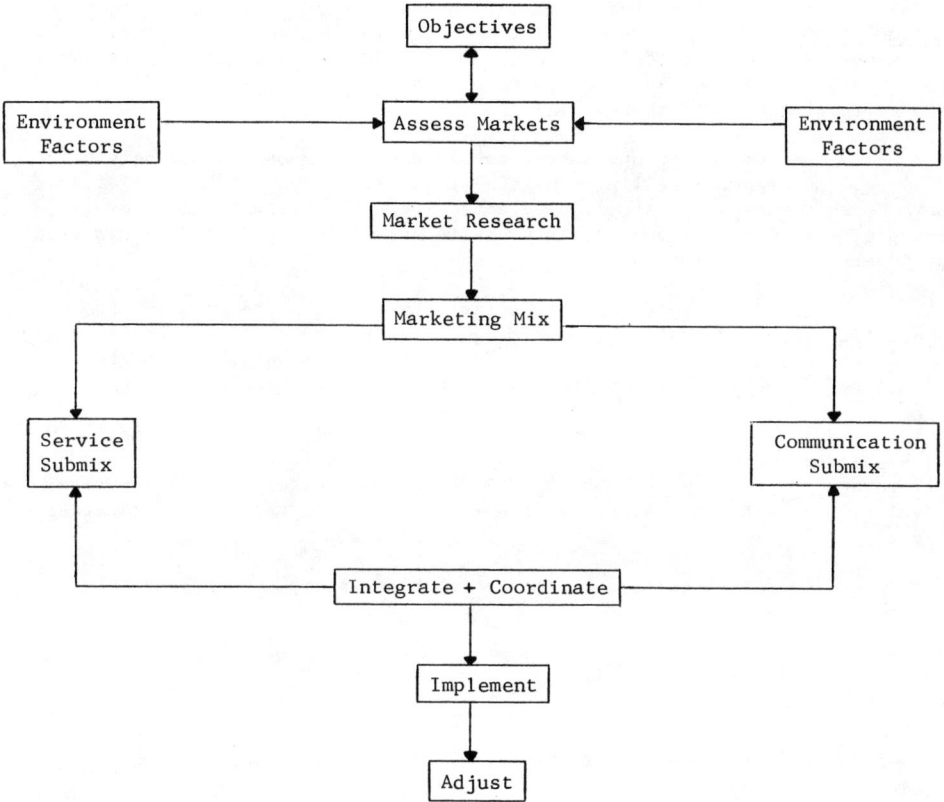

```
                          ┌──────────────┐
                          │  Objectives  │
                          └──────┬───────┘
                                 ↕
┌──────────────┐         ┌──────────────┐         ┌──────────────┐
│ Environment  │────────→│Assess Markets│←────────│ Environment  │
│   Factors    │         └──────┬───────┘         │   Factors    │
└──────────────┘                ↕                 └──────────────┘
                          ┌──────────────┐
                          │Market Research│
                          └──────┬───────┘
                                 ↕
          ┌──────────────────────────────────────────┐
          │              Marketing Mix                │
          └──┬─────────────────────────────────────┬──┘
             │                                     │
      ┌──────┴───────┐                      ┌──────┴────────┐
      │   Service    │                      │ Communication │
      │   Submix     │                      │    Submix     │
      └──────┬───────┘                      └───────┬───────┘
             │                                      │
             │      ┌──────────────────────┐        │
             └──────┤ Integrate + Coordinate├───────┘
                    └──────────┬───────────┘
                               ↓
                        ┌──────────────┐
                        │  Implement   │
                        └──────┬───────┘
                               ↓
                        ┌──────────────┐
                        │   Adjust     │
                        └──────────────┘
```

[a] Adapted from Mark E. Stern, op. cit., p. 13.

191

(1) The planner must explicitly set forth the basic objectives of the plan. He must anticipate the dynamic needs and wants of potential subscribers and stimulate demand for his service;

(2) In order to determine whether the marketing objective is achievable, the planner has to assess market opportunities. This is a determination of the market potential for the service which satisfies a certain set of anticipated subscriber wants and needs. Furthermore, it is an assessment of the complex environment in which the organization will operate;

(3) The assessment of market opportunities and appropriate marketing research provide inputs which help determine the programs for attaining the objectives. A marketing mix is devised for a specific set of strategies consisting of two submixes: the service submix; and the communications submix: The service submix includes such functions as timing, individual service strategies, quality, and pricing. A continuing assessment must also be made as to whether the service meets the current needs and wants of the subscribers.

The communications submix involves both personal and nonpersonal selling. Nonpersonal selling consists of advertising and public relations, both of which have separate subprograms. The advertising branch, for example, must consider copy quality, media selection, and the dissemination of advertising information;

(4) The service and communications submixes are received from specialists and integrated by marketing management to achieve a higher degree of effectiveness in the total marketing effort. It is at this time that the marketing strategy to be employed is selected and the plan is structured;

(5) Once marketing management agrees that the plan is consistent with the desired objectives, the plan should be submitted to top management for review, revision, and approval. A reason for review at the corporate level is the fact that marketing is but one aspect of the total organizational effort;

(6) At this stage the marketing plan is implemented and the results monitored.

MARKET FACTORS

The investigation of the nature of the market for the H.M.O. includes: (a) identifying the target markets; (b) considering potential subscriber needs and desires; and (c) weighing the possible effects of environmental factors.[27]

---

[27]
Stern, op. cit., p. 21.

Once the markets and their component parts have been identified, the marketing staff performs marketing research[28] to determine the enrollment potential of each target area.[29]

Identifying the Markets

The subscriber, his wife, and dependents all count as members. The H.M.O. subscriber is drawn from labor union, corporation, government, self-employed, and retired groups. The first three markets must be tapped extensively in order to secure sufficient enrollment.[30]

The Subscriber

The consumer is interested in obtaining as much medical care as is needed for the maintenance of health. If he enrolls in an H.M.O., he would like a contract that provides as much in the way of benefits as is consistent with high quality service.[31]

The subscriber expects to receive the benefits of the whole range of scientific medicine for prevention of disease and for treatment of all types of illness or injury when he subscribes to the H.M.O.'s comprehensive coverage.[32] This may include the full spectrum of outpatient care, extended care, home health service, drug coverage and mental health services.[33]

Personal Interest. Most patients naturally desire good technical care, but they insist nonetheless that without the personal interest of the practitioner the program cannot be satisfactory.[34] In one way or another, many subscribers of prepayment plans have reported disappointment with the degree of personal interest shown by the group doctor and with the availability of his services when requested.[35] Conversely, other patients in different situations have emphasized their gratification with the interest

---

[28]Marketing Research will be discussed in detail in the next major section of the text.

[29]Stern, op. cit., p. 22.

[30]Greer Williams, "Kaiser Plan: The Prepaid Group Practice Model and How It Began," Modern Hospital, February 1971, p. 74.

[31]Oscar N. Serbein Jr., Paying for Medical Care in the United States, (New York: Columbia University Press, 1953), p. 339.

[32]Ibid.,p. 340.

[33]Ernest W. Saward, The Relevance of Prepaid Group Practice to the Effective Delivery of Health Services, (U.S. Dept. of Health, Education and Welfare, 1969), p. 12.

[34]Eliot Freidson, Patients' Views of Medical Practice, (New York: Russel Sage Foundation, 1961), p. 209.

[35]E.R. Weinerman, "Patients' Perceptions of Group Medical Care," American Journal of Public Health, LIV, (June 1964), p. 886.

that they felt was being taken in them.[36] Member physicians must be aware that their behavior usually constitutes the crucial variable for the patient.[37] Doctors must understand that the subscriber may be alienated by impersonal treatment that he seeks personal involvement from "his" doctor - even if he is a man he has never met before.[38]

Personal interest is important in other areas. The health center complex often employs aides, receptionists, and nurses. These workers are important in organizing the flow of work and so mediate between patient and doctor.[39] As agents through whom the subscriber must pass before he reaches the physician, they can color the patient's relation to the doctor.[40]

No patient wants to feel like a nameless number.[41] Personal identity can be an issue for him. Therefore, a satisfactory program must seem to take enough personal interest in the subscriber so that he feels no threat to his identify as a person.[42] The issue of "personal interest" illustrates the importance of consumer attitudes. Whether rational or not, these views profoundly affect the degree to which the program is successful.[43]

Subscriber Education. To bridge the unfamiliar and teach subscribers how to make the most of the new service structure, the H.M.O. marketing staff must become involved in subscriber education.[44] Few subscribers of other plans are thoroughly familiar with the provisions of their contracts or even the risks they face.[45]

Effective subscriber information consists of the presentation and explanation of facts. Meetings and discussion groups are useful. So are carefully prepared printed materials that describe the plan and discuss the

-----

[36]Eliot Freidson, op. cit., p. 77.

[37]Ibid.

[38]E. R. Weinerman, "Attitudes Toward Group Medical Care," Hospital Management, XCVI, (July 1963), p. 43.

[39]Eliot Freidson, op. cit., p. 78.

[40]Ibid., p. 79.

[41]J. G. Greenberg and M. L. Rodburg, "The Performance of Prepaid Group Practice," Harvard Law Review, LXXXIV, (February 1971), p. 941.

[42]Eliot Freidson, op. cit., p. 52.

[43]E. R. Weinerman, op. cit., p. 43.

[44]Avram Yedida, Planning and Implemantation of the Community Health Foundation of Cleveland, Ohio, (Washington,D.C.: Department of Health, Education and Welfare, 1969), p. 82.

[45]T. R. Martin, Group Health Insurance from the Consumer Viewpoint, Dissertation, Stanford University, 1957, p. 95.

concepts on which it is based.[46] Furthermore, these bulletins should describe the available health services and how they can be most effectively utilized - in a simple language.[47]

Preventive Medicine. The H.M.O. must maintain active programs to educate and encourage subscribers to utilize the preventive services of the plan.[48] "In general, the public is not adequately informed of the potentialities of preventive medicine which is the cornerstone of an H.M.O."[49] Subscribers must be encouraged to receive periodic physical checkups to enable detection and treatment of disease or disturbed function at an early stage.[50] With its compact cluster of medical talent and equipment, an H.M.O. is better designed than other kinds of practice to detect and treat sickness before it becomes serious or chronic. This is especially true because doctors have stake in health rather than sickness.[51] The member pays a fixed sum per year whether he is well or sick. Naturally, it is to the physician's advantage to keep him healthy.[52]

Consumer Expectation. The public wants benefits and coverage which will provide the most health service for the health insurance dollar.[53] In practice, subscribers of H.M.O.'s and prepaid health insurance programs expect more than they receive. This expectation gap occurs when people expect their plan's medical care to be available, accessible, and comprehensive at any and all times - which is impossible.[54]

Thus, enrollees must be made aware of the capabilities and limitations of the health center. He must be taught that he can come with full confidence and that his case will be handled usually under one roof, with all kinds of specialists at hand for consultation, without having to wait days to be treated. But, he must also be taught that he will not receive as personalized care, if he fails to make an advance appointment.[55]

[46]Avram Yedida, op. cit., p. 82.

[47]Albert Deutsch, "Group Medicine - Part 3," Consumer Reports, XXII March 1957, p. 135.

[48]W.P. Dearing, Assured Health Services with Quality, National Conference of Health, Welfare, and Pension Plan, Ninth Annual Workshop, 1963, p. 336.

[49]George Rosen, Preventive and Educational Services in Medical Care, Mimeographed Paper, 1954, pp. 5-6.

[50]Albert Deutsch, op. cit.,

[51]Ibid., p. 138.

[52]Ibid., p. 135.

[53]Francis R. Smith, "Why Can't the Prepayment Plans Give the Public What it Wants,?" Modern Hospital, XCV No. 6, 1960, p. 90.

[54]Saward, op. cit., p. 3.

[55]Albert Deutsch, "Group Medicine - Part 2," Consumer Reports, XXII (February 1957), p. 85.

The value of subscriber education is best summarized by Leo Petit.[56] "On-going subscriber education is more than general health service information; it is vital for good subscriber relations."

Consumer Participation. That consumer representation in H.M.O.'s is advantageous to subscribers has been asserted by advocates of consumer plans as well as by governmental and university authorities.[57] By studying health plans in which consumers are entitled to decide policies related to the health care they receive, and contrasting them with programs in which subscribers lack any effective voice, there is evidence that consumer participation causes plans to offer better programs.[58]

The majority of individuals enrolled in H.M.O.'s have little voice or representation.[59] To solicit enrollees directly for comments and suggestions for improvement of services is, therefore, bound to create a more sensitive indication of consumer views than to wait until subscribers were discontented enough to make specific complaints.[60] Furthermore, each subscribing group can select a Health Committee from its membership to act as its official spokesman in direct dealings with the H.M.O.[61]

In some plans, consumers have initiated valuable proposals dealing with enrollment and eligibility policy, provisions of extra benefits, handling of complaints,[62] and concern for cost.[63]

Social Class. Social class is an important variable because it includes both economic and cultural standings. It involves more than the ability to pay. It is also associated with the subscribers' sense of being and their expectation of the way others will treat them.[64]

---

[56] R.I.G.H.A. Interview, op. cit., December 6, 1971.

[57] See: Prepayment for Medical and Dental Care in New York State, New York State Departments of Health and Insurance, 1962, p. 5 and Health Care for California, State of California, Department of Public Health, Berkeley, 1960, p. 31.

[58] J. L. Schwartz, Consumer Participation in Policy Making in Prepaid Health Plans: Effect on Program Patterns and Types of Service, Dissertation, University of California at Berkeley, 1965, p. iii.

[59] Ibid., p. 42.

[60] Ibid., p. 260.

[61] Albert Deutsch, op. cit., p. 83.

[62] J.L. Schwartz, "Consumer Sponsorship and Physician Sponsorship of Prepaid Group Practice Health Plans: Some Similarities and Differences," American Journal of Public Health, LV (January 1965), p. 98.

[63] Health Care for California, op. cit., p. 31.

[64] Eliot Freidson, op. cit., pp. 123-124.

In some programs, a criterion of plan selection is social status. Subscribers regard the accessibility of medical care as a goal, regardless of its economic merits. They consider membership in an H.M.O. to be a symbol of social independence and possibly a step upward from their previous situations.[65] Moreover, members of the middle class are more likely to be future oriented, prepared to forego present satisfactions in order to achieve future rewards.[66] This patient also is more informed and uses his accumulated knowledge to assess and analyse the H.M.O.[67]

In contrast, the lower classes seem less sensitive about their status and are generally more passive in their approach to plan selection.[68] These people are subject to some limitations which affect their behavior.[69] The views of this group are generally limited by fear, ignorance, and misunderstanding, as well as by different types of reactions to life situations.[70] Furthermore, actions are usually confined to the needs of the moment with the future being allowed to take care of itself.[71]

Lay Referral. "The lay referral structure .... consists in a network of consultants, potential or actual, running from the intimate and most informal confines of the nuclear family through successive more select, distant, and authoritative persons until the 'professional' is reached."[72] Cultural differences between the lower and middle class referral structures are apparent. The lower class system reports more frequent associations with parents, relatives, and close friends. The middle class, on the other hand, feels more secure in their own views and thus have less need of lay consultation.[73]

The use of referral groups for expansion of membership is usually confined in the employment unit.[74] A key person in the firm or union who

---

[65] Burton Wolfman, "Medical Expenses and Choice of Plans," Monthly Labor Review, LXXXIV (July 1961), pp. 1189-90.

[66] George Rosen, "Provision of Medical Care," Public Health Reports, LXXIV (March 1959), p. 200.

[67] Eliot Freidson, op. cit., p. 149.

[68] Ibid., pp. 210-11.

[69] E. Ginzberg, Occupational Choice: An Approach to a General Theory, (New York: Columbia University Press, 1951), p. 133.

[70] R.I.G.H.A. Interview, December 6, 1971.

[71] George Rosen, op. cit, p. 206.

[72] Eliot Freidson, op. cit., pp. 146-47.

[73] Ibid., pp. 150-51.

[74] Greenberg and Rodburg, op. cit., p. 946.

has frequent interaction with employees - especially new ones, must be located. His strategic position must then be exploited by the marketers so as to establish good internal public relations. In this way, employees can be pursuaded to subscribe to the H.M.O. and not the alternate plan.[75]

       Dual Choice. A common pattern in the enrollment programs of voluntary prepayment programs and H.M.O.'s is that of dual choice.[76] This is the health plan consumer's chance to choose between two or more competing programs.[77] These plans permit subscribers to enroll voluntarily and voluntarily retain their membership through periodic[78] renewal options.[79] Thus the person, who does not like the program, has a fair opportunity to opt for another type of coverage.[80]

       It must be realized that choice is not made on the basis of general ideological commitment, but specific attributes of the plans.[81] However, once established in a prepayment scheme, few subscribers seem to shift from one plan to the other.[82] Historically, the major criterion of any shifting has been the consumer's perception of choice of physician or lack of it.[83]

       Therefore, the philosophy underlying dual choice is one of competition[84] and such an element ... "can produce a wholesome group of satisfied, loyal subscribers."[85]

----

[75] R.I.G.H.A. Interview, December 6, 1971.

[76] E. R. Weinerman, op. cit., p. 881.

[77] Greer Williams, op. cit., pp. 93-94.

[78] These renewal options occur at one to three year intervals.

[79] Avram Yedida, "Dual Choice Programs," American Journal of Public Health, XLIX, (1959), p. 1475.

[80] Avram Yedida, op. cit., p. 81.

[81] Charles A. Metzner and Rashid L. Bashshur, "Factors Associated with the Choice of Health Care Plans," Journal of Health and Social Behavior, VIII (December 1967), p. 293.

[82] "APHA Conference Report," Public Health Reports, LXXIV, (March 1957), p. 222.

[83] W. MacColl, Group Practice and Prepayment of Medical Care, (Washington: Public Affairs Press, 1966), p. 242.

[84] Williams, loc. cit.

[85] Yedida, loc. cit.

Free Choice of Physician. Many consumers object to the H.M.O. system because they cannot use the services of their present doctor.[86] Therefore, in an H.M.O. members are given the next best thing; that is, a choice of personal physician, or better still, two or three. They can then make appointments with their "own" doctors and enjoy all the benefits of a personal physician relationship.[87] Subscribers of many plans indicate time and again that the opportunity of having free choice of physician is an important factor in their selection of plan.[88]

The H.M.O., however, cannot give members their "absolute" choice of doctor - there are limitations. Choice must be confined to member physicians.[89] Moreover, under conditions of physicians' overload of duties, free choice is limited by the doctors' inability to serve all who desire his attention.[90] This is not to say that the personal relationship between practitioner and patient is diminished; the latter can immediately obtain the attention of his "other" personal physician.[91]

Growth through Experience. The only real way to acquaint members with a new mode of delivery of health services is to allow them to experience it in action.[92] Since no one can experience a program that does not yet exist, growth during the early stages of operation is inevitably slow. The first persons to subscribe will likely be alert, progressive, conceptualizing individuals. Once the plan is established, others tend to accept it as part of their community, because it has the approval of others by which they can appraise its real advantages to themselves.[93]

Diffusion of information will be slow at first but, since it is dependent on hearsay, should accelerate. It is those with the least social contact that are most difficult to reach. Thus, the information produced in the oral network is an ally of innovation, subject to meeting the recognized needs of the various publics.[94]

---

[86]Martin (dissertation), op. cit., p. 103.

[87]Ibid., p. 133.

[88]See: Wolfman, "Medical Plans," p. 1188, and Weinerman, "Patients' Perceptions of Care," p. 882.

[89]Martin (dissertation), op. cit., p. 132.

[90]Richard Magraw, Address to: AMA Second National Congress on the Socio-economics of Health Care, March 22, 1968.

[91]Martin (dissertation), op. cit., p. 104.

[92]See: R. L. Bashshur, C. A. Metzner, and Carla Worden, "Consumer Satisfaction With Group Practice, The CHA Case," American Journal of Public Health, LVII (November 1967), pp. 1992-94. AND Martin (dissertation), op. cit., p. 104.

93Avram Yedida, op. cit., p. 82.

[94]Metzner and Bashshur, "Factors of Health Care Plans," pp. 298-99.

The staff can then develop smoothness of function through their own experience. "As this occurs, the subscribers recognize that they are receiving high quality, courteously rendered, private care within a framework of coordinated specialty services and prepayment. To the extent that these advantages are genuine, loyalty is the subscriber's natural response. Loyal subscribers communicate their satisfaction to other persons. In doing so, they make the most significant of all contributions to member recruitment and education."[95]

Legal Environment. The "Group Health and Welfare News"[96] outlines general legislation concerning the formation and administration of H.M.O.'s.

Legal obstacles to the formation of prepaid group practice plans still exist in more than 20 states. Many states retain common law rules which prohibit the use of the corporate form for the practice of medicine.

The original purpose of these laws was to prevent commercial exploitation by profit-oriented entities. Such belief has lost its validity with the rise of the nonprofit health services corporation. "So long as the corporate organization retains its nonprofit status, and refrains from exercising any control over the manner in which the physician treats his patients, there can be no rational basis for applying the rule."

"Blue Shield" statutes prevalent in 18 states and enacted in the 1930's also impede the formation of H.M.O.'s. The laws restrict administrative and economic control of health services plans to the medical profession. This presents an immovable barrier to the formation of consumer and community oriented organizations.

In many states where incorporation and operation of H.M.O.'s is permitted, regulation takes the form of insurance principles. Generally, Insurance Commissions are granted the authority to control. This tends to impede H.M.O.'s by ignoring the distinctions between prepaid plans and insurance companies[97] - the latter is engaged in indemnity payment while prepayment furnishes direct services.

New York State Situation. In July 1971, Governor Rockefeller of New York signed into legislation, a law which authorized the formation of nonprofit medical corporations.[98]

---

[95]Avram Yedida, op. cit., pp. 82-83.

[96]"Over Twenty States Have Legal Bars to Group Practice," Group Health and Welfare News, XIII, (February 1972), pp. 1-6.

[97]Four ways in which regulations are obstructive include:
(1) Requiring large amounts of contingency reserves;
(2) Setting unreasonably low rates;
(3) Limiting the percentage of assets which can be used for organizational expenses;
(4) Determining that investments be limited to securities for life insurance companies.

[98]"The Non-Profit Medical Corporations Act," Newsletter - Medical Societies' Reference Committee, p. 1.

The purpose was to encourage the formation of such corporations to expand the health care options available to the consumer. "This legislation provides a vehicle for the development of health maintenance organizations in New York State."[99] Furthermore, a council, with a subscriber majority, was strongly recommended as "a mechanism to provide consumer input into policy matters."[100]

The subscriber recruitment problem is summarized well by Greenberg and Rodburg.[101] "Evidence of the growth of membership in prepaid group practice suggests that it has been generally uneven and slow. Assuming no major change in the roles of government and legislation, the future of prepaid group practice will depend primarily on three factors: its ability to cover a broad spectrum of society, its ability to satisfy consumers of medical care, and its acceptability to health professionals, especially physicians."

MARKETING RESEARCH

McCarthy[102] defines marketing research as developing and analyzing the "facts" that help marketing managers do a better job of planning, executing, and controlling. Marketing research also supplies management with analytical tools based on logic, mathematics, and statistics.[103]

Data Collection

Primary Data Collection. When the data for a marketing problem cannot be found in any existing source, the researchers must undertake original data collection. This calls for direct contact with consumer (actual and potential), salesmen, middlemen, or other primary information sources.[104]

The most common method of gathering primary marketing information is through surveys. Surveys can produce information on characteristics,

---

[99]New York's Approach to Prepaid Comprehensive Group Practice - Considerations for Applicants, (New York State Department of Health, July 1971), p. 1.

[100]Ibid., p. 3.

[101]Greenberg and Rodburg, "The Performance of Group Practice," pp. 933-34.

[102]E. Jerome McCarthy, Basic Marketing: A Managerial Approach, (Homewood, Illinois: Richard D. Irwin, Inc., 1971),p. 90.

[103]William J. Stanton, Fundamentals of Marketing, (New York: McGraw Hill Book Company, 1967), pp. 38-39.

[104]Philip Kotler, Marketing Management: Analysis, Planning and Control, (Englewood Cliffs, N.J.: Prentice-Hall Inc., 1967), pp. 200-201.

attitudes, opinions, and motives. They are an effective way of securing data for planning service features, advertising copy, promotions, and other marketing variables.[105]

Secondary Data Collection. Researchers usually try to find the data they need in existing sources.[106] It is economical to do so when there is a plentiful supply of secondary information that is available immediately.[107] The major sources of secondary information are: governmental (federal, state, and local), trade associations and trade press, periodicals, textbook literature, institutions, and commercial services.[108]

Interrogiation methods - The market researcher faces many alternate methods for primary data collection. He must decide among survey methods, research instruments and interview techniques.[109] For the purpose of this chapter, we will demonstrate the interviewing techniques discussed by Buzzell et al.[110]

There are three methods used for collecting data by interrogation:

(A) - Personal interviews - advantages:

1) They allow the use of a more representative sample. Not everyone can be reached by telephone and a great number of people will not respond to a mail survey.

2) More questions can be asked. The respondent has to face the interviewer directly and thus is more apt to answer a greater number of questions.

3) More complex measurement methods can be used as the responses are generally more reliable.

4) Verification of responses can be established. Less distortion occurs, especially in those responses whichcan be readily verified by the interviewer.

Disadvantages:

1) This method is quite costly.

---

[105]Philip Kotler, Marketing Decision Making: A Model Building Approach, (Chicago: Holt, Rinehart and Winston, 1971), pp. 580-581.

[106]Ibid., p. 198.

[107]E. Jerome McCarthy, op. cit., pp. 96-97.

[108]Paul E. Green and Donald S. Tull, Research for Marketing Decisions, (Englewood Cliffs, N.J.: Prentice-Hall, Inc. 1970), pp. 85-86.

[109]Ibid., p. 581.

[110]Robert D. Buzzell, Donald F. Cox and Rex V. Brown, Marketing Research and Information Systems, (New York: McGraw Hill Book Co., 1969), pp. 150-154.

2) It is subject to interviewer, bias, error, and cheating.

3) it is subject to response bias.

(B) - Telephone interviews - advantage:

1) They can be conducted quickly and at a relatively low cost.

Disadvantages:

1) Sample bias is quite high as some people cannot be reached by phone and others have unlisted numbers.

2) The degree of "permissible complexity in measurement method" and total information obtainable are more limited than in personal interview.

(C) - Self-administered questionnaires - advantages:

1) They avoid interviewer bias.

2) This method is usually less expensive to administer.

Disadvantages

1) The sample is not likely to be representative.

2) They must be very carefully designed and pretested or confusion and misunderstanding result.

As an illustration of marketing research, a personal interview study was used in combination with a questionnaire. More particularly, group personal interviews were utilized. This method has several advantages:

1. The group environment provides a social mechanism for the release of respondents' inhibitions.[111]

2. The group approach contributes a wider range of responses.[112]

3. The scope provided by the group interview makes it useful as a clarification step for a subsequent questionnaire.[113]

4. The group interview activates forgotten details which would otherwise have not been recalled.[114]

---

[111]Robert K. Merton, Marjorie Fiske and Patricia L. Kendall, The Focused Interview, (Glencoe, Illinois: The Free Press, 1956), pp. 141-147.

[112]Ibid.

[113]Raymond L. Gordon, Interviewing, (Homewood, Ill.: The Dorsey Press, 1969), p. 55.

[114]Robert K. Merton, et al., op. cit.

5. Respondents in groups try harder to contribute.[115]

6. "Interstimulation" broadens the base of respondents' thoughts.[116]

Use of Computer. Various statistical tools for analysing complex relationships in multivariate data used in the marketing research can be more easily accomplished by the computer. Regression and correlation analyses, discriminant analysis, factor analysis,[117] cluster analysis and multidimensional scaling all become simple techniques when computer-programmed.[118] According to Philip Kotler, ..."these developments will lean the future of marketing toward a more analytical frame of mind with heavier emphasis on planning. If the marketer at the same time maintains a creative and innovative temperament and a people empathy, he cannot help but be extremely effective in the market place."[119]

H.M.O. Research Objective. The initial task of the research project was to gather demographic information for the potential target markets. (See Table IV - 1 for Long Island area data.) These data direct the task of the marketing mix; more time, effort, and funds should be applied to those target markets with the highest potentials.[120]

Research Design

Green and Tull[121] define research design as the specification of methods and procedures for acquiring the information needed. It is the total framework of the project that stipulates what information is to be collected, from which sources, by what procedures.

---

[115]George H. Smith, Motivation Research in Advertising and Marketing, (New York: McGraw Hill Book Company, 1954), pp. 60-64.

[116]Ibid.

[117]A computer-based factor analysis is the analytic tool used in this investigation.

[118]Philip Kotler, "The Future of the Computer in Marketing," Essentials of an Effective Marketing Program, ed. by John L. Kraushaar and Lous H. Varzimer, (Braintree, Mass.: D.H. Mark Publishing Co., 1970), pp. 21-22.

[119]Philip Kotler, "The Future of the Computer in Marketing," Journal of Marketing, XXXIV No. 1, (January 1970), pp. 13-14.

[120]Rhode Island Group Health Association (RIGHA), Providence, R. I., interview with Leo Petit and Dale Hoover, Director of Operations and Director of Enrollment, respectively, December 6, 1971.

[121]Green and Tull, op. cit., p. 73.

TABLE IV - 1

NASSAU-SUFFOLK POPULATION CHARACTERISTICS

Total Population[a]	2,539,577.00
Total Employment[b]	698,000.00
Average Family Size[c]	3.48
Nonaffiliated Employees[d]	310,424.00
Union Affiliated Employees[e]	252,676.00
Government Employees[f]	134,900.00
Income Per Household[g]	$12,969.00

Group Composition. Two major group populations were interviewed. The first was made up of employee groups from six companies in the Long Island area.[122] The other was composed of patient groups from the wards of local hospitals. It was assumed that these groups would be representative of Long Island sentiment toward H.M.O.'s and health care.

Pilot studies done in Martin's research,[123] suggest that a group of eight should be used in each interview situation. The participating companies were therefore asked to select from among their employees eight[124] who had considerable experience[125] with health plans.

---

[a]Local Government Employment in Selected Metropolitan Areas and Large Countries, U.S. Dept. of Commerce, Bureau of the Census,1970.

[b]A Handbook of Statistical Data, State of New York: Dept. of Labour, 1970.

[c]General Population Characteristics of New York, U.S. Dept. of Commerce, Bureau of the Census, Nov. 1971.

[d]This figure is secured by deducting "Union Affiliated Employees" and "Government Employees" from "Total Employment."

[e]A Handbook of Statistical Data, op. cit., 1970.

[f]Estimated from Employees Benefits Factbook, Harry Gersh Editor, (New York: Fleet Academic Editions, 1970), p. 76.

[g]Long Island Factbook, Nassau-Suffolk Planning Commission, 1969.

[122]The six companies remain anonymous by request.

[123]T.R. Martin (dissertation), op. cit., p. 94.

[124]The eight employees were composed of males or females; union or union affiliated.

[125]Martin's research indicates that health plan members who had little or no experience with their plans were a poor source of ideas about health insurance.

Six hospital groups of eight patients each were also interviewed. These discussions took place in Long Island hospital wards.

Subscribers in Blue Cross, Blue Shield, H.I.P. union plans, company plans, and private health plans were all represented in the surveys. Also represented were both sexes, different occupations, and varied income levels. A breakdown of the respondent groups by sex, employment, and income are included in Tables IV - 2, IV - 3, and IV - 4.

Interview Format. During the group interviews, the researcher conducted preliminary lectures concerning all aspects of health care and prepaid plans. It was at this time that the complex variables included in the questionnaire were discussed. An open question period followed and this was used by the respondents to gain insight into the concepts presented. Subsequently, the prestructured questionnaire was administered.

Company Interview Techniques. Long Island firms from different industrial classifications (to insure wide representation) were chosen. Local management was then asked to select respondents on the basis of their previous health plan experience.[126]

In companies with union representation, the interviewer made his position known to organizers to convince them that he was not a management spy or an agent sent in by national headquarters. Management, on the other hand, had to be assured that he was not involved in an investigation of their abilities to handle the union.[127]

To insure the validity of the interview and questionnaire responses, the interviewer posed questions to all workers that were not threatening in nature so as to have evoked defensive reactions.[128]

Hospital Interview Techniques. Interviews with hospitalized patients were conducted with two thoughts in mind:[129] "One that was appropriate to the maintenance of the marketing stance and which provided the interviewer a link with his own discipline - the other established and maintained a mode of communication with his host's culture."[130]

Data Collection Procedures. The existing sources were first scanned to determine the demographics of the target markets. Then all

---

[126]See: William C. Lawton, "Sociological Research in Big Business," Pathways to Data, ed. by R. W. Habenstein, (Chicago: Aldine Publishing Co., 1970), pp. 153-57.

[127]See: Lewis A. Dexter, Elite and Specialized Interviewing, (Evanston: Northwestern University Press, 1970), pp. 28-9.

[128]Donald F. Roy, "The Role of the Researcher in the Study of Social Conflict," Human Organization, XXIV (Fall, 1965), p. 262.

[129]Hans O. Maukach, "Studying the Hospital," Pathways to Data, ed. by R. W. Habenstein (Chicago: Aldine Publishing co., 1970), pp. 197-203.

[130]Ibid., p. 302.

TABLE IV - 2

BREAKDOWN OF RESPONDENT GROUPS BY SEX

		Respondents	Male	Female
	A	8	6	2
	B	8	2	6
Company	C	8	5	3
	D	8	4	4
	E	8	8	0
	F	8	4	4
	A	8	6	2
	B	8	7	1
Hospital	C	8	4	4
	D	8	3	5
	E	8	3	5
	F	8	6	2
Totals		96	58	38

TABLE IV - 3

RESPONDENTS BY EMPLOYEE TYPE[a]

		Respondents	Employed	Union	Union	Government	Retired
Company	A	8	0	6	2	0	0
	B	8	0	5	3	0	0
	C	8	0	4	4	0	0
	D	8	0	0	8	0	0
	E	8	0	2	6	0	0
	F	8	0	5	3	0	0
Hospital	A	8	2	1	3	2	0
	B	8	1	2	2	1	2
	C	8	1	2	3	1	1
	D	8	0	4	2	2	0
	E	8	3	0	3	0	2
	F	8	1	2	2	2	1
Totals		96	8	33	41	8	6

[a]
If female is housewife; her husband's employment noted.

TABLE IV - 4

HOUSEHOLD INCOME OF RESPONDENTS

		Respondents	Less than $7,500	$7,500 - $12,500	$12,500 - $17,500	$17,500 -
Company	A	8	0	5	2	1
	B	8	2	3	3	0
	C	8	0	3	4	1
	D	8	2	4	2	0
	E	8	0	3	5	0
	F	8	2	2	3	1
Hospital	A	8	1	3	2	2
	B	8	3	2	2	1
	C	8	1	2	3	2
	D	8	1	5	1	1
	E	8	3	2	2	1
	F	8	1	6	1	0
Totals		96	16	40	30	10

literature pertaining to health plans were studied. These materials yielded 39 health plan characteristics which were mentioned as plan selection criteria.[131]

The demographic and health plan characteristics were then incorporated into a questionnaire which was administered after each of the group interviews. Subsequently, the questionnaire results of the 96 respondents were collected and analyzed.

Data Analysis. Two factor analyses, FORTRAN IV Programs[132] were utilized to derive a smaller set of factors from the 39 inter-correlated characteristics (variables). Factor analysis is a statistical procedure for trying to discover a few basic factors that may underlie and explain the inter-correlations among a larger number of variables. The technique is based on the assumption that the inter-correlations occur because a few basic factors are shared in common by the different variables in different degrees.[133]

Ninety-six questionnaire respondents rated the 39 plan choice criteria. Then, the factor analyses Programs were used to explain the derived inter-correlations in terms of a smaller set of basic choice factors.[134]

The purpose of this factor analytic procedure was to highlight the vital choice criteria used by potential subscribers. In this way, service and communications vehicles can be developed that stress only characteristics which merit attention -- thus economizing on marketing effort.

Results

The factor analyses programs produced two near-identical ten factor solutions. Factor identifications, compositions and their respective loadings are summarized for both programs in Tables IV-5---14.

Factor loadings resemble correlation coefficients. For example, "The Importance of Peer Recommendation" in Table V - 5 is positively related to the extent of 0.7448 or 0.5400 to Factor 1, and so forth. However, this output does not reveal the identify of the factor -- only an educated

[131]The 39 health plan characteristics correspond to questions 4-42 in the Questionnaire used.

[132]FORTRAN IV Programs were selected because they were time-saving, accurate, and available. The Programs used were: William A. Scott, "Scalescore and Scale Analysis," January 1970; and Kenneth M. Warwick, "Factor Analysis and Equamax Rotations," January 1972.

[133]Harry H. Harmon, Modern Factor Analysis, (Chicago: The University of Chicago Press, 1967), pp. 22-25.

[134]Ibid., pp. 6-11.

TABLE IV - 5

FACTOR 1

THE EFFECT OF THE LAY REFERRAL SYSTEM ON MEMBERSHIP

Components	Loadings	
	Warwick Program	Scott Program
37. Importance of Peer Recommendation	0.7448	0.5400
26. Membership Eligibility Criteria	0.7343	0.6500
38. Importance of Co-Worker Recommendation	0.7275	0.7000
29. Dual Choice Option	0.7192	0.6500
40. Importance of Conversion Mechanism	0.5414	0.4300
27. Size of Membership	0.5414	0.4300

TABLE IV - 6

FACTOR 2

CONSUMER PARTICIPATION IN THE PLAN

Components	Loadings	
	Warwick Program	Scott Program
13. Determinants of Staff Salaries	0.7841	0.6000
41. Availability of Financial Statements	0.5213	0.4200
31. Membership Participation in Administration and Planning	0.4808	0.5200
33. Periodic Member Meetings	0.4597	0.5200

TABLE IV - 7

FACTOR 3

PLAN RECOMMENDATION THROUGH SUBSCRIBER EDUCATION

Components	Loadings	
	Warwick Program	Scott Program
35. Importance of Plan Reputation	0.6909	0.5100
34. Continuing Subscriber Education	0.5971	0.3000
36. Importance of Expert Recommendation	0.5830	0.4700

TABLE IV - 8

FACTOR 4

HEALTH CENTER APPEARANCE AND ATMOSPHERE

Components	Loadings	
	Warwick Program	Scott Program
21. Health Center Appearance	0.9161	0.7500
20. Health Center Atmosphere	0.8884	0.7200
19. Accessibility of Care	0.4228	0.3300

TABLE IV - 9

FACTOR 5

VOLUNTARY ENROLLMENT INTO A HIGH QUALITY PLAN

Components	Loadings	
	Warwick Program	Scott Program
23. Voluntary Enrollment	0.7606	0.3200
22. Technologically Current Equipment	0.6578	0.5700
12. Qualifications of Health Center Personnel	0.4142	0.4000
11. Qualifications of the Medical Staff	0.4010	0.4000

TABLE IV - 10

FACTOR 6

ENVIRONMENTAL EFFECTS ON FREE CHOICE OF PHYSICIAN

Components	Loadings	
	Warwick Program	Scott Program
42. Impending Federal Health Legislation	0.7085	0.3700
30. Free Choice of Physician	0.5976	0.3700
18. Accessibility of Health Center	0.5343	0.4100
39. Place of Work Promotion by Employers	0.4994	0.2800

TABLE IV - 11

FACTOR 7

COVERAGE OF A PREVENTIVE PLAN

Components	Loadings	
	Warwick Program	Scott Program
08. Comprehensive Coverage of Plan	0.8244	0.5500
09. Extra Benefits Perceived	0.7474	0.4500
11. Merits of Preventive Medicine	0.4672	0.3000
07. Cost per Member (single or group)	0.4328	0.2400

TABLE IV - 12

FACTOR 8

QUALITY OF MEDICAL CARE ITSELF

Components	Loadings	
	Warwick Program	Scott Program
07. Quality of Care Provided	0.7619	0.4900
14. Health Center Hours of Operation	0.6533	0.3200
11. Qualifications of Medical Staff	0.5257	0.3500
09. Personal Interest in Patient by Physician	0.5206	0.4300

TABLE IV - 13

FACTOR 9

SOCIO-ECONOMIC-ETHNIC MEMBERSHIP COMPOSITION

Components	Loadings	
	Warwick Program	Scott Program
28. Socio-Economic-Ethnic Composition	0.8050	0.5200
24. Health Center Facilities (Status)	0.8005	0.5300
25. Religious Denomination of Hospital Affiliate	0.4357	0.3600
04. Cost per Member	0.3190	0.1400

TABLE IV - 14

FACTOR 10

PERSONAL INTEREST SHOWN BY ALL STAFF MEMBERS

Components	Loadings	
	Warwick Program	Scott Program
10. Personal Interest Shown at Health Center	0.6896	0.4500
15. Appointment Lag	0.6807	0.3700
09. Personal Interest Shown by Physicians	0.3924	0.3100

215

interpretation can be made. The major clues to the nature of any factor are the loadings. By arranging them from high positive to high negative,[135] interpretation is made on what describes the order.[136] This is how the factor names were obtained. A summary of various data from an analyses done by the Warwick program is contained in Appendix V - C.

The service and communications submixes of the marketing mix are based on the aforementioned ten factors. Furthermore, through interrelation of the background questionnaire responses with the set of factors; service, advertising, promotion and public relations measures can be derived.

THE MARKETING MIX

Since the H.M.O. services are intangible, the task of determining the marketing mix ingredients for a total marketing program requires more sophistication than for product marketing firms.[137] Furthermore, the development of the marketing mix is an important prerequisite for tapping the target markets.[138] Generally, each target market segment requires a unique marketing mix.[139]

The marketing mix for an H.M.O. has two components:[140] the service submix and communications submix.

Service Submix

There are three methods in which the H.M.O. service can be sold to the consumer: (1) by convincing him to adjust his medical demands to the characteristics of the plan; (2) by adjusting the characteristics of the service to the subscribers' needs; (3) by some combination of the two.[141]

---

[135] Kenneth M. Warwick, op. cit.

[136] Ibid.

[137] William J. Stanton, op. cit., pp. 575-76.

[138] E. Jerome McCarthy, op. cit., p. 44.

[139] John M. Rathwell, "What is Meant by Services?," Journal of Marketing, (October 1966), p. 32.

[140] Generally, the marketing mix is decomposed into three constituent parts: the service, communications, and distribution submixes. No problems of physical distribution exist in the case of an H.M.O. and the channels of distribution are simple. Consequently, no detailed distribution submix is required.

[141] Ibid., pp. 48-52.

216

The strategy which uses knowledge of the nature of demand is called
market segmentation.[142] Here, the heterogeneous target group is divided into
homogeneous segments.[143] In this way, underlying demands of each segment
can be identified and the H.M.O. service designed accordingly.[144]

Service Planning

Management will determine the scope of the services to be offered,
the pricing, and the safeguards to be installed to assure quality[145] and
subscriber satisfaction.

Communications Submix

Communication consists of both personal and nonpersonal components.
More specifically, personal and nonpersonal selling. The former involves
sales messages and subscription drives undertaken by sales representatives;
the latter, advertising, sales promotion, and public relations.[146]

The task of a marketing communications system is to direct the
selling message from the source toward the potential subscriber and other
purchasing influentials. Environmental and social factors (noise)[147] can
distort or divert the message unless marketing research provides the necessary
information to improve the effectiveness of the communications.[148] A marketing communications system for an H.M.O. is shown schematically in Figure -
V - 3.

Personal Selling

Personal selling is defined as a face-to-face presentation to one
or more prospective customers or customer's agents for the purpose of making
sales.[149]

---

[142] Wendell Smith, "Product Differentiation and Market Segmentation as
Alternative Strategies," Journal of Marketing, (July 1956), p. 3.

[143] William J. Stanton, op. cit., p. 77.

[144] Wendell Smith, op. cit., pp. 4-5.

[145] Donald D. Parker, "Improved Efficiency and Reduced Cost in Marketing,"
Journal of Marketing, (April 1962), pp. 18-19.

[146] Mark E. Stern, op. cit., pp. 59-63.

[147] Noise refers to those factors which reduce the effectiveness of the
communications process by interfering with the transmission or reception
of the message.

[148] See: (1) E. Jerome McCarthy, op. cit., pp. 517-520.

[149] "Report of the Definitions Committe," Journal of Marketing, XIII
(October 1948), p. 212.

FIGURE IV - 3[a]

A MARKETING COMMUNICATIONS SYSTEM FOR H.M.O.

Message Channel

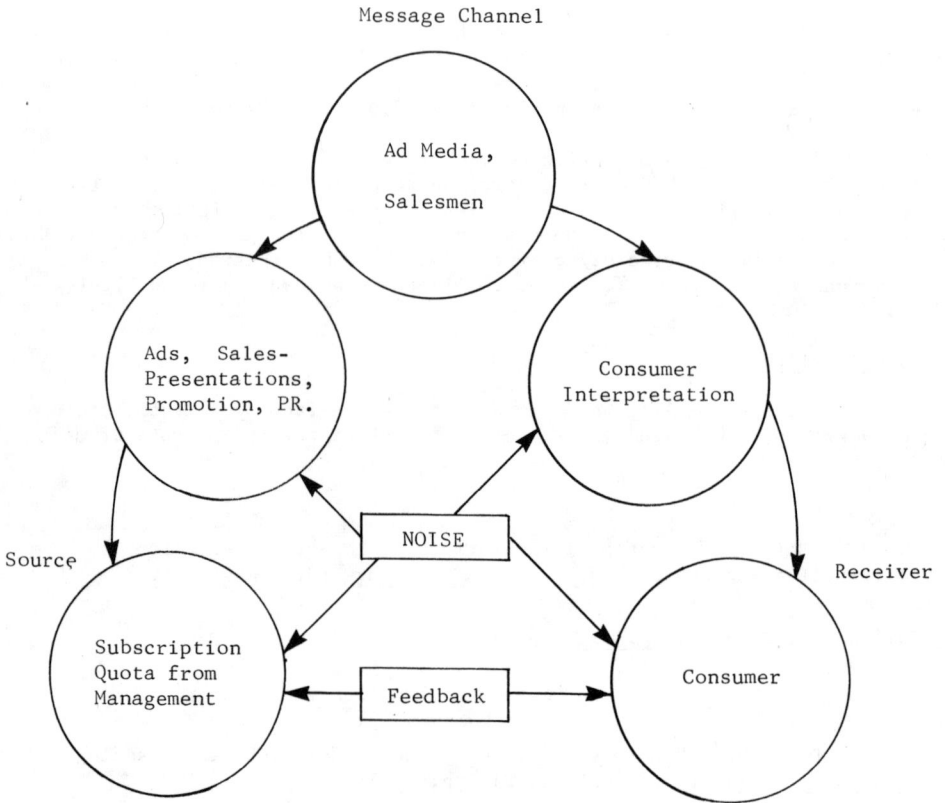

[a]Adapted from William J. Stanton, op. cit., p. 498.

The close association between the production and consumption of the H.M.O. service results in a personal relationship between subscriber and provider.[150] A salesman, therefore, is a very important aspect of the marketing mix. He is trained to adapt the marketing effort to the special circumstances of each target market segment and, in the extreme, to each potential subscriber. Furthermore, face-to-face selling provides immediate feedback which guides the salesman to adapt to unexpected conditions in the market.[151]

The success of a service enterprise is related directly to the quality of the personal selling effort.[152] This fact is substantiated by empirical studies which indicated that personal influence was more important in marketing of services than any of the mass media programs.[153]

Therefore, to upgrade the personal selling effort, H.M.O. sales management must emphasize three factors: (a) development of a consumer-centered attitude; (b) training in basic personal selling skills; (c) and inculcating consumer confidence in the likelihood of receiving fair treatment and quality service.[154]

Nonpersonal Selling

Advertising is any paid form of nonpersonal presentation and promotion of ideas, goods, or services by an identified sponsor.[155] Sales promotion includes those sales activities that supplement both personal selling and advertising, coordinating them and helping to make them more effective.[156]

The promotional program of an H.M.O. has two major objectives. (1) to portray the service benefits in as appealing a manner as possible; (2) to build a good reputation and image.[157] A major part of image building can be promoted at the health care center. Health education, exhibits, counselling services, and various clinics[158] all should be visible to the H.M.O. subscriber at the health center.

---

[150]Donald D. Parker, The Marketing of Consumer Services, Dissertation, (Seattle: University of Washington, 1958), pp. 258-59.

[151]E. Jerome McCarthy, op. cit., p. 516.

[152]Donald D. Parker (dissertation), op. cit., p. 259.

[153]Elihu Katz and Paul Lazarsfeld, Personal Influence, (Glencoe, Ill.: The Free Press, 1955), Chapter V.

[154]Donald F. Mulvihill, Improving Personal Selling in Small Business, (Washington: Small Business Administration, 1956).

[155]"Report of Definitions Committee," p. 205.

[156]Ibid., p. 214.

[157]William J. Stanton, op. cit., pp. 580-81.

[158]Some of the counselling services and clinics include: drug-abuse; nutrition; family-planning; prenatal care; and adolescent guidance.

Effective publicity and public relations also contribute to promotion and, at relatively low cost.[159] The virtues of the H.M.O. service will be extolled as far as its "newsworthiness" will permit. Such publicity will take the form of service announcements and customer testimonials. Indirect publicity can also be used by the H.M.O. to highlight the basic need for preventive, comprehensive health care -- an important factor in the H.M.O. service mix.[160]

Another form of H.M.O. public relations could involve a key person within the firm or union who is well known by the employees -- especially new ones. Such an unofficial ambassador can help sell H.M.O. benefits in an informal and "nonpressured" manner.[161]

SERVICE SUBMIX PROGRAM

Doctor's Care[162]

A typical plan can provide physician care and related services in the Regional Medical Group facility and in the Health Care Center or affiliated hospitals, with home calls when necessary. Such services as diagnoses, treatments, checkups, surgery, cost-price prescriptions, short-term physical therapy, limited, short-term mental health care,[163] maternity care,[164] eye care, diagnostic and laboratory tests, X-ray tests and treatments, visiting nurses, emergency ambulances, outpatient treatment, and specialist consultation can be all included in the H.M.O. service mix. Other long-term services and dental care can be included at extra cost.

Hospital Benefits[165]

A H.M.O. can provide for hospital care for all inpatient services necessary for the diagnosis and treatment of illness or injury. This covers: hospital room and board, including general nursing care and meals; use of operating rooms, special treatment rooms, and intensive care units; anesthetics and oxygen; diagnostic, laboratory, and X-ray tests; casts and medications; administration of blood and intravenous solutions; private duty nursing when necessary; short-term physical therapy; and inpatient drugs and

---

[159] E. Jerome McCarthy, op. cit., p. 516.

[160] Cutlip and Center, op. cit., pp. 330-31.

[161] RIGHA Interview, December 6, 1972.

[162] Adapted from the service schedules of Group Health Association, Inc. (GHA) and Rhode Island Group Health Association (RIGHA).

[163] See: Subsection on "Mental Illness Benefits."

[164] See: Subsection on "Maternity Benefits."

[165] Adapted from GHA and RIGHA service schedules.

medicines. (The H.M.O. physicians in the Regional Medical Groups make the necessary hospital arrangements.)

In cases of drug addiction, alcoholism, long-term mental illness, or any chronic condition requiring care in other than a general hospital, eligibility for institutionalization at the expense of the H.M.O. usually will cease when final diagnosis has been completed and the medical staff has recommended specialized institutional care unless special contractual agreements have been made.

Maternity Benefits[166]

Comprehensive care for each pregnancy can be provided by the H.M.O. Services falling under the blanket coverage include: complete obstetrical care, including prenatal care, delivery, and post-natal care; "Cesarian Section" and care of other complications; care of newborn child during mother's confinement; hospitalization including anesthetics and all necessary hospital services; and laboratory and X-ray tests at the Health Care Center.

Mental Illness Benefits[167]

Upon referral by a H.M.O. physician, treatment of acute mental illness and emotional disorders which in the opinion of the medical staff, are subject to significant improvement through short-term therapy can be provided. The scope of H.M.O. mental health care encompasses; professional services in office, hospital care during the acute phase; and any psychological testing available at the Health Care Center.

Other Health Services[168]

The typical medical care coverage is augmented by special elements taking the form of exhibits, lectures, clinics, and counselling services. Exhibits depicting new medical technology and methods; educational lectures by the medical staff and guest experts; nutrition, family-planning, first aid, and baby care clinics; and counselling for guidance, drug-abusement and alcoholism can all be made available to the subscriber at the Health Center.

Staff Education

The subscriber has some needs that are not explicitly included in the H.M.O. service package. Marketing research reveals that all groups desire various forms of intangible service. One area which is of extreme importance is that of "personal interest of all staff members."[169]

---

[166]Ibid.

[167]Ibid.

[168]S. R. Garfield, "The Delivery of Medical Care," Scientific American, CCXXII (April 1970), pp. 15-23.

[169]See: Table IV - 14

The H.M.O. should have a policy of staff education to insure effective, personalized attention from all staff members. The interview is one medium for the improvement of the subscriber-staff relations and therefore medical, nursing, and staff education should include specific training in interviewing skills and, understanding of psychological reactions to illness.[170]

Both verbal and nonverbal communication are parts of health professional and patient interaction. The words and gestures used by physician, nurse, or health center employee are thus potent forces for therapeutic success or failure.[171]

Training in effective interviewing involves skill in attentive listening as a means of creating a climate in which the patient can communicate freely. The staff must demonstrate real interest in the member and his problem to establish rapport. But emotional detachment is also needed for self-control to permit effective treatment.[172]

In these ways, the H.M.O. staff, from physician to receptionist, can be trained to take enough personal interest in the subscriber so that he will feel no threat and will feel welcome and secure. Furthermore, these training techniques also contribute to higher quality care and thus, can bring the H.M.O. more recognition and public esteem.[173]

Quality of Care

The subscriber is interested in a health plan that provides as much in the way of benefits as is consistent with high quality service and reasonable cost.[174] Marketing research supports this claim since all market segments interviewed perceived high quality care as an essential plan characteristic.[175]

But, comprehensive coverage and staff education are only a part of the picture. The H.M.O. must also provide high quality care conveniently. The Regional Medical Group's hours of operation should be adequate, house calls should be available if needed, and 24-hour emergency service should be provided. In routine cases, appointments should be made at least a week in advance, but short-term notice consultations can be arranged -- though not necessarily with the member's regular physician. Furthermore, the center

---

[170]Lewis Bernstein and Richard H. Dana, Interviewing and the Health Professions, (New York: Appleton-Century-Crofts, 1970), pp. 22-23.

[171]Ibid., pp. 25-26.

[172]Ibid., pp. 30-38.

[173]R. H. Blum, The Management of the Doctor-Patient Relationship, (New York: McGraw-Hill Book Company, 1960), pp. 58-61.

[174]Oscar Serbein, Jr., op. cit., p. 339.

[175]See: Table IV - 12.

should be accessible by private or public transportation and parking facilities should be readily available.

Staff members working closely together in a group become thoroughly familiar with the ways their colleagues care for members.[176] "The life of a successful H.M.O. will, as a matter of course, foster this multifaceted exchange through regularly scheduled conferences. Such meetings are one of the important keys to the promotion and maintenance of quality care in H.M.O.'s."[177]

Subscriber Education

H.M.O. management will discover that the success of the plan will ultimately depend on the satisfaction and loyalty of the subscribers. Thus, to achieve and maintain member loyalty, the H.M.O. must continuously inform potential and actual subscribers about the character of the program, its intent, its mechanics, its advantages and its disadvantages.[178]

Our marketing research shows that only self-employed and nonunion affiliated consumers of above average incomes thought enough of subscriber education to consider it an important plan choice criterion.[179] This finding points out a problem in union and government employee education. Moreover, in many situations, potential subscribers have revealed that although they were aware of the H.M.O. option of dual choice, they had no clear understanding of what benefits the pre-payment plan offered, or how these benefits compared with those of other plans.[180]

In group enrollment situations, such as union and government employees, educational meetings should be scheduled with personnel and their representatives. Material should be introduced in an orderly fashion, at a pace designed to promote comprehension of the objectives and methods of the plan.[181] Similarly, for individual enrollments, workshops and neighborhood meetings can be sponsored to provide educational materials dealing with the philosophy, history, objectives, and services of the program.[182]

At the subscription meetings, verbal and visual explanation of the principles and processes of the health plan should be augmented by printed matter for study at home. H.M.O. programs described in these meetings are

---

[176]Avram Yedida, op. cit., pp. 69-70.

[177]Ibid., p. 70.

[178]Yedida, loc. cit.

[179]See: Table IV - 7.

[180]Ann S. Bush, Group Practice: Planning and Implementing a Community-wide Prepayment Plan, (New York State Health Planning Commission, May 1971), pp. 88-89.

[181]Avram Yedida, op. cit., pp. 76-77.

[182]Ann S. Bush, op. cit., p. 92.

usually new to the consumers, and the thoughtfully designed pamphlets service to remind them of pertinent points, to clarify details, to explain relationships, to lay a foundation for further thought, and provide a reference for the future use of the services.[183]

Some subjects, which experience shows caused difficulties in other plans, merit special emphasis in the educational program. Misconceptions concerning preventive medicine, subscriber expectation, free choice of physician, dual choice, voluntary enrollment, conversion, and the Health Center all should be clarified in the H.M.O.'s educational activities and literature.[184]

Subscribers should be encouraged to receive periodic physical checkups as preventive treatment. At the same time, enrollees can be made aware of the range of benefits of the plan along with the capabilities of the Medical Groups and the Health Center. In this way, no expectation gap will occur and possible dissatisfaction can be eliminated.[185]

Subscribers must also understand that they are allowed their choice of primary physicians within the plan and change of doctor can be accomplished if desired. The objective of such a policy is to place the primary physician in the Regional Medical Group in much the same relationship to the subscriber as he would be in private practice.[186] The factorial study revealed that this element is of particular interest to females and employees with lower incomes.[187]

Furthermore, potential enrollees and employee group representatives are informed that each person joining the program does so voluntarily.[188] There is freedom of choice in the initial selection process and periodic opportunities to change program, if so desired.[189] Also, if a group subscriber wishes to leave the group, he may be able to convert his membership in the H.M.O. to individual coverage as may be in effect at the time of his application for conversion.[190]

---

[183] Avram Yedida, op. cit., pp. 79-80.

[184] See: pp. 231-237.

[185] See: Saward, op. cit., p. 3; and Deutsch, "Group Medicine - Part 2," p. 85.

[186] Ann S. Bush, op. cit., p. 91.

[187] See: Table IV - 10 and Avram Yedida, op. cit.,p. 80.

[188] See: Table IV - 9.

[189] Ann S. Bush, op. cit., pp. 88-90.

[190] RIGHA Interview, December 6, 1971.

Another area of concern, especially for the majority of female subscribers, is that of the health center -- its appearance and atmosphere.[191] The H.M.O. should have a pleasantly styled building with adequate facilities for parking and accessibility by public transportation. Interior decor should be attractive and the facilities furnished with up-to-date equipment. Moreover, staff education should be geared to developing warm and cordial reception and, at the same time, de-emphasizing the clinical atmosphere.[192]

The active support and cooperation of management leaders and union officials of subscribing groups is essential to the education process.[193] In many cases, these executives can cooperate the educational process and feed materials into their organizations which can eventually influence subscription decisions.[194]

Consumer Participation

Some H.M.O. programs include a level of involvement by the consumer and his community.[195] The factorial study reveals that those consumers with above average incomes and nonunion affiliation desire such active participation in administrative, economic, and planning affairs.[196] Collectively, they can participate in policy-making by attending meetings, making suggestion, actually voting on proposals, and, perhaps even having a voice in the election of one or more H.M.O. directors.[197] Moreover, each group selects a Health Committee from its membership to participate in such matters as handling of complaints, enrollment and eligibility policy-making, and premium-costing.[198] Such participation subsequently leads to better designed benefit mixes.[199]

[191] See: Table IV - 8.

[192] Group Health Association of America (GHAA) Washington D.C., interview with Herman Schmidt, Field Director, February 1972.

[193] Ann S. Bush, op. cit., p. 97.

[194] GHAA Interview, February 1972.

[195] Ann S. Bush, op. cit., pp. 92-93.

[196] See: Table IV - 6.

[197] Schwartz (dissertation), op. cit., p. 206.

[198] Albert Deutsch, "Group Medicine - Part 2," p. 83.

[199] Anne K. Somers, Editor, The Kaiser - Permanente Medical Care Program: A Symposium, (New York: The Commonwealth Fund, 1971), pp. 42-43.

The communications mix decision involves the evaluation of alternative media and message content and alternative audiences.[200] (The mix is
intended to direct the selling message from the H.M.O. to the health care
consumer or purchasing influential as is shown in Figure V - 4.[201])

Personal Selling Skills

For successful operation of an H.M.O., high quality personal selling
is needed.[202] The H.M.O. salesman must have the technical knowledge of
everything about the service, its application, its benefits, and its limitations. He must have knowledge of the potential subscriber's business -- the
organizational, technological, financial and policy facets. He should, in
fact, be trained to be an expert in the enrollee's firm and be able to relate
the H.M.O. advantages to the company's situation so that they are recognized
as being beneficial. He should have knowledge of the consumer as an individual -- of each person who directly or indirectly influences decisions, of
how that person perceives, thinks, and acts.[203]

Personal selling proficiency can be improved if the H.M.O. salesman
is trained to develop a consumer-centered attitude. The person who meets and
talks with potential members is taught to display an empathic attitude and a
sincere desire to understand the needs of the target group.

Personal selling -- the nonunion affiliated organization and
government employees. These firms and agencies are approached at
the top management level to arrange for a group presentation.[204] At this
time, the well-equipped salesman shows how the H.M.O. service would be
beneficial to the organization as a whole and to employees at all levels (in
uses and terms that are understood by management personnel).[205] The salesman
then stresses those plan factors which research has shown to be most attractive to company executives, such as: quality of care, plan cost of the
comprehensive coverage, personal interest, member participation, subscriber
education, and free choice of physician.[206]

---

[200]S. Watson Dunn, Advertising: Its Role in Modern Marketing, (New York:
Holt, Rinehart and Winston, Inc., 1961), pp. 42-43.

[201]E. Jerome McCarthy, op. cit., pp. 517-20.

[202]Parker (dissertation), op. cit., p. 259.

[203]George D. Downing, Sales Management, (New York: John Wiley and Sons, Inc.
1969), pp. 54-55.

[204]William C. Lawton, op. cit., pp. 153-54.

[205]Harvard Community Health Plan, Boston, Mass., interview with Roger Birnbaum,
Assistant Director, March 1972.

[206]These factors correspond to factor numbers 8, 7, 10, 2, 3 and 6, respectively

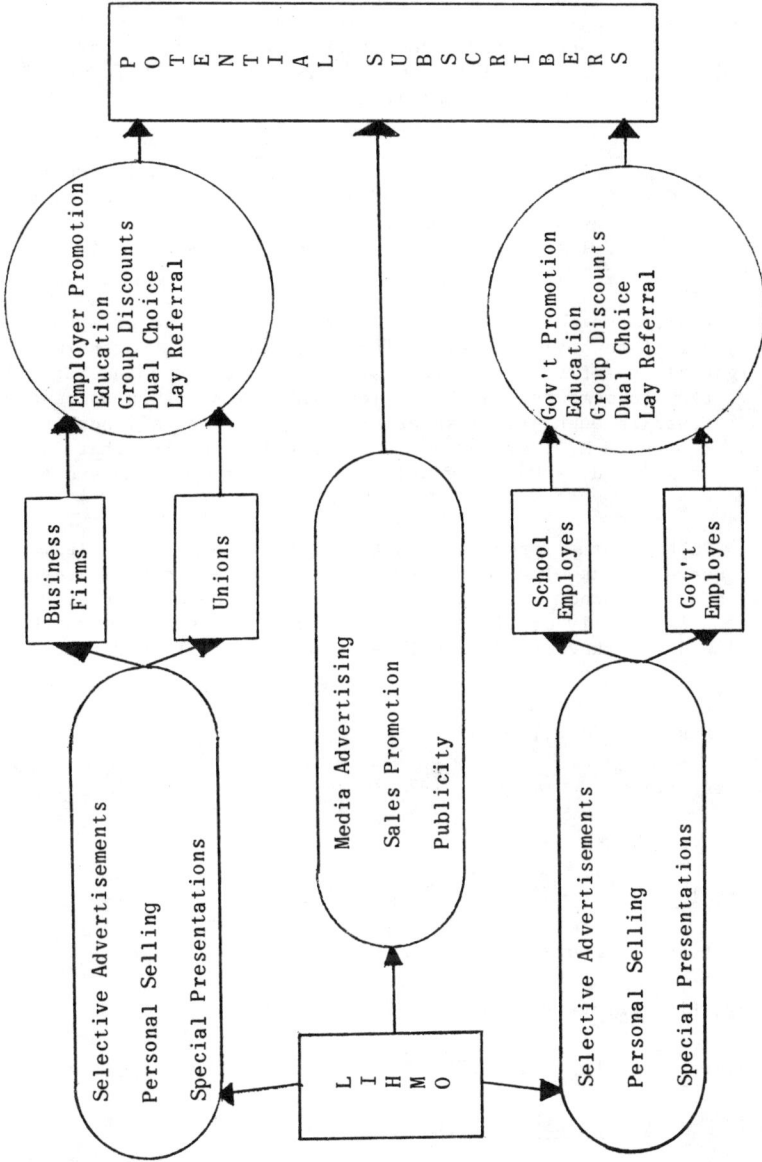

FIGURE IV - 4[a]

LIHMO MARKETING CHANNELS AND COMMUNICATORS

POTENTIAL SUBSCRIBERS

Business Firms

Unions

Employer Promotion
Education
Group Discounts
Dual Choice
Lay Referral

School Employes

Gov't Employes

Gov't Promotion
Education
Group Discounts
Dual Choice
Lay Referral

Selective Advertisements
Personal Selling
Special Presentations

Media Advertising
Sales Promotion
Publicity

Selective Advertisements
Personal Selling
Special Presentations

LIHMO

[a]Adapted from Philip Kotler and Gerald Zaltman, "Social Marketing: An Approach to Change," Journal of Marketing, XXXV (July 1971).

In general, management and government are both interested in finding solutions to the problems of health care delivery,[207] and thus they are involved by the salesman in responsible efforts to improve the health situation of their people.

When involved in the group presentation the salesman should make a verbal and visual explanation of the principles and processes involved in the H.M.O. plan and present printed matter accentuating factors most important to the audience, as he distributes membership application forms.[208] A typical printed sales-aid is shown in Exhibit IV - 1.

Personal Selling and Union-affiliated Organizations. Slightly different tactics are required for firms having strong union representation; the union leadership is first contacted.[209] The salesman then describes the benefits of including H.M.O. as one alternative in a dual choice arrangement -- being careful to first clarify his role so as to avoid possible hostility or suspicion.[210]

Labor management are a particularly responsive group because unions typically negotiate health benefits for their members. Furthermore, the union organization structure is well suited to the dissemination of educational information to members.[211] Union leadership support is necessary and it can be attained through artful sales presentation.[212] All possible union benefits from the H.M.O. are expounded -- keeping in mind that labor executives are usually quite knowledgeable of many forms of comprehensive health care.[213]

In the formal presentation to union members, the salesman must know his audience.[214] The blue collar worker is basically conservative and passive in his approach to plan selection.[215] Moreover, research indicates that action is usually confined to the needs of the moment with the future being allowed to take care of itself.[216] Simple verbal and visual

---

[207]Ann S. Bush, op. cit., p. 97.

[208]RIGHA interview, December 6, 1971.

[209]Lawton, loc.cit.

[210]Dexter, loc. cit.

[211]GHAA interview, February 1972.

[212]Harvard Plan Interview, March 1972.

[213]GHAA interview, February 1972.

[214]Donald F. Roy, op. cit., p. 262.

[215]Eliot Freidson, op. cit., p. 149.

[216]George Rosen, "Provision of Medical Care," p. 206.

EXHIBIT IV - 1[a]

AN H.M.O. SALESMAN'S PRINTED SALES-AID

Wouldn't you like to have your health supervised by a doctor who is backed by a team of other medical specialists?

If you are enrolled in the Harvard Community Health Plan — the new and unique pre-paid comprehensive health plan conceived by the Harvard Medical School — you choose your own doctor from the doctors participating in the Plan. The medical group provides total care 24 hours a day, seven days a week.

Your doctor and the team of specialists are from Beth Israel Hospital, Boston Hospital for Women, Children's Hospital, and Peter Bent Brigham Hospital.

If you are enrolled in this Plan, you see your doctor in a modern "one-stop" family health center — the Harvard Community Health Center — at Kenmore Square, Boston. Without leaving the building, you can have a physical checkup, X-rays, eye examination, and laboratory tests. And equally important, the Center contains and maintains your family's medical records. The Center also operates a 24-hour emergency call service. A doctor is always available.

Your doctor and the medical staff guide your family's complete health care ... days ... nights ... even on weekends. Your records are always up-to-date and available. Adults choose a specialist in internal medicine and children choose a pediatrician as "their" doctor from among the doctors in the Plan. Then he is backed up by the specialists ... in surgery, obstetrics, eye, ear, nose and throat, skin conditions, X-ray and mental health.

Enrollees in this Plan benefit from the association with the Harvard Medical School and the participating hospitals ... and you don't have to be sick to benefit. The Harvard Community Health Plan tries to keep you well. Preventive medicine is emphasized. For example — an annual physical is not only covered, it is encouraged.

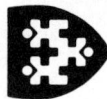

SUMMARY OF BENEFITS

In the Health Center

Doctor office visits, check-ups, eye examinations	You pay $1 per visit
Lab and X-ray services, nursing services, counseling services, prescribed physical therapy, immunizations and injections, casts and dressings	No charge

In a Participating Hospital

Physicians' and surgeons' services, including operations and specialists' consultation	No charge
Room and board in semi-private accommodations — general nursing — use of operating room — anaesthesia	No charge
Laboratory and X-ray services	No charge
Radiotherapy	No charge
Drugs and medications	No charge
Prescribed special duty nursing	No charge
Blood transfusions, if blood is replaced	No charge

In the Home

Doctors' home calls, when indicated in the judgment of physician (within designated home call service area)	You pay $5 per visit
Organized home health care services, when arranged by Plan-affiliated physician, not including meals, housekeeping and personal comfort items.	No charge

"YOU DON'T HAVE TO BE SICK TO BENEFIT"

Harvard
Community
Health Plan

690 Beacon Street
Boston, Massachusetts 02215
For further information,
call: 261-3100 and ask for
a Health Plan Representative

[a]Courtesy of Harvard Community Health Plan; reproduced by permission.

descriptions are supplemented with printed leaflets accentuating the generally accepted plan characteristics which motivate blue collar action. Such principles as personal interest, quality of care, socio-economic-ethnic member composition, lay referral, voluntary enrollment, and free choice of physician are emphasized in the pamphlets along with enrollment application forms. This recommendation is based upon the factorial study which showed that factors 1, 5, 6, 8, 9, and 10, were important to this market segment.

      Personal selling and other groups. Direct personal selling is not economically feasible for the individual and family enrollment situations. However, H.M.O. representatives reflect the stature of the organization by their very actions. Opinions are formed on the basis of impressions left by H.M.O. personnel in their dealings with the public. Therefore, H.M.O. employees perform indirect personal selling by exhibiting tact, diplomacy, and social poise in day-to-day relations with the population.[217]

      Personal selling, both direct and indirect, consists in individual, face-to-face communication -- in contrast to the impersonal nature of advertising, sales promotion, and public relations. Consequently, personal selling has the advantage of being more flexible in operation. Objections and questions can be uncovered and answered immediately. However, the personal seller cannot reach a wide range of prospects, as well as can nonpersonal promotional devices.[218]

Nonpersonal Selling

      Even a well qualified salesman stands little chance of enrolling subscribers, if the prospect knows little or nothing about the H.M.O. and its service. Therefore, personal selling is supported and its productivity enhanced by nonpersonal selling activities which include advertising, sales promotion, and public relations.[219]

      Advertising. Numerous factors influence the content of the advertising program. Environmental factors[220] are uncontrollable, while short-run goals in tune with long range objectives, are controllable. Examples of environmental factors affecting H.M.O. programming are: market size and characteristics, available media, nature of the communication channels, social habits and customs, and legal constraints. These factors are reassessed from time to time because changes can influence the content of the program.[221]

---

[217]See: William J. Stanton and Richard H. Buskirk, Management of the Sales Force, (Homewood, Illinois: Richard D. Irwin, Inc., 1969), p. 16. and Thomas R. Wotruba, Sales Management, (New York: Holt, Rinehart and Winston, Inc., 1971), pp. 4-6.

[218]William J. Stanton, op. cit., pp. 519-23.

[219]Mark E. Stern, op. cit., pp. 74-75.

[220]See: pp. 232-233 and 236-237.

[221]Albert W. Frey and Jean C. Halterman, Advertising, (New York: The Ronald Press Company, 1970), pp. 72-76.

The most important controllable advertising factor is the determination of objectives.[222] Producing direct and immediate action is the
primary objective of H.M.O. advertising. The initial message advanced is
aimed at the acceptance of the prepaid comprehensive health care concept.
Then, awareness is created in the consumers reached by the advertising, of
the features, benefits, and characteristics of the H.M.O. itself. The
message should be designed to create an image of high quality and efficiency.
This is aimed at gradual build-up in the acceptance of the H.M.O. concept
and in subscriptions to H.M.O.

An additional advertising objective is that of market segmentation.[223] Specialized message are directed to the various market targets.
That is: advertisements stressing quality of care, comprehensive-preventive
coverage, personal interest, member participation and subscriber education,
are generally directed toward executive groups; those emphasizing socio-
economic-ethnic considerations, voluntary enrollment into a high quality
plan, and the effect of the lay referral system attract general employees;
while free choice of physician, member participation, and Health Center
atmosphere interest many female consumers; and so on.

Advertising and the agency. These objectives are encompassed in
advertising copy themes which must be written effectively and forcefully.[224]
This is a highly professional task better left to an independent advertising
agency. An example of an agency advertisement for an H.M.O. is found in
Exhibit V - 2.

The advertising agency provides the specialized knowledge, skills,
and experience needed to produce effective advertising campaigns. It contributes a quality and range of service greater than any single H.M.O. could
afford or would need to employ for himself.[225]

The agency chosen may have to be educated in the background of
H.M.O.'s -- their services, policies and benefits.[226] Then, those tasks the
agency is best equipped to handle are assigned, and those which the H.M.O.
itself can carry out most effectively, are not delegated.[227] The agency is
made responsible for the preparation of copy, art, and related work while the
H.M.O. management proposes the strategies. Both parties work together in the
area of media selection but the agency contracts for the space in the media.[228]

---

[222]Richard D. Crisp, How to Increase Advertising Effectiveness, (New York:
   McGraw-Hill Book Company, Inc., 1963), pp. 14-23.

[223]C. H. Sandage and Vernon Fryburger, Advertising Theory and Practice,
   (Homewood, Illinois: Richard D. Irwin, Inc., 1967), pp. 223-25.

[224]Victor P. Buell, op. cit., p. 13-19.

[225]C. H. Sandage and Vernon Fryburger, op. cit., pp. 625-27.

[226]Richard D. Crisp, op. cit., pp. 60-61.

[227]Albert W. Frey and Jean C. Halterman, op. cit., pp. 119-20.

[228]Albert W. Frey and Kenneth R. Davis, The Advertising Industry, (New York:
   Association of National Advertisers, 1958), pp. 374-76.

EXHIBIT V-2ᵃ
An H.M.O. Advertisement Designed by an Agency

THE BENEFICIARY'S ABC

INSURED SERVICES

The Québec plan is universal - it covers all residents of Québec, without exception. It insures:

A all medically required services dispensed by a physician for diagnostic, therapeutic or rehabilitative purposes, such as:

- doctor visits (patient's home, doctor's office or hospital)
- anaesthetic services
- surgical services
- obstetrical services - including pre-natal and post-natal visits
- psychiatric services

B oral surgery services performed by dental surgeons in hospital

C services rendered by optometrists, including eye examinations.

PAYMENT OF FEES

For payment of fees the Health Insurance Act defines three categories of health professionals:

A THE *OPTED-IN* HEALTH PROFESSIONAL

As a beneficiary you have *nothing to pay* when you consult an *opted-in* health professional; his fees will be paid in full by the Québec Health Insurance Board and will be remitted directly to him.

B THE *OPTED-OUT* HEALTH PROFESSIONAL

As a beneficiary you will be reimbursed by the Board for the cost of insured services dispensed by an *opted-out* health professional on presentation of the prescribed claim form. These forms will be supplied by the Board to all opted-out health professionals. Therefore, you will be required to pay the health professional directly. However, the latter may not charge more for his services than the amount the Board will reimburse.

C THE *NON-PARTICIPATING* HEALTH PROFESSIONAL

You must pay the full amount charged for insured services dispensed by a *non-participating* health professional and the cost of these services *will not* be reimbursed by the Board. The non-participating health professional is obliged to notify his patient in advance that he does not participate in the health insurance plan.

Every resident of Québec is entitled to reimbursement of the cost of insured services he receives outside Québec. In such case he forwards invoices for fees paid, or unpaid claims, to the Board. The Board then supplies him with a special claim form to be completed and returned justifying the payment claimed.

When this claim form is duly completed and returned to the Board, reimbursement is made to the resident if he has paid the fees. Should he not have paid the fees claimed, the Board will issue payment by cheque to the joint order of beneficiary and health professional. This cheque will always be sent to the beneficiary who must endorse it before forwarding it to the health professional.

In either case, the amount of the reimbursement or of the payment may not be in excess of the amount provided by the Québec Health Insurance Plan for these insured services.

THE HEALTH INSURANCE CARD

The Board issues a health insurance card to every person - man, woman and child - who resides in Québec and who is registered with the Board. This card enables the health professional to identify the patient and to prepare claims for submission to the Board.

A *You are registered* with the Board and *you have not yet received your health insurance card.* There is no need to be worried! - you will receive it in the near future. In the meantime, you are eligible for services insured under the plan and dispensed by both opted-in and opted-out health professionals. Should you require such services, you simply supply the health professional with your name, address and your date of birth.

B *You are not registered* with the Board. You are, nevertheless, eligible for insured services dispensed by an opted-in or an opted-out health professional. Register as soon as possible since registration is an obligation for all Québec residents.

C To register, either yourself or one of your dependents, complete an application coupon or write to the following address stating your name, address, date of birth and sex:

REGISTRATION CENTER
QUÉBEC HEALTH INSURANCE BOARD
P.O. Box 6600
Québec 2 (Québec)

For information by telephone, dial:

Metropolitan Québec 529-6531
Metropolitan Montréal 878-9261

For information by mail, write to:

«RENSEIGNEMENTS»
QUÉBEC HEALTH INSURANCE BOARD
P.O. Box 6600
Québec 2 (Québec)

ᵃCourtesy of the Quebec Health Insurance Board: reproduced by permission.

The agency-H.M.O. arrangement is such that the parties must work closely together. The relationships and responsibilities must be clearly understood and carefully spelled out in an atmosphere of mutual trust.[229]

Media Selection

The advertising medium is the carrier of the advertising message.[230] The H.M.O. and its agency will probably develop a plan that makes use of several kinds of media for economically delivering the advertising message to the appropriate market targets.

The first step of planning is to outline the primary media objectives.[231] For an H.M.O., these are: (1) to reach employees fertile for group enrollments; (2) to concentrate the greatest weight of advertising at the work place where employees can be contacted in their informal groups; (3) to provide advertising continuity and fairly consistent level of impressions throughout the year, except for extra weight during open enrollment periods;[232] (4) to deliver advertising impressions to employees in direct relation to enrollment potentials; (5) to use media which will help strengthen the copy strategy which puts emphasis on combinations of the researched plan choice factors; (6) to attain the greatest possible frequency of advertising impressions consistent with the needs of such coverage at the work place.

The secondary media objectives include:

(1) to reach individual consumers with special emphasis on self-employed and retired groups;

(2) to concentrate the greatest weight of advertising in new areas where populations are in a state of mobility and have not as yet established a personal physician relationship;[233]

(3) to provide advertising at a fairly consistent level throughout the year except for extra weight during the plan's inception period;

(4) to use media which will help strengthen the copy strategy which puts emphasis on combinations of the plan choice factors derived from marketing research;

(5) to attain the greatest possible frequency of advertising impression consistent with the need for broad coverage of the target population.

---

[229]Albert W. Frey and Jean C. Halterman, op. cit., p. 122.

[230]C. H. Sandage and Vernon Fryburger, op. cit., p. 431.

[231]S. Watson Dunn, op. cit., p. 432.

[232]The time in which employees can make a new selection of health plans in their dual choice arrangement.

[233]Harvard Plan interview, March 1972.

Once the H.M.O. and the agency finalize the media objectives; the types, classes, vehicles, and combinations of media are selected.[234] For the Long Island case; company, industry and local newspaper media are very often used. Only during open enrollment periods or in the case of the advent of new services are large circulation newspapers and local radio stations to be utilized. Union, company and industry newspapers can be used extensively. Employees identify with the working community through these media. Moreover, these newspapers are usually conveniently distributed at little or no cost at the work place. Also, such media generally have relatively low rates per target audience member reached.[235]

Local newspapers, with reasonable rates, present a considerable variety of material to provide interesting fare for a wide range of readers. They provide intensive coverage of the community and surrounding areas in which they circulate. Furthermore, they allow H.M.O. to tie in with local events or to cooperate with local community centers -- which are of special interest to newly arrived consumers. Also, local newspapers will often provide free space and are more receptive to printing publicity handouts.[236]

Large circulation newspapers and local radio stations, though much more expensive,[237] perform necessary functions. They reach the group employee away from his working environment and generally reinforce the efforts of the other chosen media but the cost per impression is very high.

Sales Promotion

Sales promotion is intended to intensify and accelerate the acceptance of the H.M.O. services by ultimate subscribers.[238] It serves as a bridge between advertising and personal selling -- to supplement and coordinate efforts in these two areas. Under direct H.M.O. control, sales promotion stimulates the potential subscriber to act and reinforces the demand created by the other elements of the communications submix.[239]

Wedding and Lassler[240] classify sales promotional services into three groups: direct forcing promotions; indirect forcing promotions; and point-of-purchase promotions.

Direct forcing promotions. Promotions that provide the consumer with an additional obvious value fall into this category.[241] Here, the H.M.O. uses such offers as group enrollment rates, early subscription

---

[234]S. Watson Dunn, op. cit., p. 434.

[235]Adapted from C.H. Sandage and Vernon Fryburger, op. cit., pp. 460-61.

[236]Adapted from Albert W. Frey and Jean C. Halterman, op. cit., pp. 303-06.

[237]Ibid.

[238]Ibid., pp. 40-41.

[239]William J. Stanton, op. cit., pp. 514-17.

[240]Nugent Wedding and Richard S. Lassler, Advertising Management, (New York: The Ronald Press Co., 1962), pp. 10-14.

[241]Ibid., p. 10.

deductions, gifts, premiums, special price deals, and, to a great extent, inherent plan benefits. In Exhibit IV - 3, the inherent benefits of an H.M.O. are compared with the Blue Cross-Blue Shield plan. Such a promotion can be invaluable in the effort to gain additional subscriptions.

Indirect forcing promotions. These aids produce results by providing special incentives to intermediaries rather than to potential subscribers.[242]

Point-of-purchase promotions. For an H.M.O., this subdivision should be called point-of-education promotions. At the work place, sales presentations are reinforced by promotional booklets which stress relevant blends of researched plan choice factors. Visual aids are also employed and they reflect an image of modern technology and efficiency.

The Health Center and Regional Group Centers are involved in other promotional efforts. These take the form of health exhibits, lectures, clinics, and counselling services. All these educational vehicles draw subscribers and friends into an environment conducive to promotion of H.M.O. subscription.

Other promotional materials are distributed at the Health Center or through direct mail to subscribers. General health education materials, guides to the optimum use of the H.M.O. service, schedules of Health Center events, financial statements and prospectus, and a monthly news bulletin are available. The bulletin summarizes the roles of the other available educational devices and generally keeps the member current with H.M.O. affairs. Exhibit V - 4 shows an example of such a bulletin.

Public relations. P.R. involves the use of a variety of tools to build good relations between the H.M.O. and certain important sections of the public in conjunction with a public relations agency. This takes the form of expert support, employer promotion, customer testimonials, location of influential employee spokesmen, and institutional advertising. Such advertisements are designed to create a proper attitude toward the H.M.O. and to build a favorable image of the organization among employees, experts in the field of health care, and the general public.

The objectives of public relations advertising are twofold -- image building and action inducing. H.M.O. and the P.R. agency promote comprehensiveness, quality of care, personal interest -- or factors associated with an image of tactful competence and efficiency. In this way the intangible nature of the H.M.O. service can be perceived by the public as more real and tangible.

CONCLUSIONS

The basis for selecting particular marketing strategies is the total effect that these strategies have upon the H.M.O.'s overall marketing success.

---

[242]Albert W. Frey and Jean C. Halterman, op. cit., p. 41.

EXHIBIT IV - 3^a

COMPARISON OF AN H.M.O. WITH BLUE CROSS-BLUE SHIELD PLANS

COMPARE THE RHODE ISLAND GROUP HEALTH ASSOCIATION PLAN
with BLUE CROSS-BLUE SHIELD
for STATE EMPLOYEES

BENEFIT	BLUE CROSS-BLUE SHIELD	RIGHA
Physicians Services Out of Hospital		
.. Office visits to physician	Not covered until you have paid $100 or $200. Then pays 80%.	Provided by physician you choose at Health Center. No Charge.
a) Surgical Services	Same as above.	Provided without charge to patient.
2. Visits to other specialists.	Same as above.	Provided without charge when arranged by a member of RIGHA Medical Staff.
3. Preventive Medicine, Physical Check-ups, etc.	Not Covered.	Provided without charge by physician at Health Center.
4. Eye exams and prescriptions for glasses.	Not Covered.	Provided without charge when arranged by Health Center.
5. Pediatric Services.	Not covered unless treating illness or injury, (same as above #1)	Provided without charge by specialists at the Health Center.
6. Laboratory Tests.	Same as #1 above.	Provided without charge.
7. Post Hospital Physician Services	If covered, same as #1.	Provided without charge.

a
Courtesy of Rhode Island Group Health Association (RIGHA); reproduced
by permission.

236

EXHIBIT IV - 4ᵃ

A TYPICAL H.M.O. BULLETIN

computers have their own requirements

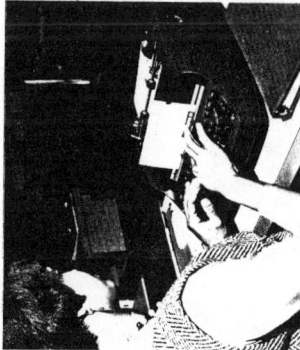

An employee of the Data Reduction Unit transcribes on a substitute document, using "machine-language", the information contained on a claim form.

Computers were invented to enable man to increase his efficiency and to do a larger volume of work in a shorter time. Historians will probably refer to our era as that of the computer. This highly perfected instrument makes it possible for man to reach beyond his own limitations, provided however that he does not lose sight of certain guidelines which he must respect if the computer is to react adequately to his orders.

Data fed into a computer must correspond exactly, in quantity and quality, to the instructions given to the computer and the slightest variance is likely to bog down the entire data processing operation. A low rate of error in handling and reducing data might very well give disastrous results. At the Québec Health Insurance Board where considerable use is made of computers, the Data Reduction Unit will help to illustrate the situation. This group of more than two hundred employees is responsible for translating into "machine language" all the information contained on claims from health professionals. The error rate in this operation may be considered minimal as it is less than 0.2% (two tenths of one percent).

The computer "servant" is essential to an organization such as the Board, especially when one realizes the volume of transactions carried out each day. However, the "servant" is an exacting one, and must be so, if the Health Insurance Plan is to be administered in keeping with the Health Insurance Act and Regulations, with the agreements concluded between the Minister of Social Affairs and each of the bodies representing the health professionals.

a popular documentary film

The documentary film on Health Insurance, which the Board makes available to interested groups, free of charge, is receiving considerable popularity in Québec colleges. Eleven CEGEPS have shown or are about to show this film to their students.

This 30 minute documentary was produced to inform the spectator on all facets of Health Insurance : history, the creation of the Board, the enacting of legislation on Health Insurance in Québec.

Any person desiring to obtain a copy of the film, in French or in English, is invited to contact Miss Alice Perreault, Publicity Service, Québec Health Insurance Board, P.O. Box 6600, Québec 2.

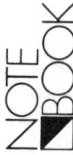

NOTE BOOK

On Wednesday, March 31st, Dr. Jean-Baptiste Gagnon, M.D., of the Professional Affairs Division of the Board will be a guest of the "Association coopérative féminine de Sainte-Louise-de-L'Islet". Dr. Gagnon will present the documentary film on Health Insurance and take part in a panel discussion on the same subject at the monthly meeting of this group.

On Monday, April 5th, Dr. Gustave Auger, M.D., of the Professional Affairs Division will present the documentary film on the Health Insurance to a meeting of the members of "Club Lions Québec-Métro".

ᵇ Courtesy of the Quebec Health Insurance Board; reproduced by permission.

Techniques for programming the marketing mix have been presented and these techniques having been substantiated by marketing research.

Integration and Coordination

Integration is necessary because interactions among the several marketing functions exist and require that coordination be accomplished in order to maximize the total effectiveness of the marketing plan -- the basis of this entire study. Figure V - 5 illustrates how the elements can be integrated and coordinated into the total marketing process. It is at this point that the marketing plan for the H.M.O. can be implemented.

Adjustments

The marketing plan does not purport, by any means, to be the whole answer to the enrollment problems that plague most health maintenance organizations in America. It is simply intended to provide a basis for promoting the H.M.O. as economically and rapidly as possible.

This chapter focussed on the initial enrollment of subscribers. Future adjustments in the plan must be made. When the initial enrollment process is over, substantial changes would be required, although the basic marketing principle will change very little.

Once the plan is established, diffusion of information should accelerate. Loyal subscribers will communicate their satisfaction to other consumers. In doing so they will make a significant contribution to further member recruitment and education. Then the marketing plan will be adjusted to build upon these favorable actions.

FIGURE IV - 5[a]

LIHMO MARKETING -- INTEGRATION AND COORDINATION SYSTEM

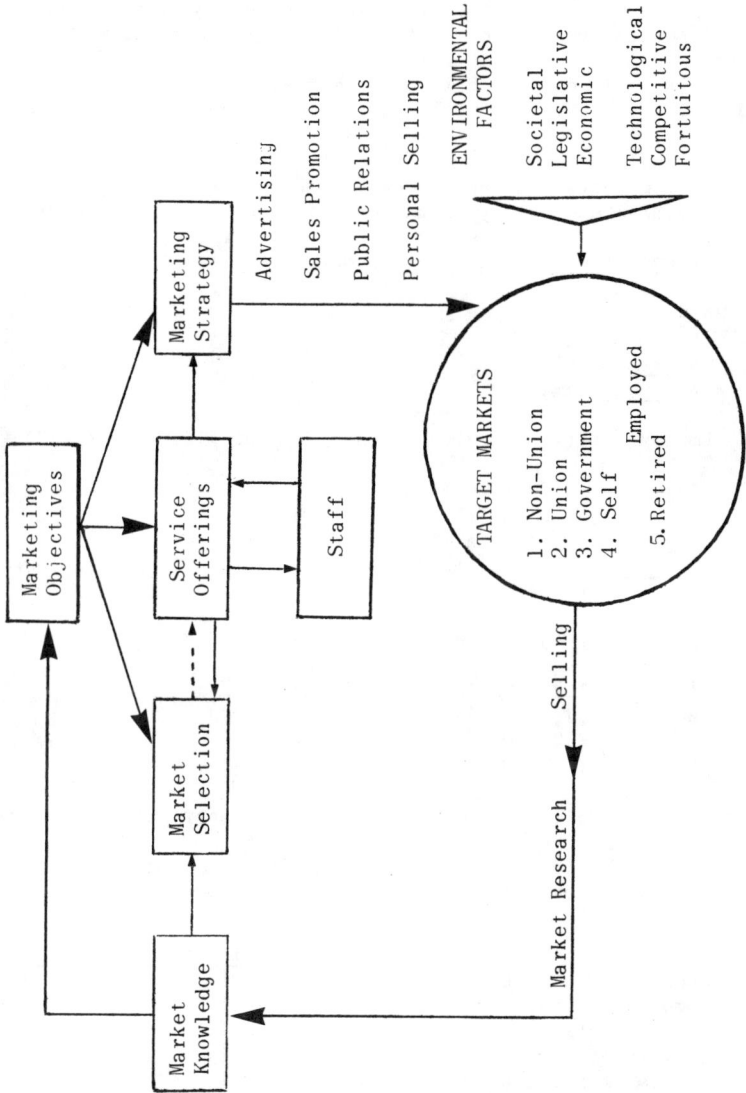

Marketing Objectives	
Marketing Strategy	Advertising
	Sales Promotion
	Public Relations
	Personal Selling
Service Offerings	
Staff	
Market Selection	
Market Knowledge	

ENVIRONMENTAL FACTORS

Societal
Legislative
Economic

Technological
Competitive
Fortuitous

TARGET MARKETS

1. Non-Union
2. Union
3. Government
4. Self   Employed
5. Retired

Market Research   Selling

[a]Adapted from George D. Downing, op. cit., p. 19.

APPENDIX IV - A

SAMPLE QUESTIONNAIRE

Instructions

This is a survey of a sample of Long Islanders. It is designed to find out what your experience has been with medical care and what qualities you would desire from a nonprofit prepaid health care plan.

It is important that you answer every question. Even if you have had no previous experience with a prepayment plan, your responses are important and valuable.

Note that it is not necessary for you to write your name. In this way it is guaranteed that your answers will be kept anonomous and confidential.

I. Background (Put an X in the appropriate space)

1. Sex:

   A _____ Male
   B _____ Female

2. Employment (if unemployed, that of your wife or husband):

   A _____ self-employed
   B _____ union affiliated employment
   C _____ nonunion affiliated employment
   D _____ governmental employment (municipal, state, federal)
   E _____ retired

3. Approximate Annual Household Income:

   A _____ less than $ 7,500
   B _____ $7,500 - $ 12,500
   C _____ $12,500 - 17,500
   D _____ $17,500 +

2. Health Plan Qualities: (simply circle the appropriate number)

Rate the following items on a 1-5 point scale (i.e. 1 - being very important in your choice of a plan --- 5 - being unimportant)

		Very Important	Neutral	Unimportant
4. Subscription cost		1 2	3 4	5
5. Comprehensiveness of plan		1 2	3 4	5
6. Extra benefits		1 2	3 4	5
7. Quality of care		1 2	3 4	5
8. Merits of Preventive Medicine		1 2	3 4	5
9. Personal interest of physician		1 2	3 4	5
10. Personal interest of Health Care Center personnel		1 2	3 4	5

240

		Very Important		Neutral		Unimportant
11. Qualifications of medical staff		1	2	3	4	5
12. Qualifications of Health Center personnel		1	2	3	4	5
13. Medical staff salary determinants		1	2	3	4	5
14. Accessibility of Health Center		1	2	3	4	5
15. Accessibility of care		1	2	3	4	5
16. Appointment lag		1	2	3	4	5
17. Clinic hours		1	2	3	4	5
18. Emergency service		1	2	3	4	5
19. House calls						
20. Health Center atmosphere		1	2	3	4	5
21. Health Center appearance		1	2	3	4	5
22. Technologically current equipment		1	2	3	4	5
23. Health Center facilities (library, labs)		1	2	3	4	5
24. Religious denomination of hospital affiliate		1	2	3	4	5
25. Membership eligibility		1	2	3	4	5
26. Voluntary enrollment		1	2	3	4	5
27. Size of membership		1	2	3	4	5
28. Socio-economic-ethnic composition		1	2	3	4	5
29. Dual choice		1	2	3	4	5
30. Free choice of physician		1	**2**	3	4	5
31. Member participation in admin. and planning		1	2	3	4	5
32. Vehicle for complaints		1	2	3	4	5
33. Periodic member meetings		1	2	3	4	5
34. Continuing subscriber education		1	2	3	4	5
35. Plan reputation		1	2	3	4	5
36. Expert recommendation		1	2	3	4	5
37. Peer recommendation		1	2	3	4	5
38. Co-worker recommendation		1	2	3	4	5
39. Place of work promotion by employer		1	2	3	4	5
40. Conversion		1	2	3	4	5
41. Availability of financial statements		1	2	3	4	5
42. Impending federal legislation		1	2	3	4	5

This is the end of the questionnaire. Thank you for filling it out. Feel free to ask the interviewer any questions you desire answered.

BIBLIOGRAPHY

TEXTS AND DISSERTATIONS

Alderson, Wrae and Shapiro, Stanley J. Marketing and the Computer,
    Englewood Cliffs, N.J.: Prentice-Hall, Inc., 1963.

Bernstein, Lewis and Dana, Richard H. Interviewing and the Health
    Professions, New York: Appleton-Century-Crofts, 1970.

Blackenship, A.B. and Doyle, J.B. Marketing Research Management,
    American Management Association, 1967.

Blum, R. H. The Management of the Doctor-Patient Relationship, New York:
    McGraw-Hill Book Company, 1960.

Buell, Victor P. ed., Handbook of Modern Marketing, New York: McGraw-Hill
    Book Company, 1970.

Buzzell, Robert C., Cox, Donald F. and Brown, Rex V. Marketing Research and
    Information Systems, New York: McGraw-Hill Book Company, 1969.

Cordtz, Dan. "Change Begins in the Doctor's Office," Fortune, LXXXI
    (January 1970).

Crisp, Richard D. How to Increase Advertising Effectiveness, New York:
    McGraw-Hill Book Company, Inc., 1963.

Cutlip, Scott M. and Center, Allen H. Effective Public Relations,
    Englewood Cliffs, N.J.: Prentice Hall, Inc., 1965.

Dexter, Lewis A. Elite and Specialized Interviewing, Evanston: Northwestern
    University Press, 1970.

Downing, George D. Sales Management, New York: John Wiley and Sons, Inc.,
    1969

Duff, R. S. and Hollingshead, A.B. Sickness and Society, New York: Harper
    and Row, 1968.

Dunn, S. Watson, Advertising: Its Role in Modern Marketing, New York:
    Holt, Rinehart and Winston, Inc., 1961.

Freidson, Eliot. Patients' Views of Medical Practice, New York: Russel
    Sage Foundation, 1961.

Frey, Albert W. and Davis, Kenneth R. The Advertising Industry, New York:
    Association of National Advertisers, 1958.

Frey, Albert W. and Halterman, Jean C. Advertising, New York: The Ronald
    Press Company, 1970.

Gersh, Harry, ed., Employees Benefits Factbook, New York: Fleet Academic
    Editions, 1970.

Ginzberg, E. Occupational Choice: An Approach to a General Theory,
    New York: Columbia University Press, 1951.

Gordon, Raymond L. Interviewing, Homewood, Illinois: The Dorsey Press, 1969.

Green, Paul E. and Tull, Donald S. Research for Marketing Decision,
    Englewood Cliffs, N.J.: Prentice-Hall, Inc., 1970.

Harmon, Harry H. Modern Factor Analysis, Chicago: The University of
    Chicago Press, 1967.

Johnson, Eugene M. An Introduction to the Problems of Service Marketing
    Management, Wilmington, Delaware, 1964.

Katz, Elihu and Lazarsfeld, Paul. Personal Influence, Glencoe, Ill.:
    The Free Press, 1955.

Konrad, Evelyn. Computer Innovations in Marketing, American Management
    Association, 1970.

Kotler, Philip. "The Future of the Computer in Marketing," from Essentials
    of an Effective Marketing Program ed. by John L. Krawshaar and
    Louis H. Varzimer, Braintree, Mass.: D. H. Mark Publishing Co.,
    1970.

_____. Marketing Decision-Making: A Model Building Approach,
    Chicago: Holt, Rinehart and Winston, 1971.

_____. Marketing Management: Analysis, Planning and Control,
    Englewood Cliffs, N.J.: Prentice-Hall Inc., 1967.

Lawton, William C. "Sociological Research in Big Business," from Pathways
    to Data, ed. by R. W. Habenstein, Chicago: Aldine Publishing Co.,
    1970.

MacColl, William A. Group Practice and Prepayment of Medical Care,
    Washington: Public Affairs Press, 1966.

Martin, T. R. Group Health Insurance from the Consumer Viewpoint,
    Dissertation, Stanford University, 1957.

Maukach, Hans O. "Studying the Hospital," from Pathways to Data ed. by
    R. W. Habenstein, Chicago: Aldine Publishing Co., 1970.

McCarthy, E. Jerome. Basic Marketing: A Managerial Approach, Homewood,
    Illinois: Richard D. Irwin, Inc., 1971.

Merton, Robert, Fiske, Marjorie and Kendall, Patricia. The Focussed Interview,
    Glencoe, Illinois: The Dorsey Press, 1969.

Miller, Ernest C. Marketing Planning: Approaches of Selected Companies,
    American Management Association, 1967.

Mulvihill, Donald F. Improving Personal Selling in Small Business,
    Washington: Small Business Administration, 1956.

Parker, Donald D. The Marketing of Consumer Services, Dissertation, Seattle: University of Washington, 1958.

Sandage, C. H. and Fryburger, Vernon. Advertising Theory and Practice, Homewood, Illinois: Richard D. Irwin, Inc., 1967.

Schwartz, S. L. Consumer Participation in Policy-Making in Prepaid Health Plans: Effect on Program Patterns and Types of Service, Dissertation, University of California at Berkeley, 1965.

Seltz, David D. Successful Industrial Selling, Englewood Cliffs, N.J.: Prentice-Hall Inc., 1958.

Serbein, Oscar N. Jr. Paying for Medical Care in the United States, New York: Columbia University Press, 1953.

Smith, George H. Motivation Research in Advertising and Marketing, New York: McGraw-Hill Book Company, 1954.

Somers, Anne K. ed., The Kaiser-Permanente Medical Care Program: A Symposium, New York: The Commonwealth Fund, 1971.

Stanton, William J. Fundamentals of Marketing, New York: McGraw-Hill Book Company, 1967.

Stanton, William J. and Burkirk, Richard H. Management of the Sales Force, Homewood, Ill.: Richard D. Irwin, Inc., 1969.

Stephenson, Howard, Ed., Handbook of Public Relations, New York: McGraw-Hill Book Company, 1971.

Stern, Mark E. Marketing Planning: A Systems Approach, New York: McGraw-Hill Book Company, 1966.

Urwick, Lyndell. The Elements of Administration, New York: Harper and Row Publishers, Inc., 1944.

Wedding, Nugent and Lassler, Richard S. Advertising Management, New York: The Ronald Press Co., 1962.

Wortruba, Thomas R. Sales Management, New York: Holt, Rinehart and Winston, Inc., 1971.

PERIODICALS, CONFERENCES AND REPORTS

"APHA Conference Report," Public Health Reports, LXXIV, (March 1957).

Bashshur, R. L., Metzner, C. A. and Worden, Carla. "Consumer Satisfaction With Group Practice, The CHA Case," American Journal of Public Health, LVII (November 1967).

Bush, Ann S. Group Practice: Planning and Implementing a Community-Wide Prepayment Plan, New York State Health Planning Commission, (May 1971).

Dearing, W. P. "Assured Health Services With Quality," National Conference of Health, Welfare, and Pension Plan, Ninth Annual Workshop, 1963.

Deutsch, Albert. "Group Medicine - Part 2," Consumer Reports, XXII (February 1957).

_____. "Group Medicine - Part 3," Consumer Reports, XXII (March 1957).

"The Diminishing Service Dollar," NADA Magazine, XXVIII No. 10 (1956).

Drucker, Peter F. "Long Range Planning: Challenge to Management Science," Management Science, V, No. 3 (1959).

Faltermayer, Edmund K. "Better Care at Less Cost Without Miracles," Fortune, LXXXI (January 1970).

Garfield, S. R. "The Delivery of Medical Care," Scientific American, CCXXII (April 1970).

General Population Characteristics of New York, U. S. Dept. of Commerce, Bureau of the Census, November 1971.

Greenberg, J. G. and Rodburg, M. L. "The Performance of Prepaid Group Practice," Harvard Law Review, LXXXIV (February 1971).

A Handbook of Statistical Data, State of New York: Dept. of Labor, 1970.

Health Care for California, State of California Dept. of Public Health, Berkeley, 1960.

Heim, Ronald and Gatty, Ronald. "The Application of Factor Analyses to Marketing Research," New Brunswick, N.J.: Rutgers Department of Agricultural Economics, Technical AES, (December 1961).

Kirsch, Arthur D. and Banks, Seymour. "Program Types Defined by Factor Analysis," Journal of Advertising Research, (September 1962).

Kotler, Philip. "The Future of the Computer in Marketing," Journal of Marketing, XXXIV (January 1970).

Kotler, Philip and Zaltman, Gerald. "Social Marketing: An Approach to Planned Social Change," Journal of Marketing, XXXV (July 1971).

Local Government Employment in Selected Metropolitan Areas and Large Countries, U.S. Dept. of Commerce, Bureau of the Census, 1970.

Long Island Factbook, Nassau-Suffolk Planning Commission, 1969.

Magraw, Richard. Address to: AMA Second National Congress on the Socio-Economics of Health Care, March 22, 1968.

Massy, William F. "Applying Factor Analysis to a Specific Marketing Problem," Proceedings of the Winter Conference of the American Marketing Association, Boston, (December 1963).

245

McNary, William S. "P.R. and the Health Industry," Public Relations Journal, X, No. 9 (1954).

Metzner, Charles A. and Bashshur, Rashid L. "Factors Associated With the Choice of Health Care Plans," Journal of Health and Social Behavior, VIII (December 1967).

Mott, F. D. "The Success of Group Health Plans," AFL-CIO American Federationist, October 1963.

Mukherjee, B. N. "A Factor Analysis of Some Qualitative Attributes of Coffee," Journal of Advertising Research, V (June 1965).

New York's Approach to Prepaid Comprehensive Group Practice - Considerations for Applicants, New York State Dept. of Health, July 1971.

"The Non-Profit Medical Corporations Act," Newsletter - Medical Societies' Reference Committee, 1971.

"Over Twenty States Have Legal Bars to Group Practice," Group Health and Welfare News, XIII, (February 1972).

Parker, Donald D. "Improved Efficiency and Reduced Cost in Marketing," Journal of Marketing, (April 1962).

Pilgrim, F. J. and Kamen, J. M. "Patterns of Food Preferences Through Factor Analyses," Journal of Marketing, XXIV (October 1959).

Prepayment for Medical and Dental Care in New York State, New York State Departments of Health and Insurance, 1962.

Rathwell, John W. "What is Meant by Service?," Journal of Marketing, (October 1966).

"Report of the Definitions Committee," Journal of Marketing, XIII (October 1948).

Reynolds, William H. and Wofford, George T. "A Factor Analysis of Air. Traveler Attitude," Proceedings of the American Marketing Association, Chicago: AMA, June 1966.

Rosen, George. Preventive and Educational Services in Medical Care, Mimeographed Report, 1954.

_____. "Provisions of Medical Care," Public Health Reports, LXXIV (March 1959).

Roy, Donald F. "The Role of the Researcher in the Study of Social Conflict," Human Organization, XXIV (Fall 1965).

Saward, Ernest W. The Relevance of Prepaid Group Practice to the Effective Delivery of Health Services, U.S. Dept. of Health, Education, and Welfare, 1969.

Schwartz, S. L.   "Consumer Sponsorship and Physician Sponsorship of
         Prepaid Group Practice Health Plans: Some Similarities and
         Differences," American Journal of Public Health, LV (January 1965).

Smith, Francis R.   "Why Can't the Prepayment Plans Give the Public What It
         Wants?," Modern Hospital, XCV No. 6, (1960).

Smith, Wendell,   "Product Differentiation and Market Segmentation as
         Alternative Strategies," Journal of Marketing, (July 1956).

Stephenson, William.   "Public Images of Public Utilities," Journal of
         Advertising Research, (December 1963).

Stoetzel, Jean.   "A Factor Analysis of the Liquor Preferences of French
         Consumers," Journal of Advertising Research, I (December 1960).

Twedt, D. W.   "A Multiple Factor Analysis of Advertising Readership,"
         Journal of Applied Psychology, XXXVI (June 1952).

Vidich, A. and Bensman, J.   "The Validity of Field Data," Human Organization,
         XIII (Spring, 1954).

Weinerman, E. R.   "Attitudes Toward Group Medical Care," Hospital Management,
         XCVI (July 1963).

_____.   "New Ideas in Health Service," Proceedings of the Los Angeles
         Conference on Health and Welfare, (February 1955).

_____.   "Patients' Perceptions of Group Medical Care," American Journal
         of Public Health, LIV (June 1964).

Williams, Greer.   "Kaiser Plan: The Prepaid Group Practice Model and How it
         Began," Modern Hospital, February 1971.

Wolfman, Burton.   "Medical Expenses and Choice of Plans," Monthly Labor
         Review, LXXXIV (July 1961).

Wood, Albert J.   "New Dimensions in Marketing Research for Banks," Banking,
         LI (April 1959).

Yedida, Avram.   "Dual Choice Programs," American Journal of Public Health,
         XLIX (1959).

_____.   Planning and Implementation of the Community Health Foundation
         of Cleveland, Ohio, Washington: Department of Health, Education and
         Welfare, 1969.

Zaltman, Gerald and Vertinsky, Ilan.   "Health Service Marketing: A Suggested
         Model," Journal of Marketing, XXXV (July 1971).

INTERVIEWS

Connecticut General Insurance Company, Hartford, Conn., telephone
        interview with Fran Brissette, Health Insurance Representative,
        March 1972.

Group Health Association of America (GHAA) Washington, D. C., interview
        with Herman Schmidt, Field Director, February 1972.

Harvard Community Health Plan, Boston, Massachusetts, interview with
        Roger Birnbaum, Assistant Director, March 1972.

Rhode Island Group Health Association (RIGHA), Providence, R. I., interview
        with Leo Petit and Dale Hoover, Director of Operations and
        Director of Enrollment, respectively, December 6, 1971.

CHAPTER V

THE MANPOWER PLAN

Jack Abeshouse

INTRODUCTION

Objectives of the Plan

General Objective

The success of any organization, whether it be industrial, commercial, service or institutional; whether profit oriented or not, depends to
the largest degree upon the caliber and motivation of its personnel. But
good personnel is no more than a reflection of good organizational structure
and especially competent leadership, for "..... leadership is the fulcrum on
which the demands of the individual and the demands of the organization are
balanced."[1] "Without leadership, an organization is only a muddle of men and
equipment; leadership is the human factor which binds the group together,
motivates it towards goals and transforms potential into reality."[2]

The growing complexity of life itself and of medical practice in
the 1970's demands that health care, one of society's most essential services,
be organized more efficiently and be better coordinated than in the past.
Prepaid group practice in some form of Health Maintenance Organization is
one means for achieving these ends.

Although official recognition has now been achieved for this form
of prepaid group practice,[3] the question still remains as to how these
entities, when formed, are going to be staffed and how they are going to be
managed, not only from the medico-technical viewpoint, but also from the
administrative and financial standpoints. One objective of this manpower

---

[1]W. G. Bennis, "Revisionist Theory of Leadership," Harvard Business Review,
Jan.-Feb. 1961, p. 150.

[2]Keith Davis, Human Relations at Work, (New York: McGraw-Hill, 2nd ed.,
1962, p. 103.

[3]Medical Economics: Hard Evidence that HMO's Really Work, June 7, 1971,
pp. 222-233.

plan is to aid in creating a living, working organization of skilled people dedicated to the ideals of promoting and enhancing the general health of the community through prepaid group practice in a Health Maintenance Organization.

Specific Objectives

Most people tend to think of health services in terms of doctors, nurses, and pharmacists. This highly trained core of professionals is a key visible element of the health services work force, but they account for just one third of the total health-service personnel.[4] The other two-thirds include practical nurses, attendants, nurse's aids, technicians of many and varied skills, therapists trained in rehabilitative procedures; and a wide range of supportive personnel concerned with record-keeping, administration, food-handling, supplies, housekeeping, maintenance and related tasks. These jobs require unskilled labor, semi-skilled and high skilled professionals, and together they constitute the dynamic and vital elements of the total work force of the health-care delivery system.[5] Proper utilization of these peoples' skills is essential both to the quality of the health care to be rendered by the H.M.O. and to the morale and efficiency of all employees. This chapter has as its other objective the establishment of a workable manpower structure and a set of practical procedures for the administration of the H.M.O.'s personnel resources.

Initial Organization

Founder's Group

The success of the H.M.O. will depend upon the structure of the enterprise and the caliber of its leadership and the workers. Before the H.M.O. can function it must be manned by competent people. In the formative stages, a key figure may emerge, an entrepreneurial type who will provide the motivating power; who will plant the seed of the idea and create the climate for the seedling to emerge. This man, be he a local industrialist, doctor, politician or business executive, will gather a small nucleus of people with whom he can discuss the promotion of the idea and whom he can induce to join him in the venture.

The founders' committee may conceive of several tentative organizations based on probabilities of public acceptance, then having selected one upon which to base the initial organization,[6] will have plans for modification that could be introduced after the organization has been operating for one, three, and five years, or as subscriber enrollment reaches predetermined levels.

4
U.S. Dept. of Labor, Manpower Administration. Job Descriptions & Organizational Analysis for Hospitals & Related Health Services, U. S. Supt. of Documents, June 1971.

5 Ibid.

6 See Chapter II of this study on details of organization.

Initial Arrangement

The first arrangement will of course be modest, because there will
be no way of determining in advance how successful the subscriber recruiting
campaign might be. It may not even be possible to operate the H.M.O. as a
prepaid group practice entity until there are at least several thousand subscribers because the ratio of physicians to subscribers is usually around
one per thousand.[7]

For manpower planning purposes, an H.M.O. with a subscribership
of between 30,000 and 50,000 members, might have a table of organization as
shown in Figure V - 1.

At the head of this organization is an unpaid Board of Directors
or Trustees, a group of well-qualified, public-spirited citizens responsible
for setting broad policy. The President and Chief Executive Officer functions
in much the same way as the head of any enterprise, with the authority vested
in him by the Board of Directors.

The two basic operating segments shown in Figure V - 1 are:

The Regional Medical Groups (1)

The Medical Center (or hospital) (2)

Regional Medical Groups (1)

Located at spots convenient to public transportation and with
adequate parking facilities, each typical Regional Medical Group (RMG)
operates in a building containing a number of medical administrative offices,
treatment and waiting rooms. This facility may be owned jointly by the
participating partners, each of whom are licensed to practice medicine.
Under the single roof of this local clinic would be the family-practice G.P.,
the pediatrician, the internist, the obstetrician-gynecologist and possibly
an analytical test laboratory for the more routine work-ups.[8]

Specialists such as orthopedists, ear-nose-and throat men,
ophthalmologists, dermatologists, neurologists, surgeons and so forth could
visit each location once or twice per week according to pre-arranged schedule,
or, if the case were more urgent, the patient could be referred to the H.M.O.
Medical Center, the base of operations for the specialists. As any one
Regional Medical Group grows in enrollment to where the services of a full-
time resident specialist would be needed one could be appointed. Figure VI -
2 shows the relationships between the RMG's and the Medical Center.

The Regional Medical Groups (RMG's) would be legally constituted
partnerships organized to provide high quality comprehensive health care to

---

[7] H.I.P. of Greater New York, brochure on Information for Physicians
Interested in a Prepaid Group Partnership Practice with HIP Affiliation,
Feb. 1971.

[8] Ibid.

FIGURE V - 1

H.M.O. PLAN INC. TABLE OF ORGANIZATION

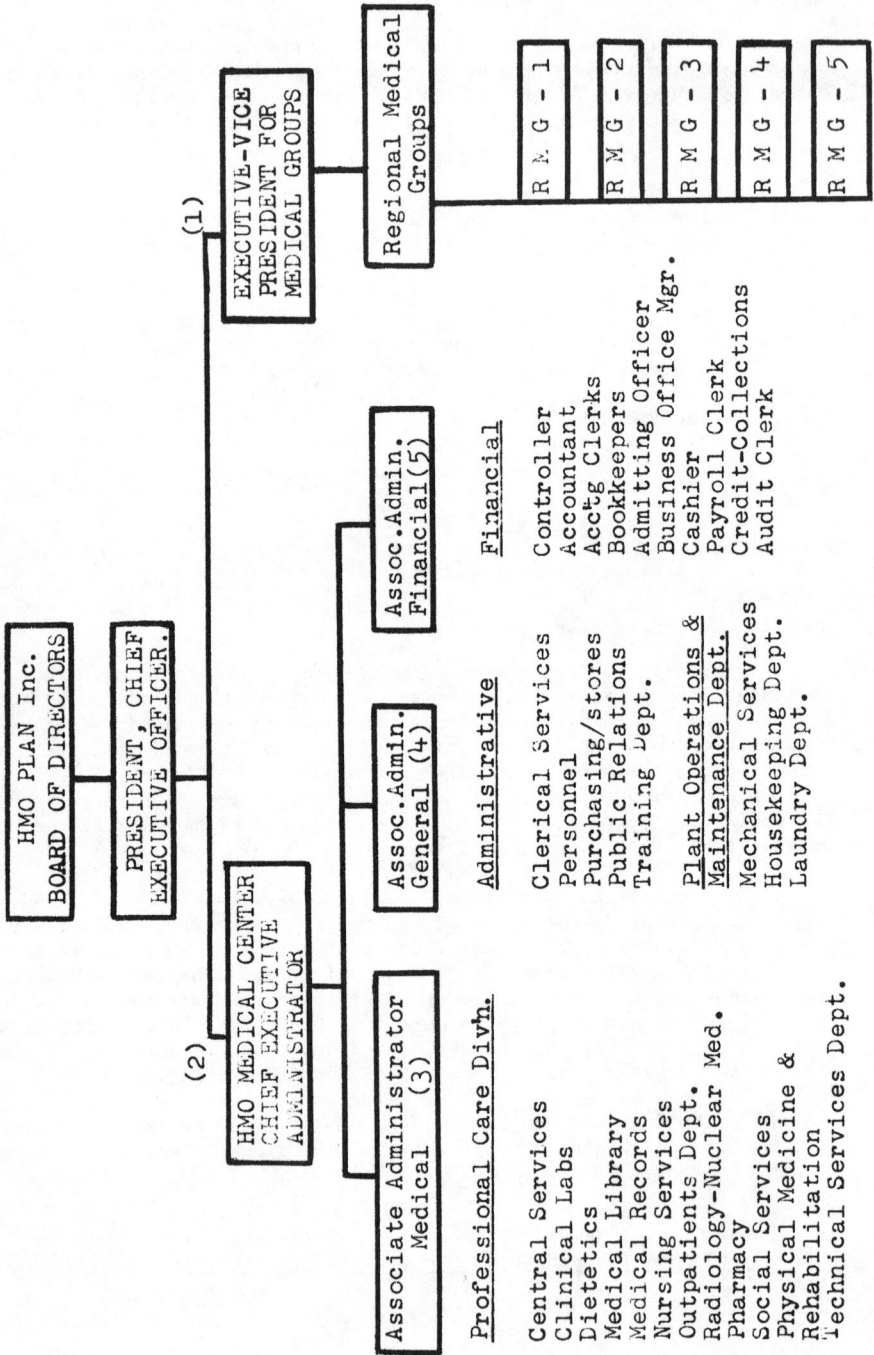

FIGURE V - 2

DIAGRAMATIC SCHEME FOR THE RELATIONSHIP BETWEEN THE H.M.O.
MEDICAL CENTER AND DISPERSED REGIONAL MEDICAL GROUPS

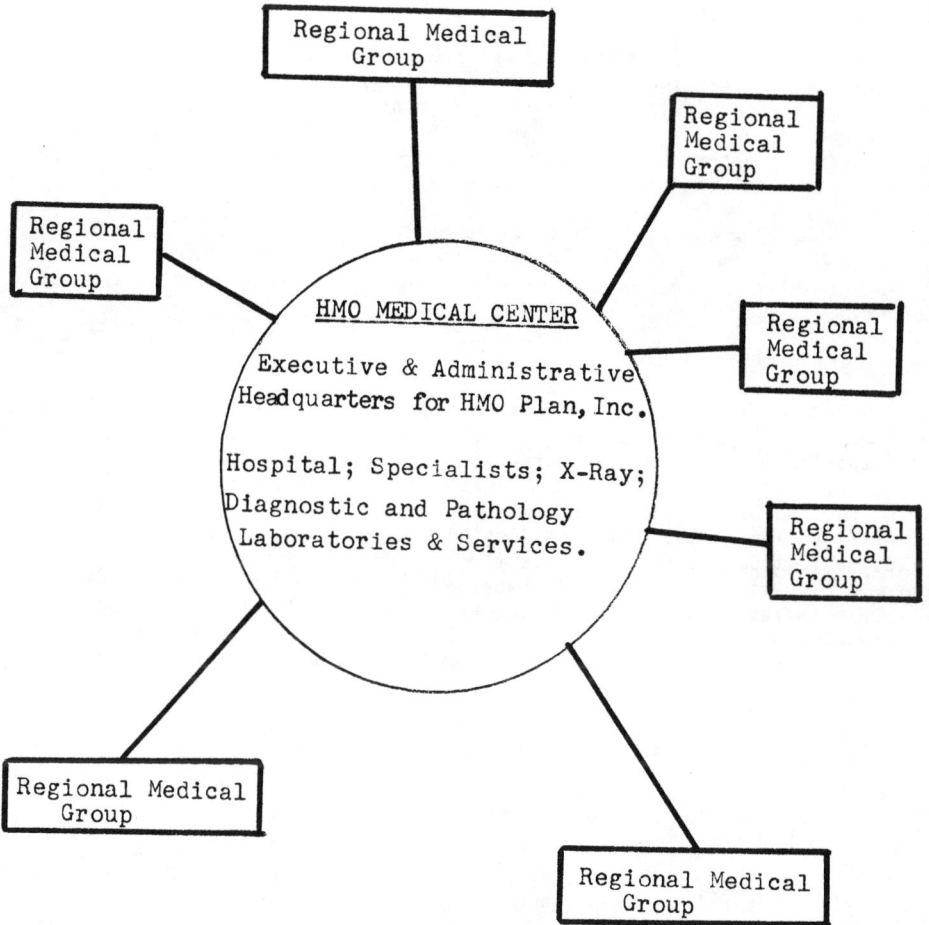

253

a segment of the enrolled population on a prepaid basis. All physicians
affiliated with a RMG may be either partners, or are employees under written
contract to the partnership.[9] According to this plan, each Regional Medical
Group will be led by a Medical Director who would be elected to that position
according to the provisions of the Medical Group Partnership Agreement.[10]

The Medical Directors of each Regional Medical Group shall, in turn,
elect one of their number as Executive Vice-President for Medical Groups to
represent the medical practitioners at the highest level of management.
While the President of H.M.O. Plan Inc., does not necessarily need to be a
medical doctor, it is of course mandatory that the Executive Vice-President
for Regional Medical Groups be one.

H.M.O. Medical Center[11]

The establishment, operation and administration of a modern hospital
is an extremely expensive and complex undertaking. The marketing of a
health maintenance plan would be made more difficult without the provision
for hospital care under the plan's auspices. Therefore, it is a requirement
that a medical center capable of providing good, but not super-specialty type
service, ultimately be included in the organization.

The plan contemplates that the Medical Center will be under the direc-
tion of a Chief Executive Administrator to whom will report three Associate
Administrators, (3, 4 & 5 in Figure V - 1) for Medicine, Administration and
Finance.[12]

Interrelationships

Shown at the head of the structure in Figure V-1 is the H.M.O. Plan
Inc., a nonprofit corporation controlled by a Board of Directors or Trustees.
The corporation enters into subscription contracts with either groups or
individuals to provide them with medical care. It then contracts with the
H.M.O. Medical Center Inc., a nonprofit organization which develops and owns
the hospital facilities. The distinction between H.M.O. Plan Inc., and
H.M.O. Medical Center Inc., is more formal than substantive, since their
Boards of Trustees would probably overlap. The functions of the two are
quite dissimilar; however; the H.M.O. Plan Inc. is primarily concerned with
the membership enrollment, finances and administration, whereas H.M.O.
Medical Center, Inc. is mainly concerned with inpatient health services.

---

[9]See Appendix A for Specimen Agreement for a Regional Medical Group.

[10]See Appendix A, Article VI, Sect. 1, pp. 8-9.

[11]Figure V - 2 shows the geographical relationship between the H.M.O.
Medical Center and the dispersed Regional Medical Groups.

[12]The detailed functions of these Administrators are given on page 318.

The Plan obtains professional medical services from the Regional Medical Groups located at spaced population centers, on a negotiated, contractual capitation basis. Physicians of the Regional Medical Groups care for patients principally in nonhospital, group-practice facilities. Each RMG is an independent organization which elects its own officers who lead negotiations and participate actively in the entire medical care program. In operation, negotiations between the Plan and the Groups would be at arm's length, yet hopefully in a spirit of cooperation, because of joint management control.

STAFFING THE HEALTH MAINTENANCE ORGANIZATION

Timing

Getting Started[13]

Since it is not the direct concern of this chapter to determine who will provide initial funding for the H.M.O. to get started before regular income is available to meet payroll and operating expenses, it will be assumed that funds are available to cover the first year of operation.

The first step would be for the founders and organizers of the H.M.O. to appoint an experienced Hospital and Medical Services Administrator who will be the temporary head of H.M.O. Plan Inc., but who will ultimately head the H.M.O. Medical Center. Typically, this executive will have a graduate degree in Hospital Administration and have had experience in the selection of executive personnel. His first task will be to hire a small clerical/secretarial staff to handle correspondence and the usual secretarial duties while he, along with the President and Trustees, is recruiting medical staff to join in the formation of Regional Medical Groups. He will also hire a marketing specialist to plan and implement a campaign for attracting and enrolling subscribers[14] and a personnel manager to work on formalizing the job specifications, qualification requirements and performance evaluation standards for all positions in the organization.

As each intermediate step is achieved in the H.M.O. master plan, from establishing the Regional Medical Groups, the enrollment of subscribers and the commencement of actual health service, the acquisition of personnel with the prerequisite skill will be undertaken.

Thus, getting started is a complex matter requiring an ordering of priorities by the founders. As shown in Figure V - 3 the starting period may last as long as four months while a rudimentary staff is recruited, indoctrinated and they proceed with their tasks to find and acquire other workers to form the nucleus of the operating units.

---

[13]See Figure V - 3, a Time-Event (Gantt) chart for a diagramatic plan of the sequences of organizing activities for the H.M.O. Plan Inc.

[14]
See Chapter V for details of the Marketing Plan.

FIGURE V - 3

TIME-EVENT CHART SHOWING SEQUENTIAL ORGANIZING
ACTIVITIES - H.M.O. PLAN INC.

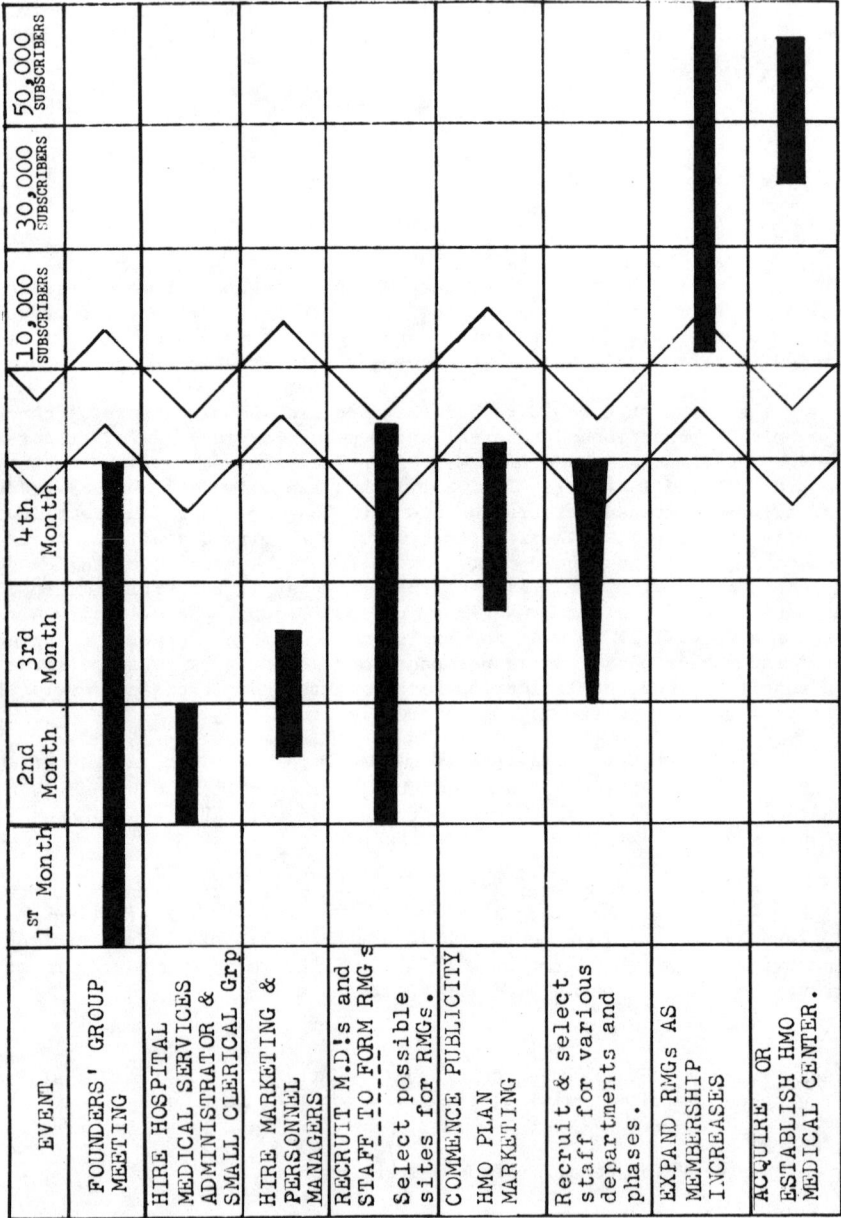

EVENT	1ST Month	2nd Month	3rd Month	4th Month	10,000 SUBSCRIBERS	30,000 SUBSCRIBERS	50,000 SUBSCRIBERS
FOUNDERS' GROUP MEETING							
HIRE HOSPITAL MEDICAL SERVICES ADMINISTRATOR & SMALL CLERICAL Grp							
HIRE MARKETING & PERSONNEL MANAGERS							
RECRUIT M.D's and STAFF TO FORM RMG s							
Select possible sites for RMGs.							
COMMENCE PUBLICITY HMO PLAN MARKETING							
Recruit & select staff for various departments and phases.							
EXPAND RMGs AS MEMBERSHIP INCREASES							
ACQUIRE OR ESTABLISH HMO MEDICAL CENTER.							

The Initial Operating Phase

Having acquired sufficient enrolled subscribers to permit operations to commence, the formation of one or more Regional Medical Groups can proceed.

A Medical Group should have the following personnel:[15]

1. A Physician as Medical Director in charge of medical policy administration. (He would be responsible for both the medical direction of the Group and the supervision of the quality of medical care);

2. A minimum of one family physician per 1,000 members enrolled, plus at least one and preferably two pediatricians and access to one physician in each of the major specialties; (Family physicians and pediatricians are the primary physicians who serve as the portal of entry for enrollees into the RMG. Primary physicians may serve in only one RMG; specialists may serve in more than one. Every person or family enrolled in the RMG selects one of the family physicians of the RMG as his personal physician, and also selects a pediatrician for his children. Not more than two specialists in any clinical field should be included until the first two average 20 hours of service a week to RMG subscribers.)[16]

3. A sufficient number of qualified nurses, practical nurses, nurse's aides, physical therapists, X-ray and laboratory technicians commensurate with good medical practice;

4. A full-time lay administrator responsible to the Medical Director for the functioning of the nonmedical aspects of the RMG, and sufficient personnel to maintain business and office services in an orderly manner; (appointment making, accounting, bookkeeping services, reception, telephone operation, secretarial, medical records and other clerical and maintenance functions must be provided.)

H.M.O. Revenue and Staff Ratios

For purposes of this study, an initial enrollment of 50,000 subscribers is assumed, made up of 12,500 families with an average of four person per family. Current premium rates for medical coverage of the type envisaged for H.M.O. for the family unit specified above would be about $38.00 per month. Twelve thousand five hundred monthly subscriptions at $38.00 would give the H.M.O. an approximate gross revenue of $475.00 per month or $5,700,000 per year.

Table V - 1 contains an estimate of expenses of a Medical Group in the Greater New York area, caring for 50,000 enrollees.[17] Note that there

---

[15] HIP Brochure: Information for Physicians, op. cit, p. 6.

[16] Ibid.

[17] Ibid.

is a difference of $2,632,500 between the estimated gross revenues and the estimated gross expenses. These funds will be allocated to provide hospital care for subscribers. In the early stages before the H.M.O. Medical Center becomes operative, H.M.O. Plan Inc.,will purchase hospital coverage from an insurance carrier such as Blue Cross so that inpatient service will be available despite the lack of the Plan's own hospital.

Table V - 2 shows the staff requirements of nonphysician personnel needed for Medical Groups of 10,000-15,000 and 20,000 enrollees.[18] The statistics in the column for 50,000 enrollees are projected estimates only. Variations of these estimates would arise depending on whether the 50,000 were members of four, five or eight separate RMG's. A larger staff is required to maintain eight separate RMG's than would be to maintain only four or five. At each RMG there would need to be at least one receptionist-telephone operator, a bookkeeper, assistant administrator, one porter-handy man, one housekeeper. The more enrollees serviced at each RMG, the less it costs per enrollee for overhead and administration.

TABLE V - 1

ANNUAL ANTICIPATED EXPENSES OF A GROUP FOR 50,000 ENROLLEES[19]

Type of Expense	Amount per Enrollee	Total for 50,000 Enrollees
Nonphysician salaries, costs	$18.00	$900,000
Rent, light, heat, phone	3.50	175,000
Insurance	.75	37,500
Equipment	.40	20,000
Supplies & Services	3.60	180,000
Legal & Audit	.25	12,500
Maintenance & Repair	.25	12,500
Special Services, claims, subscriber relations	1.30	65,000
Other operating expenses (debt service, etc.)	1.30	65,000
Physician Salaries for 48 M.D.'s	32.00	1,600,000
	$61.35	$3,067,500

[18] Ibid.

[19] Ibid.

TABLE V - 2

ESTIMATED NON-PHYSICIAN PERSONNEL NEEDED FOR MEDICAL
GROUPS OF 10,000-15,000-20,000 AND 50,000 SUBSCRIBERS[20]

Duty	Group of 10,000	Group of 15,000	Group of 20,000	50,000* Members
Administrator	1.0	1.0	1.0	5.0
Secretaries (plus medical records)	3.5	5.0	7.0	12.0
Bookkeeper	0.5	1.0	1.5	5.0
Switchboard operator	1.5	1.5	2.0	5.0
Registered nurses	3.0	3.0	4.0	8.0
Nurse's Aides, medical asts.	6.0	8.5	10.0	20.0
Nurse clinicians	2.0	2.0	3.0	6.0
Receptionists (appointments)	4.0	5.0	6.0	10.0
Clerks	2.0	3.0	4.0	10.0
X-ray technicians	1.5	1.5	1.5	3.0
Laboratory technicians	1.5	2.0	2.5	5.0
Physiotherapists	0.5	1.5	2.5	4.0
Maintenance man	1.0	1.0	1.0	●3.0
Housekeeper	1.0	1.0	1.5	5.0
	29.0	37.0	47.5	101.0

*Based on an assumption of service at five different RMG's.

[20] Ibid.

259

The statistics given in Table V - 2 for the columns headed "Group of 10,000-15,000-20,000" assume that a single RMG is involved. The column headed "50,000 Subscribers" assumes that about five different RMG's cover those members. In the developmental stages of H.M.O., it is not expected that only one medical group will be established with an enrollment approaching the sizes shown in Table V - 2. Rather, there will be several smaller groups dispersed at convenient locations for the benefit of the subscribers. Thus, the employee ratios will naturally vary from the figures cited above until the groups stabilize at these levels. The discretion of the Medical Director of each RMG will permit of variations in staff make-up. These figures reflect the experience of Health Insurance Plan of Greater New York medical groups during 1970 and no doubt this experience will rather closely parallel what H.M.O. will also do.

Table V - 3 shows how the much larger California Region of the Permanente Medical Group has composed its roster of doctors. It is likely that any group of similar size would have essentially the same roster.

TABLE V - 3

AVERAGE NUMBER OF FULL-TIME AND FULL-TIME EQUIVALENT
PHYSICIANS PER 100,000 MEMBERS: THE PERMANENTE
MEDICAL GROUP, NORTH CALIFORNIA REGION[21]

Specialty	Physicians per 100,000 Members
Medicine (incl. General Practice)	32.5
Pediatrics	17.5
Obstetrics-Gynecology	9.0
Surgery	9.0
Urology	1.5
Orthopedics	4.0
Radiology	4.0
Pathology	1.5
Ophthalmology	3.0
Allergy	1.5
Anaesthesiology	2.5
Dermatology	3.0
Neurology	0.5
Neurosurgery	1.0
Psychiatry	1.5
Otolaryngology	3.0
Total	95.0

[21] American Medical News, September 13, 1971.

Staffing the Organization

The Board of Directors or Trustees

The Board of Directors (or Trustees, whichever name is selected), can either be a showcase of prestige, a shadow king, or it can be an organ of review, appraisal, appeal; the "Supreme Court" of an organization, which has to discharge the final judicial function in respect to major problems. It gives final approval to the objectives of the organization, and makes the measurements it uses to evaluate progress towards its stated objectives. It looks critically at the capital structure and expenditures as proposed by the operating executives and watches the spirit of the organization as it develops.[22]

The Board cannot and must not be a governing body involved in day to day operations. Only in a crisis does it become a body of action, and then only to remove existing executives who have failed, or to replace those who have retired, resigned or died. Once the replacement has been made, the Board again becomes an organ of review.[23]

A Board of Directors typically consists of between ten and 20 members (depending upon the size of the organization), whose qualifications may include those with civic or local government background and those with legal, financial, academic, industrial-managerial, political, public relations and, of course, medical experience. Membership on the Board is largely honorary, with the rewards for such work being prestige and the personal satisfaction of providing the benefits of one's special talents in performing a vital public service.

Since efforts will be made to obtain large groups of subscribers from major employers in the area, in the early days of soliciting, a position on the Board might be offered to a high management official of such a firm as an inducement for the firm to join the H.M.O. Plan, Inc. Precedent for this has long been established both with the Kaiser-Permanente plan as well as with Health Insurance Plan of Greater New York. In the case of the latter, officers of several labor unions whose members are subscribers to the plan, have been elected to the Board. In this way there is direct and immediate communication between the Plan and responsible representation of its clients.

In 1970, there were 27 members on the Board of Directors of H.I.P. of Greater New York, composed as follows:[24]

Medical background	11 members
Labor union officials	7
Government-political	3
Industrial-financial-Institutional	6
	27

---

[22]Peter F. Drucker, The Practice of Management, Harper, 1954, p. 178.

[23]Ibid.

[24]HIP of Greater N.Y. 1970 Annual Report.

The Board would select a President-Chief Executive Officer under whose guidance the H.M.O. would develop not only in terms of efficient organization, financial strength and volume of subscribers enrolled, but also in the quality of health care delivered at reasonable cost.

The President and Chief Executive Officer

It is necessary for the chief executive to be a man who thinks through the purpose and business of the organization, by developing and setting over-all objectives. He makes the basic decisions needed to reach these objectives. He communicates the objectives and the decisions to his managers whom he educates into viewing the organization and its business as a whole so that they too can develop their own objectives and contribute to the totality of the business. The President measures performance and results against the objectives and he reviews and revises objectives as conditons demand.

The President-Chief Executive Officer makes the decisions on senior management personnel and assures himself that future managers are being developed all down the line. He makes the basic decisions on company organization and knows what questions to put to his managers and makes sure they know what the questions mean. He coordinates the various "product lines," divisions, facilities, activities, within the total organization and arbitrates conflicts within the group and either prevents or settles personality clashes. Like an orchestral conductor, he guides, coaxes, inspires, whips the players into a harmonious whole for the ultimate goal of making a beautiful performance. Like the captain of a ship, he takes personal command in an emergency.

A vital function which the President, and only he can do, is assume responsibility for capital expenditure planning and raising capital. In the case of a Health Maintenance Organization, he must keep abreast of the various governmental sources of funds available for such essential public services and be able to develop appropriate, provable data which would qualify his organization for a share of such Federal, State or County assistance. Weak presentation of the facts, or lack of knowledge of the route through the complex maze of public institutional finance will certainly impede the viability of the organization.

Since undue reliance upon governmental financial assistance can be hazardous to the fiscal health of the organization because government programs take years to make a final settlement of each year's reimbursable share of hospital costs, alternate sources must be pursued by the President to tide him over. Saint Francis Hospital, San Francisco, according to Forsyth and Thomas[25] had not in 1971 yet obtained final settlement for any fiscal period under either Medicare or Medicaid since the inception of both of these programs in 1966 and more than half a million dollars remain outstanding.

Thorough knowledge of such legislation, both enacted or proposed and pending, as the Hill-Burton Act for assistance in hospital construction

---

[25]G. C. Forsyth & D. C. Thomas, "Models for Financially Health Hospitals," Harvard Business Review, July-August 1971, Vol. 49, No. 4, pp. 107-8.

finance, or the Javits Bill, the Kennedy Bill, Griffiths Bill, or the AMA Medicredit Plan, must be at the command of the President of the H.M.O.

At least once a month or more often as may be required, the President must prepare the agenda for the monthly meeting of the Board of Trustees and be ready to answer their questions and relay Board decisions to his managers.

This narration of the long list of duties and responsibilities of the Chief Executive Officer is not exhaustive; much depends on the man himself and the type of people he has to work with. His own energies, his special interests, training and background will shape much of his work load.

Chief, H.M.O. Medical Center[26]

This position is variously known as Hospital Superintendent, Executive Director, Hospital Administrator, Executive Vice-President and in general he administers, directs and coordinates all activities of the hospital to carry out its objectives in the provision of health care, furtherance of education and research, and participation in community health programs.

He is responsible for the operation of the hospital, for the application and implementation of established policies, and for liason among the governing authority (Board of Trustees), the President, the medical staff and various departments of the hospital, the Regional Medical Groups and the commercial aspects of the plan.

He organizes the functions of the hospital through appropriate departmentalization and the delegation of duties. He establishes formal means of accountability from those to whom he has assigned duties; regularly schedules inter-departmental and departmental meetings where appropriate, to maintain liason between the medical staff and other departments; names appropriate departmental representatives to the multidisciplinary committee of the hospital.

He prepares reports for, and attends meetings with the President and Board of Trustees regarding the total activity of the hospital as well as governmental developments which affect health care. He provides for personnel policies and practices that adequately support sound patient care and maintain accurate and complete personnel records.

He reviews and acts upon the reports of authorized inspecting agencies; implements the control and effective utilization of the physical and financial resources of the hospital. He employs a system of responsibility accounting, including budget and internal controls. He participates, or is represented, in community, State, and national hospital associations and professional activities which define the delivery of health care services and aid in short and long range planning of health services and facilities. He pursues a continuing program of formal and informal education in health care, administrative, and management areas to maintain, strengthen and broaden his

---

[26]U. S. Dept. of Labor, Job Descriptions, op. cit., pp. 23-24.

concepts, philosophy, and ability as a health care administrator. He
delegates administrative responsibilities to Associate Administrators and to
department heads.

He should have graduated from an accredited college or university,
with graduate work in an accredited program in hospital administration. His
education and experience requirements must be of a high order for this is a
very demanding, high level position.

Associate Administrators[27]

Three Associate Administrators will be appointed to manage the
following functional groups:

Medical & Professional Care Services. This executive is responsible for all
services performed in the treatment and care of the patient, whether in
direct contact with the patient or not. The outpatient and pharmacy departments, clinical and diagnostic laboratories, food services, operative
surgeries, nursing services and similar functions are under his supervision.
The occupant of this position should be a licensed medical doctor.

General Administration and Operational Services Administrator. This executive
supervises general clerical services, the personnel department, purchasing
and stores, public relations, the training department, housekeeping and
laundry services. His position is akin to both plant and office manager in
an industrial setting.

Financial Administrator. (Controller) Directs and coordinates hospital
activities concerned with financial administration, general accounting, patient
business services and financial and statistical reporting. He may have
administrative responsibility for the data processing function and for
administrative systems and procedures. He devises and installs new or
modified accounting systems to provide complete and accurate records of
hospital assets, liabilities, and financial transactions. He evaluates
accounting and patient business service procedures to plan methods for
insuring timely receipt of payments on patient accounts, reducing costs of
accounting operations, and expediting flow of work. He compiles information
about new equipment, such as cost and labor saving features, application to
hospital accounting procedures, and storage requirements. He prepares or
directs subordinates in preparing hospital budgets based on past, current
and anticipated expenditures and revenues. He directs compilation of data
and preparation of financial and operating reports for planning effective
administration of hospital activities by management. He prepares detailed
analyses of financial statements to reflect variances in income, expenditures,
and capital asset values from previous periods; makes recommendations to the
administration concerning means of reducing hospital operating costs and
increasing revenues, based on knowledge of market trends, financial reports
and industry operating procedures.

He participates in discussions with the finance committee concerning such matters as equipment purchases and construction of additional

---

[27]Ibid.

facilities. Arranges for audits of hospital accounts. Computes and records depreciation on buildings, equipment and real estate holdings. Examines insurance policies to ascertain that hospital assets are properly insured against loss. He is responsible for preparation of cost reimbursement reports to government and private third party agencies.

He supervises the account(s) bookkeepers(s) admitting clerks, cashier, business office manager, payroll clerk, credit and collections and audit clerks.

A Bachelor of Science degree in accounting or a Bachelor of Business Administration degree with a major in accounting is a minimum requirement. Certification by State Board as a Certified Public Accountant may also be required. A minimum of three to five years' experience as an accountant is required plus from six to nine months' on-the-job training to become thoroughly familiar with hospital policies and procedures would be deemed advisable.

Executive Vice-President for Medical Groups

According to the plan, the Medical Directors, or their nominees (who shall in any case be a partner in a RMG), of the various Regional Medical Groups, will cast votes at a special meeting called for the purpose of electing one of their number to the position of Executive Vice-President for Regional Medical Groups. Nominations for this position shall be made at a partnership group meeting preceding the meeting at which the election is held. Candidates must be partners.

The holder of this position will be the chief spokesman and representative of the medical doctors who are the partners in the Regional Medical Groups. He will express the majority opinions of and represent the partners in both the professional as well as the business aspects of their negotiations with the H.M.O. Plan, Inc.

Breaches of professional practice or other such matters will be reviewed by a committee of partners chaired by the Executive Vice-President for Regional Medical Groups.

Professional Level

The recruiting of the physicians might present more difficulties than other personnel and the usual charges by those in private practice against group practice and its alleged impersonal attitudes, will need to be overcome. The best chance for attracting physicians will probably be in approaching the younger man just completing his residency, military service or post-graduate training. Working with an H.M.O. will give such a young physician a taste of private practice in a group setting.

Table V - 4 shows the percentage distribution by length of service in the Permanente Medical Group, North Carolina Region.[28] From these

---

[28] *American Medical News*, September 13, 1971.

figures it appears that almost half of the region's physicians would be younger people probably gaining more experience before attempting to set up a practice of their own. By joining a well established group practice and earning a fairly high salary right away, the young doctor can build up financial reserves to help launch him independently later.

TABLE V - 4

PERCENTAGE DISTRIBUTION OF PHYSICIANS BY
LENGTH OF SERVICE WITH A MEDICAL GROUP[29]

Permanente Medical Group; North Carolina
Region.

Years Service with PMG	Per cent of Physicians
0 - 5	48%
6 - 10	25
11 - 15	10
16 - 20	13
21 - 25	3
26 - 30	1
	100%

Source: AMA News, Sept. 12, 1971.

The academic year, 1971 has seen the commencement of the first undergraduate class in Medicine on Long Island. The State University of New York at Stony Brook has inaugurated a Medical School and it would be highly recommended if an affiliation with the faculty and student body could be arranged with a Long Island based H.M.O. so that the nucleus of professionals could be used to provide patient service in the early days of its functioning. There is precedent for the use of medical teaching staff for H.M.O. patient services for this has been done under the Yale Health Plan, the Harvard Health Plan and the Community Health Foundation of Cleveland, Ohio were faculty of the Western Reserve University School of Medicine provide part-time services in the treatment of subscribers to the plan.[30]

General Functions of Physicians in the Group

When a subscriber enrolls in the H.M.O. he will select one of the RMG's as his "home base" for medical services, preferably one closest to

---

[29]Ibid.

[30]Avram Yedida, U. S. Dept. of H.E.W. Planning and Implementation of Community Health Foundation of Cleveland, Ohio, Case Study, 1969 Public Health Service.

266

his residence. He can select one of the general or family doctors as his primary physician for general supervision of his family's health, including health counseling and advice, periodic health examinations, diagnosis and treatment of illness which does not require referral to the relevant specialist for that ailment.

If, in the primary physician's opinion, the services of a consultant are required, he arranges for consultation and laboratory services at the main H.M.O. medical center. The reports of the examination are sent back to the "home base" RMG primary physician for him to interpret to the patient and his family.

Specialists render only those services for which they are qualified, and make a complete report to the referring physician. The opinion given to the patient following consultation will usually be based on joint discussion between the family physician, pediatrician or obstetrician-gynecologist or other specialist.

Under the plan, each specialty has a Chief, Board Certified in his specialty who is active in and responsible for the clinical work of his department. His assistants must be at least Board Eligible, that is, they must have completed the prerequisite training in the specialty, have practised the specialty under certified hospital residency requirements and be eligible to take the Specialty Board examination for full qualification.[31]

The Chief of each service will maintain his principal office at the main H.M.O. Medical Center where he will be available for consultation with patients referred to him by physicians in the various RMG's. He may also visit local RMG's when required for special purposes or when work loads become heavier than usual at any clinic.

In general, the work week of physicians in an RMG will be divided as follows:[32]

Medical Department

1. RMG physicians will have office sessions of approximately 25 to 30 hours each week. This will include one evening a week or Saturday morning.

2. Depending on the size of the RMG, physicians will be on back-up call one evening a week from 5 p.m. to 8 a.m. Calls will be screened and only those requiring a special house call or who need to be hospitalized will be referred to the physician on call. They will also be on call one weekend periodically depending upon the number of general physicians in the RMG who can share his duty.

3. Internists will rotate through the RMG's "urgent visit sessions" unless the RMG employs a full-time "urgent visit physician" or part-time UVP for evenings,

_____
[31]HIP Brochure: Information for Physicians, op. cit., p. 5.
[32]Ibid.

267

Saturdays, Sundays and holidays. Urgent visit sessions
are for those who are ill and have no appointment.
These sessions are not required but are recommended
because they avoid interference with the family
physicians' appointment schedule.

4. A centralized emergency service will operate from the
    H.M.O. Medical Center where ambulance transportation
    will be located and from where it will be dispatched.

5. Each RMG's Medical Department will conduct hospital
    rounds to review the RMG's hospitalized patients.
    Internists will be assigned to chart reviews at the
    hospital on a rotation basis. Case conference will
    also be conducted at each group clinic usually once
    a week with attendance by the RMG's physicians being
    obligatory as far as possible. Peer review sessions
    may also be conducted or initiated at these times.

Pediatric Department

This will be organized very much as is the department of Internal
Medicine, except that special time will be set aside in each pediatric
session for telephone calls from mothers.

Other Specialists

The specialist's work week will vary with the size of the RMG.
Those specialists with full time responsibilities in the RMG will have much
the same schedule as the primary physicians.

Contractual Arrangements for Doctors

Four different levels of status exist for the medical practitioner
working under the auspices of the H.M.O. prepaid group practice plan.[33]

(a) partner   (b) full-time employee

(c) part-time employee   (d) Consultant specialist
                                         (fee-for-service)

In the case of (d) above, the Specialist Consultant, such a man
may be used only rarely where a particularly difficult surgical procedure
or baffling medical case is met with, requiring consultation with an eminent
specialist in the field. In such a case, a fee-for-service arrangement
without written contract would be undertaken between the H.M.O. RMG and the
Consultant.

In most plans, extra-curricular or confidential fiscal arrangements
between affiliated physicians and persons enrolled under H.M.O. contract are

---

[33]
  See Specimen Agreement, (a) Appendix A (b) Appendix B.

268

forbidden.[34] Fee-for-service care may be provided for patients not enrolled in the H.M.O. plan by physicians of the Regional Medical Group, but all income therefrom is pooled and distributed after provision for expenses, in a manner mutually agreed upon in the partnership documents.

Interns and residents on hospital staffs may not be affiliated with an RMG, except that they may serve in after hours emergency service programs, or when under the direct supervision of an RMG partner.[35]

Semi-Professional and Technical Level

A Health Maintenance Organization is labor intensive to an unusual degree. The highly trained core of professional doctors, dentists, nurses, pharmacists, while a key element in the health services work force, account for only a little more than one-third of total health service personnel. The other two-thirds, is composed mainly of practical nurses, nurses' aides, laundry workers, kitchen helpers, housekeeping-maintenance staff, attendants, laboratory technicians, administrative services and related tasks. These jobs range from unskilled labor to highly skilled professionals.[36]

The proper utilization of these workers' skills and their employment in the correct proportions, is essential to the efficient and financially responsible running of any health facility. Advances in medical science and health technology are bringing about changes in the kinds of work performed by health workers, and formalizing the techniques into many new types of jobs. Thus traditional occupational patterns in the health service industry are being altered to permit of greater specialization.

Since 1952, new jobs added in many of the larger hospitals include computer programmer, inhalation therapist, heart-lung machine operator, medical record technician, dialysis technician, communications coordinator, catheterization technician and radio-active materials specialist and many others.

Naturally, in the smaller facility it would not be possible to employ as many of the highly specialized technicians as have emerged of late and an experienced Medical Director or Administrator would decide on the proper job combinations required for their facility.

In the developmental stages of the H.M.O. Medical Center, only a relatively small percentage of the possible positions will be required to be filled because if the ratio of hospital beds to enrolled population as prescribed by the Kaiser-Permanente experience of 1.85 beds per thousand is followed, an enrollment of 50,000 members means that a hospital of 95 to 110 beds should be provided for.

Several hospitals in Nassau and Suffolk counties were contacted by telephone to inquire about the ratio of nonphysician employees to hospital

---

[34] HIP Brochure: Information for Physicians, op. cit., p. 5.

[35] Ibid.

[36] U.S. Dept. of Labor, Job Descriptions, op. cit., p. xiv preface.

beds and in general it was found that there were between 2.1 and 2.6 employees per bed.[37] The Kaiser-Permanente program employs about seven allied
health professionals and other paramedical employees for every physician,
as compared to a national ratio estimated at ten to one.[38] Thus to support
the Kaiser plan's 2,000 physicians there are approximately 14,000 other
employees, of whom 4,000 are nurses and 10,000 are other health workers.
Kaiser hospitals employ an estimated two persons per patient as compared
with 2.8 per patient in nonfederal short-term general hospitals, based on
the adjusted average daily census.

All Other Health Service Workers

Information on health service positions has been compiled in the
latest and most comprehensive source available, the U.S. Dept. of Labor,
Manpower Administration's publication, released in June 1971, entitled:
"Job Descriptions and Organizational Analysis for Hospitals and Related
Health Services." No better source can be cited, especially since the
report was compiled by the joint efforts of the U. S. Training and Employment
Service, the American Hospital Association, in cooperation with selected
hospitals throughout the United States. Full descriptions of the jobs whose
titles are listed in Table VI - 5, will be found in this government publication which is available from the Superintendent of Documents, U. S.
Government Printing Office, Washington, D. C. 20402. ($4.25 per copy post-
paid).

It might seem however, that the job descriptions and organizational
analyses as given in the U. S. Dept. of Labor guidebook are geared more
towards application in a hospital setting than in a Regional Medical Group.
But, since there is an almost perfect correlation of skills for the same
type of job in an RMG as in a hospital, the description should suffice. A
medical secretary in an RMG office would perform much the same duties as
she would in a hospital. A bookkeeper in one or other setting would similarly work under almost identical principles.

In the scaled-down version, where a smaller staff is required,
there are jobs which will be done by one person which, in a larger setting,
might be performed by several employees. For example, the business office
manager, might also handle credit approval and approval of insurance plan
payments. He might also supervise and hire the office clericals. In a
small operation, the same bookkeeping clerk might handle both accounts payable and accounts receivable; the admitting officer may also function as
cashier and release officer. In the large hospitals, such jobs as "salad
and dessert preparer," "dietetic clerk," baker, blood bank technologist,
director of volunteer services, incinerator man, speech pathologist, may be
normally required, but not so for a 100 to 200 bed facility.

---

[37] July 16, 1971, Mrs. Glenn Ass't. Administrator, Central General Hospital,
Plainview, N.Y.
Dr. Behrer, Nassau Hospital, Mineola, N.Y.
Miss Pearl Klick, Administrator, Syosset Hospital, N.Y.
Mr. D. Buckley, Director, North Shore Hospital, Manhasset, N.Y.
Mr. Potorsky, Suffolk County Hospital Affairs Office.

[38] Carnegie Commission Report on Higher Education: Higher Education and the
Nation's Health.

TABLE V - 5

CLASSIFICATION OF HEALTH SERVICE JOBS BY DEPARTMENT[39]

Executive Department

Chief Executive/Administrator
Associate Administrators:
 a. medical   b. general
Administrative assistant
Administrative secretary

Financial Management Dept.

Controller
Accountant
Accounting Clerk
Accounts Receivable/Payable clerk(s)
Admitting Officer & admitting clerk
Audit clerk
Bookkeeper
Business Office Manager
Cashier Coding, billing clerk
Credit & Collection, Insurance Liason clerk
Payroll clerk

General Clerical Department

Medical secretary
Medical stenographer
Secretary
Typist
Receptionist
Telephone Operator
Mail-room clerk;Xerox-duplicating machine
    operator
General clerk; file clerk; general office
    clerk
Clerk-typist
Messenger
Hospital guide/Page

Personnel Department

Personnel Director
Employment Manager
Job Analyst/Training Director
Personnel Assistant
Statistical clerk (could be combined with
                payroll clerk in a small
                office)

Training Department

Director/coordinator
Training programs

Instructor(s)

Public Relations Dept.

Director, P. R.
Public Information Officer
Subscriber Relations

Purchasing, Receiving,Stores

Purchasing Agent
Stock clerk
Storeman

---

[39] Job Titles listed in Table V are those most commonly used as defined in the U. S. Dept. of Labor Manpower Administration, Job Descriptions, op. cit.

TABLE V - 5 (continued)

Classification of Health Service Jobs by Department

PROFESSIONAL CARE DIVISION

Central Service Department

Director Central Service
Central Service Technician

Clinical Laboratories Dept.

Pathologist
Biochemist & Biochem. Technologist
Cytotechnologist
Hematologist & Hematology Technician
Laboratory Aides
Microbiologist & Technician
Serologist & Technician
Medical Lab. Assistant
Medical Technologist

Food Service Department

Director, Food Service
Dietitian, Administrative
Dietitian, Therapeutic
Food Production Supervisor
Cook
Dietetic Clerk
Dining Service Worker
Patient Food-Service Worker

Nursing Service Department

Director, Nursing Service
Assistant Director, Nursing
Nurse Supervisor, Day/Night
Staff Nurse (R.N.)
Licensed Practical Nurse
Nursing Aide
Orderly-Ward clerk
Surgical Technician
Operating Room Nurse
Ward Service Manager

Medical Library Department

Medical Librarian
Library Assistant

Pharmacy Department

Director, Pharmacy
Services: Chief Pharmacist
Pharmacist
Dispensary Clerk
Pharmacy Helper

Medical Records Dept.

Medical Records Librarian
Medical Records Clerk

Out-Patient Department

Director, O-P Services
Clinic Coordinator
Ambulance Driver
Ambulance Attendant

Physical Medicine & Rehabilitation Dept.

Physiatrist
Coordinator
Corrective Therapist
Educational Therapist
Occupational Therapist
Physical Therapist

Dept. of Radiology and Nuclear Medicine

Dir., Radiology, Nuclear Med.
Radiologist
Radiologic Technologist
Darkroom Attendant

Social Service Dept.

Director, Social Service
Medical Social Worker
Psychiatric Social Worker

TABLE V - 5 (continued)

Classification of Health Service Jobs by Department

Technical Services Department

Cardio-Pulmonary Technician
Dialysis Technician
Electrocardiograph/electroencephalograph
  Technician
Inhalation Therapist
Orthopedic appliance and limb specialist
Prosthetic-Orthoptist
Therapy Technician

Catheterization Technician
Heart-Lung Machine Operator
Orthopedic cast Specialist
Orthoptist
Pulmonary Function Technician
Thermograph Technician

Plant Operation & Maintenance Dept.

Director, Plant Operations
Carpenter
Dispatcher, Maintenance Services
Electrical Repairman
Electromedical equipment Repairman
Fireman, Stationary Boiler
Guard
Maintenance Mechanic
Maintenance Helper

Housekeeping Department

Director, Housekeeping Services
Housekeeping Supervisor
Housekeeping Crew Leader
Housekeeping Aide
Housekeeping Attendant
Linen Room Aide

Laundry Department

Laundry Manager
Foreman, Washing
Foreman, Finishing
Stockroom Inventory Controller
Seamstress
Washman
Extractor Man
Tumbler Operator
Flatwork Finisher
Sorter-Marker
Shaker
Presser, Hand
Presser, Operator
Porter

Physician Assistants

A nomenclature for designating emerging health professionals has
been suggested by the founder of the Medex program, Dr. Richard A. Smith.
Writing in the Sept. 6, 1971 issue of the American Medical Association
Journal, he contends that the category now generally referred to as
physician's assistant should be re-named "paraphysician."[40]

Within this category of paraphysician there should be subdivision
of primary and specialty areas:

    (a) A Primary Paraphysician would be the "Nurse clinician/
        practitioner (generalist); other names suggested for
        this function are "medex" and Osler" (a paraphysician
        generalist). An "Osler," the article states, would be
        "an individual trained to assist general practitioners
        and other primary care providers." The category is
        named after the late Sir William Osler, considered by
        many to be the father of the art of modern medicine.

    (b) The name, Flexner would be assigned to the physician's
        assistant/specialist who has been trained solely to
        assist in surgery under the supervision of a surgeon.
        The category is named after Abraham Flexner, whose
        study of U. S. medical education in the early 1900's
        revolutionized the profession.

    (c) The name, Cruzer would be the designation given to the
        professional assistant to the physician in the non-
        surgical specialties especially internal medicine-
        pediatrics. The title derives from the late Oswaldo
        Cruz, M.D. who was a Brazilian doctor who pioneered
        in the control of infectious diseases.

In addition to the physician's assistant nomenclature, other
suggested titles have been considered for health professionals in emergency
room settings, nursing and other allied health fields.[41] The nomenclature
is designed, "to give the emerging health professionals an identity which
is not confusing, and to provide them with a sense of status in the professional environment..."[42] In developing names for the new health and medical
workers, the article said, those which can be used to address such individuals at work, as well as to connote tasks they can perform, should be used.

Purchased and Part-time Services

Occasions will arise when temporary additional help will be
required. There should be provision in the financial budget to permit such

---

[40]"Health Professionals Renamed in M.D.'s Plan," American Medical News,
October 1971.

[41]Dr. Richard A. Smith, "A Strategy for Health Manpower," Journal of American
Medical Assoc., Sept. 6, 1971.

[42]Ibid.

temporary manpower to be employed when necessary. Purchased services might include the hiring of a special medical consultant on a fee-for-service basis, to treat an unusual case arising with a subscriber; or special treatment not available within the H.M.O. facilities might be necessary. These special services and needs will therefore be made available under the provisions suggested here.

Circumstances might require the services of a management consultant, structural and construction engineer or computer specialist to advise H.M.O. management on problems which might occur in any one of those areas. Funds should be allocated to permit such consultant to be engaged without difficulty.

Two vital purchased services which have not been provided for elsewhere in the overall Manpower Plan are:

(a) Legal Counsel

(b) Public Accountants-Auditors

In both instances it is more usual to retain the services of competent firms in these professions than to try to provide full, in-house service by employees, even though they may be fully qualified to do so. Broader contacts of the various members of the retained firms with a greater variety of special areas would give obvious advantages that a one or two man in-house department would not be capable of having. Further, the cost of retaining such firms would probably be less than if a legal department or a full auditing department were maintained by H.M.O. Plan, Inc. In both of these cases, the fees would be budgeted for under the provisions of "purchased services."

Voluntary Workers

In most nonprofit community hospitals, a corps of voluntary workers attends to providing supplemental services to aid and comfort the ill by performing numerous tasks to relieve the busy work load of the nurses and other staff. These workers must be organized, trained and motivated to perform the duties assigned to them.

As their title implies, these workers are unpaid, yet they should bring to the performance of their jobs, the same enthusiasm and conscientious attitude that would be expected of paid workers. Close integration of hospital activities and volunteer functions is essential.

The supervision of volunteer workers can be delegated to either the Senior Nurse Supervisor, or the Associate Administrator (General) of the hospital, depending upon the type of work to be assigned to the volunteer. At such time as the Medical Center develops to a more substantial size when the services of a staff Director of Volunteer Services can be obtained, the two officials mentioned above will have to perform the job.

Acquisition of Personnel

Recruitment. In order to obtain and maintain an effective work force, the organization must have accurate and current information on the number and qualifications of workers needed. The process of recruiting, selecting and inducting a new worker to the organization may require a considerable lead time for its proper fulfillment. Under ideal conditions, job openings should be anticipated as far ahead as possible so as to permit the proper screening and selection of the most suitable candidates and to maintain a more efficient and stable work force.[43]

For a Health Maintenance Organization, manpower planning and recruitment is directly correlated with the size of the enrollment to be served, since the members provide almost all the revenues. Therefore, the size of the work force must be kept strictly in balance with immediate needs to supply service to the subscribers.

If the organization is to be staffed effectively, management must know where to obtain those persons who are most qualified to fill each position vacancy, as well as have the means of securing applications from the best qualified personnel, even if they are already working elsewhere. It can be just as important for an organization to seek out the best manpower as it is to obtain the best grade of raw materials, equipment and finance arrangements. Frequently the most suitable personnel are the ones who are already employed and not those who may happen to be available. Aggressive recruitment of such people must be considered, especially of fully qualified people who have occupied a post for some time as second-in-charge of a department and who would like a chance to develop as head of a department in a different organization.

As the need for staff arises, a routine method of requisitioning applicants will be established whereby the details of the position to be filled can be made known to the personnel department so that recruitment can be commenced. A personnel requisition form, Figure V - 4, shows what data must be supplied so that the specified position can be recruited for. The departmental supervisor will interview the applicants already screened by the personnel department, and report his findings to that department which will then notify the applicant of the outcome.

Recruitment is typically done through:

a. Newspaper or magazine advertisement;

b. House-organ or bulletin board notice;

c. Word of mouth at meetings, conferences, conventions;

---

[43] H.J. Chruden & A. W. Sherman, Jr., Personnel Management, 3rd ed. Southwest Publ. Co. 1968, pp. 109-133.

d. Employment agencies;

e. Professional organizations and societies and their journals;

f. Referral to industry sources such as other hospitals, universities, nursing schools, colleges, high school guidance counselors, union offices, state, county or federal employment services.[44]

FIGURE V - 4

Personnel Requisition

H.M.O. Plan, Inc.
H.M.O. Medical Center, Inc.
Regional Medical Group:

Requisitioning Department:

Location:

Job Title: Date to be filled by:

Job Specifications:

Job Qualifications:

Educational Requirements:

This job reports to:

Applicants to be interviewed by:

Salary Range:

Method of recruitment:
(a) Internal referral or transfer

(b) Newspaper, magazine advertisement; which?

    When?

(c) Employment agency. Which?

Other comments:

This Personnel Requisition Authorized By: ....

Date:..........................

---

[44]The College Placement Council is undertaking a placement assistance Program for employers and college graduates and alumni to provide an information retrieval system to operate nationally. This system, known as GRAD (Graduate Resume Accumulation & Distribution) program is designed to store on magnetic tape the personal placement files of graduates seeking employment. the files are made available to an unlimited number of potential employers.

Recruitment and Selection Policy Issues

The caliber of an organization's work force largely determined its strength and success, yet the employment policies of many organizations are not formalized; they have just evolved as practices over the years and changed to suit an immediate situation. Such haphazard practice leads to abuse and injustice. There is much to be gained from the adoption of care- fully considered, stable employment policies which, "as statements of inten- tion and guides to action, can be positive instruments to shape the entire recruitment and selection program....and ensure consistency of action throughout."[45]

1. Internal/External Preference Hiring

If an opening occurs for a position, should preference be given to promote an employee to the position by transferring him/her from another department? Most organizations have a stated policy that they favor promotion from within as far as possible for the follow- ing advantages:

a. Most people expect to advance their careers to a higher pay and status; this policy fosters better morale when practiced.

b. Management can appraise the skills, knowledge and personality characteristics more accurately of those already in their employ, so there is less risk of error in placement, than for some applicant whose only contact with the organization has been an interview or two.

c. The processing of an internal placement is relatively simple.

There are also limitations and disadvantages to internal promotion, but as a generalization the most desirable policy is probably filling most vacancies from within, but going to the outside when fully qualified talent is not otherwise available. "It is also probably wise to fill a moderate percentage of the higher level managerial and professional positions by going to the outside labor market to inject new ideas into the organization."[46]

2. Public Policy: Fair Employment Practices

In the past decade, civil rights legislation and a changing climate of social responsibility have brought about a more conscious effort to engage in fairer employment practices. Evidence of this is seen by such statements included in newspaper personnel advertisements as "an equal opportunity employer" and "this position is open to all regardless of race, creed, color, or national origin."

No large employer can afford to show bias towards any ethnic group and especially in health services positions the way has been opened for all

---

[45]Dale S. Beach, Personnel: The Management of People at Work, 2nd ed. New York: MacMillan & Co. 1970, pp. 216-217.

[46]Ibid., p. 218.

to participate at their own level of competence in this important work. Of more recent origin is the movement to overcome discrimination based upon sex. Male nurses and para-medicals and female doctors are becoming more visible now and the concentrated attention of the Womens' Liberation Movement is forcing sex discrimination into public notice for the purpose of exposing the fallacy of stereotyped sex-role jobs.

Age bias, usually in favor of the young has also come under fire and to meet the problem, the U. S. Congress enacted the Age Discrimination in Employment Act of 1967 which declared its intention to protect and promote the employment of those between 40 and 65 years of age.[47]

Selection of Personnel[48]

The following steps should generally be taken in personnel selection procedure:

1. Reception in personnel office; brief discussion on purpose of visit;

2. Completion of application blank;

3. Brief review of completed application blank;

4. Selection tests; (done before main interview so that test results can be seen and evaluated by interviewer);

5. Main employment office interview;

6. Investigation of applicant's background;

7. Final selection interview by manager or department Supervisor.

8. Medical review or examination;

9. Induction

The decision to add persons to the payroll in particular departments is not a function of the personnel department. It is a duty of the operating or line management which initiates an employment requisition that is sent to the personnel department for action. When an applicant presents himself/herself for a position, an employment application blank of a type available from commercial stationers (or contained in many books on personnel practices)[49] will be completed before an interview is given. This form

---

[47]Ibid., p. 221.

[48]Ibid., p. 236.

[49]For example see Wilbert E. Scheer, Personnel Director's Handbook, Dartnell Publ. 2nd ed. 1970 or: Dale Yoder, Personnel Management & Industrial Relations 6th ed.,(Englewood Cliffs,N.J.: Prentice-Hall, 1970).

summarizes much important biographical data about the applicant and permits transmission and comparison of the information in a uniform pattern.

After an initial screening by a personnel department interviewer to clarify any details not properly attended to by the applicant, he will be given a series of selection tests, in the case of applicants for nonprofessional jobs.

Selection Tests

These are usually specially constructed by industrial psychologists and grew out of the World War I army Alpha test used to aid in the selection and placement of soldiers in duties they seemed most suited to. Testing procedures are very complex and varied and need expert understanding and interpretation when administered for certain types of positions. Reference to more technical discussion on this topic can be found in books suggested in the footnote.[50-51-52]

Upon completion of the tests, the candidate will be introduced to the departmental representative authorized to conduct the interview specifically in the area for which employment is being considered. Thus a bookkeeping candidate would be interviewed by the controller or a senior accountant; an X-ray technician would be interviewed by the radiologist.

As far as possible, the interviewer should try to maintain the standards set forth in the job specifications for that position. If it is not possible, and the candidate is still deemed acceptable, reasons for acceptance outside of the job specifications should be noted in the interviewing report. Final approval by the head of the department authorizing the employment must be signed on the application form and interview report. Concluding formalities concerning the addition to the employment rolls of the organization are performed in the personnel office after all references and background checks have been made.

At the professional and senior administrative-executive level, the procedures will vary according to the method of recruitment. Usually, resumes of educational and work-related experience of these candidates are submitted to the President who may be authorized to hire such personnel on his own authority or he may need to submit his recommendation to the Board of Trustees for confirmation.

Employee Services and Benefits

Most employers provide benefits and services that add to the advantage, convenience and pleasure of working for them. Thus, department

---

[50] W. J. Barnett, Jr., Readings in Psychological Tests and Measurements, (Homewood, Illinois: Dorsey Press, 1964).

[51] E. E. Ghiselli, The Validity of Occupational Aptitude Tests, (New York: John Wiley Sons, Inc.,1966).

[52] R. M. Guion, Personnel Testing, (New York: McGraw-Hill, 1965).

stores permit their employees to make purchases at discount, banks may lend money at more advantageous rates of interest, and airlines allow their employees and family, travel privileges at greatly reduced prices. With the H.M.O., these service benefits will be more limited due to the nature of its "product," still, there may be other forms in which benefits could be provided and some of them are shown below.

1. Food Service. Since the Medical Center will have its own kitchen to provide for patient feeding, the same facilities can also provide cafeteria service at a subsidized rate to H.M.O. employees.

2. Health and Safety. Readily available diagnosis and treatment of employees and their family would be available within the H.M.O. system without charge, or at very nominal cost.

3. Uniform and Clothing Service. Those jobs requiring uniforms or laboratory coats would have them serviced by the hospital laundry.

4. Fringe Benefits. Additional benefits such as insurance, vacation, pensions are discussed in a later section of this chapter. (See "Compensation and Incentives.")

5. Sabbatical Leave. (for physicians only). After six consecutive years of full-time service, physicians are eligible for three months sabbatical leave at the option of the RMG. The H.M.O. may wish to contribute towards this sabbatical possibly at the rate of one-half of the minimum annual guaranteed salary as used in determination of the full-time physician bonus plan and up to $500 towards the cost of transportation, books and tuition.

6. Vacations. Regular vacations and time off for study will be provided. A customary vacation for professionals is one month, after the completion of a full year of service.[53] When a physician is off duty, his practice is fully covered by other physicians associated with the RMG.

A different set of standards and personnel policies applies to the physicians, both partners and employees (nonpartners because of their professional status and the need to maintain their interest in the plan rather than have them leave to become private practitioners. Some of the usual additional benefits applicable to the doctors are not available to other employees, although it might be beneficial to extend sabbatical leaves for study purpose to the more senior staff members in the highly technical occupations, such as microbiologists, hematologists, physican therapists, and biochemists. However, the extension of subsidized sabbatical leaves to such personnel might create an unwarranted financial burden on an organization such as H.M.O. Plan, Inc. Perhaps a modified scheme could be used as an occasional reward for exceptional service.

---

[53]HIP Brochure: Information for Physicians, op. cit., p. 13.

Compensation and Incentives

An equitable wage structure, fairly administered, is a major requirement of any well-managed organization. The greater mobility of the work force and the ready availability of information concerning salaries paid for almost all types of jobs, as listed in the classified advertisements in the major newspapers, make it mandatory for salaries to be closely comparable from one job to another of the same type in a similar institution. Therefore, it is not quite as possible as formerly to obtain "cheap labor." The going rate of pay for almost all categories of jobs has been largely predetermined by the labor market, so the personnel manager must keep up to date by reference to various sources such as the National Conference Board publications on compensation and salaries, or the periodic reviews on salaries of the American Management Association.[54]

Most enterprises recognize the necessity of having a secondary compensation scheme to attract and maintain the interest and loyalty of their employees. Especially since the early 1950's, the addition of "fringe benefits packages" has become virtually a mandatory part of the compensation of employees.[55]

Prepaid life insurance, major medical insurance, more liberal vacation policies and observance of public holidays, profit-sharing, annual merit cash bonus, stock options, company matched incentive contributions, subsidized college tuition costs, pension and retirement funds, seniority privileges, are some of the types of fringe benefits used.

It would not be practicable to set forth here, what the fringe benefits package should be in the H.M.O. Plan, Inc. Since it can add from 20 to 40 per cent to the cost of the payroll, it would be the province of the Board of Trustees to determine what fringe benefits and incentives could be afforded.

Forsyth and Thomas[56] have stated that hospitals operating around the clock, seven days a week, require the equivalent of 4.6 full time employees to cover one job for all three shifts. They state that labor accounts for about 65 per cent of a hospital's total operating costs, while

---

[54] These periodic salary reviews, divided into occupational groups, types of company, geographical region, size of company, size of budget and other statistical data are available to corporate members of the American Management Association as part of their service to member companies. Similarly, the National Industrial Conference Board's services is available to corporate members whose annual dues, based on the size of the company may amount to thousands of dollars, make them eligible to receive these confidential surveys.

[55] L. G. Reynolds, Labor Economics and Labor Relations, (Englewood Cliffs,N.J.: Prentice-Hall, 1954), pp. 595-598.

[56] Forsyth & Thomas, op. cit., pp. 106-7.

282

the Statistical Profile of the Nation's Hospitals published in the current (1971 August) annual report of the Journal of the American Hospital Association gives the figure that labor constituted about 58 per cent of hospital expenses. During 1970, expenses for community hospitals reached $19.6 billion - an increase of 248 per cent over the 1960 outlay of $5.6 billion. Thus the health services payroll for 1970 amounted to about $113.7 billion.[57]

Table V - 5 shows how increases in monthly starting salaries of several random selected hospital job categories have risen in the past six years, indicating how unionization in the health services field has affected personnel costs.

TABLE V - 5

INCREASES IN MONTHLY STARTING SALARIES
FOR VARIOUS HOSPITAL JOBS[58]

Job Title	1965	1971	Per cent Increase
Registered Nurse	$425	$720	69%
Licensed Practical Nurse	370	570	54
Nurses' Aide	350	515	68
Surgical Technician	405	660	63

Source: G. C. Forsyth & D.G. Thomas, "Models for Financially Health Hospitals, Harvard Business Review, July-August 1971, pp. 106-7.

The total expenses of hospitals increased annually by about ten per cent during the period 1950 to 1965, but with the introduction of Medicare in 1966, the annual rate of increase has been fairly consistent between 17.2 and 17.7 per cent.[59] No longer are hospital workers among the lowest paid on the economic ladder.

Employee Communications

It is impossible to have human relations without communications for communication is a network which binds all of the members of an organization together. Communication is the process of passing information and understanding from one person to another, or for conducting the attention

---

[57] Journal of the American Hospital Association, Annual Statistical Issue, August 1971, p. 454.

[58] Forsyth & Thomas, op. cit.

[59] Journal of American Hospital Association, op. cit.

of another person for the purpose of speech or demonstration, so that cooperative action can occur. It serves to motivate and direct people to act, as when a supervisor induces a subordinate to perform a task.

"The significance of communication was illustrated early in history by the incident of the Tower of Babel, recorded in Genesis of the Bible. When God chose to stop the building of the Tower, he confused the workers' tongues, thereby effectively ending the project."[60]

Leadership takes effect through the process or communication in its multiple forms. Without communication there is no leadership since leadership ideas are strictly "armchair thoughts" until the leader, through communications puts them into effect. "Communication is not an end itself, but it is the process by which ends are accomplished."[61]

When a problem arises the blame is often placed on poor communications. The theory says that if communications improve, the situation should get better. Good communication is vital to good employee relations, but too little is understood about what is useful communication. All too often, mere information is passed off as communication without concern as to whether the information can and will be understood. Thus much of the information is wasted.

For the manager, skill in speaking, listening, reading, writing and conversation is vital. His environment and his job are primarily involved in language and communication continually interacting with others in conferences, interviews, and telephone conversations. A multitude of reports, letters, documents and diagrams occupy 60 to 80 per cent of his total working hours as various forms of communication.[62]

Besides the communication of instructions and specific job-related information, many other forms of communications circulate in any organization, many other forms of communications circulate in any organization and it is important that proper channels be kept open for news and information to be disseminated accurately and not left to the chances of the "grapevine." Bulletin board notices, a house-organ organized through the personnel department where departmental representatives can leave copy about people and events for inclusion in the magazine, are some of the means of making the personnel of an H.M.O. feel as though they belong to a "family" where the other members are interested in them.

The house-organ is one of the most widely used media for downward communication within an organization and for reaching the families of employees. News about employees and their families is still the backbone of the house-organ, but employees are also interested in the plans and policies of the organization which might be written about there. The house-organ affords management an opportunity of maintaining good employee

---

[60]Keith Davis, op. cit., pp. 346-7.

[61]Ibid.

[62]Dale S. Beach, op. cit., p. 580.

relations by inculcating a team or family spirit by restating the importance of the work of the organization and each employee in it and by drawing to special attention the notable achievements of individuals.[63]

Creating the family spirit is especially important in an organization where facilities are spread out over various locations. Thus the members of each Regional Medical Group would feel more closely affiliated with the H.M.O.Medical Center when they read news from there as well as the news from other Regional Medical Groups in the H.M.O. Plan.

The list of employee communications media in Table V - 6 shows how many and varied are the means by which information of all types flows around people in an organization. Not all of these media are available in all organizations, but it is rare indeed for there to be difficulty in obtaining information of the sort that is necessary for an employee to have.

TABLE V - 6

EMPLOYEE COMMUNICATIONS MEDIA[64]

Bulletin Boards - Company or departmental, prominently located and well maintained.

Employee Magazine - (house organ) For personals, news, social activities.

Company Magazine - For products, services, history, plans.

Newsletter - Digest of news and current events relating to company business.

Employee Handbook - Rules and regulations, working conditions.

Benefit Book (companion handbook) - Welfare and insurance programs.

Policy Manual - Helpful guide on official company position.

Job Manual - Departmental guide on performance of each job.

Indoctrination - Individual consultations to get new workers off to a good start.

Orientation - Group meetings of both new and old employees to influence attitude of employees towards company objectives.

Individual Counseling - On job-related and personal problems.

Performance Rating Interviews - To tell the employee how he is doing and where he may improve.

Suggestion System - To give formal recognition to good ideas.

Grievance Procedure - To resolve problems in troublesome areas.

---

[63]Wilbert E. Scheer, Personnel Director's Handbook, Dartnell Publ. 2nd ed. 1970, p. 461.
[64]Ibid., p. 462.

TABLE V - 6 (continued)

Group Meetings - To announce or explain organization changes, new
   products, financial stability, results, progress, programs.

Public Address System - For quick messages and late news.

Annual Report - To reassure employee of company growth and personal job
   security.

Performance Appraisal

Each position in an organization is filled in order to meet a
particular need in the overall plan designed to achieve the organizational
goal. In the words of the old saying that "a chain is only as strong as
its weakest link," it becomes necessary for management to maintain a system
of inspection of each link (i.e. department, supervisor, employee) so that
a uniformly efficient structure is maintained.

This system if inspection is called performance appraisal and while
regular day to day appraisals of subordinates are made in every supervisor's
mind, for equitable reasons, a more systematic approach is required in order
to assure thoughtful, thorough appraisal to be recorded for later use by the
organization in considering promotions, salary increases or any other action.

Performance appraisal is most valuable in helping management with
its forward manpower planning, but it is also useful in appraising the
appraiser's own performance as well. If the supervisor is having problems
with his staff, the trouble may lie with the supervisor's own methods of
communication, instruction or interpersonal relationships. In manpower
planning the appraisal is concerned with a person's potential ability, while
for salary review, the appraisal reviews primarily his past performance.

In the more routine types of job, performance appraisal is
measured against the basic job specification filed in the department. The
usual job behaviour criteria, lateness, cooperation, willingness to work,
utilization of time on the job, absenteeism, excessive personal telephone
use, are rated. Comments by the supervisor as to whether prior attention
has been drawn to the employee to such infractions should also be made.
These reports are then passed on to the department manager who passes them
in turn to the personnel manager, after examination and discussion with the
appraiser.

Appraisal of department managers will be the province of the
President or his delegated authority. For the more technical and professional
areas where competence, knowledge, dedication and keeping abreast of recent
developments are basic criteria for performance appraisal, the standards
will be more exacting and here, the department manager should be directly
concerned in the appraisal.

Figure V - 7 shows a typical performance appraisal form with a
simple graphic rating scale. A list of qualifications or attributes are
noted in the left hand column, designed to describe an employee in terms of
a numerical rating scale. If an employee is chronically late for work, the

appraiser would check this fact in the extreme right column under number one for "poor;" a high rating for knowledge would be checked in column five.

FIGURE V - 7

PERFORMANCE APPRAISAL FORM[65]

Simple Graphic Rating Scale

Name: Position:

Department: Location:

Appraisal Date: Appraiser:

Check rating figure for each quality: Excellent. Good. Avge. Fair. Poor

Qualification	Excellent 5	Good 4	Average 3	Fair 2	Poor 1	Other Comment
works consistently						
accepts responsibility						
shows initiative						
attendance						
cooperation						
follows instructions						
shows judgment						
neat & orderly						
learns readily						
communicates						
sense of economy						
dependable						
punctual						
knowledgeable						
time utilization						

[65]Adapted from Dale Yoder, Personnel Management and Industrial Relations, 6th ed. (Englewood Cliffs, N.J.: Prentice-Hall, N.J. 1970), p. 239.

Where specific skills relating to a particular job are concerned the data in the qualifications or attributes column could be directed to the details of that job. For example, in rating a delivery truck driver questions as to on-time deliveries, correct paper work, accurate deliveries, frequency of damages claims, care of his equipment, driving skill, accident rating are some of the points to be covered.

However, it has been said that human attributes should not be reduced to numerical simplicity for in the area of human relations, "the things that count most cannot be counted."[66] Work does not exist merely to produce more or better goods and services, but it affords the principal means by which individuals may gain satisfaction to accomplish something more than merely sustaining their own lives.

Over the years subtle changes have occurred in the attitudes towards performance appraisal and in more enlightened managements, a somewhat more meaningful and human approach has evolved. Figure V - 7 summarizes the major changes in emphasis in performance appraisal over the years.

Peer Review

For physicians, the American Medical Association[67] recently agreed on an official definition of the term "peer review" and stated that all county and state medical societies should take an active part in it. Documentation of such activity will not only be in their own interests, but also in the public interest stated a resolution passed by the AMA House of Delegates. The resolution also reaffirmed AMA's support of "voluntary

FIGURE V - 7

TRENDS IN PERFORMANCE APPRAISAL[68]

Item	Former Emphasis	Present Emphasis
Terminology	Merit Rating	Employee Appraisal Performance Appraisal
Purpose	Determine qualification for wage increase, transfer, promotion, layoff	Development of the individual; improved performance on the job
Application	For hourly paid workers	For technical, professional and managerial employees
Factors Rated	Heavy emphasis is on personal traits	Performance, results, accomplishments
Techniques	Rating scales with emphasis on scores. Statistical manipulation of data for comparison purposes	Appraisal by results, mutual goal setting, critical incidents, group appraisal, performance standards, less quantitative;

---

[66]W. E. Scheer, op. cit., pp. 32-33.

[67]American Medical News, October 1971.

[68]Dale S. Beach, op. cit., p. 334.

FIGURE V - 7 (continued)

Item	Former Emphasis	Present Emphasis
Post-Appraisal Interview	Supervisor communicates his rating to employee and tries to sell his evaluation, seeks to have employee conform to his views	Supervisor stimulates employee to analyze himself and set own objectives in line with job requirements, supervisor is helper and counselor

Chart summarizing changing emphasis in performance appraisal over the years.

mechanisms of review and education by physicians."[69] The official definition of peer review, in this case dealing only with physician peer review is: "Evaluation by practicing physicians of the quality and efficiency of services rendered or ordered by other practicing physicians." Peer review, an AMA document reported, "is the all-inclusive term for medical review efforts."[70]

While this is a relatively new development for the AMA to endorse, the peer-review system has been working effectively since 1954 as part of the system of the nonprofit San Joaquin Foundation for Medical Care in California.[71] Under this system, panels of local doctors review the medical services provided by 96 of the area's physicians to 150,000 patients covered by 12 private health insurance plans, the federal government's medicare and California's Medi-Cal program for the medically ingident. Their formula has been effective enough to inspire 17 imitators in California alone. Checks on overutilization of certain procedures (e.g. vitamin or penicillin injections) has saved between 12 and 15 per cent of the costs of these procedures and has been a restraining factor. Routine processing of all reimbursement claims by computer has been invaluable in spotting overutilization, then subject to peer review.

Skills Inventory

Many organizations coast along in the comfortable belief that all pertinent information about their employees' experience and skills is on file somewhere. Unfortunately the trouble with this assumption is that the information believed to be "somewhere" is really "nowhere" when needed at short notice and more probably not available anywhere in the organization in current, presentable form.[72]

---

[69]American Medical News, October 1971.

[70]Ibid.

[71]Business Week, "Where the Doctors Police the Doctors, September 4, 1971, p. 58.

[72]T. H. Patten, Jr. Manpower Planning & the Development of Human Resources, Wiley Interscience, 1970, p. 236.

A small organization with fewer than 100 people has little need for a formal skills inventory since a more personal knowledge of each member of the organization is usual and informal records will suffice to keep track of each person's skills. As the organization grows, it is essential to maintain more accurate and standardized records of each person's skills.

A skills inventory must be designed so that a searcher can find specific items of information without knowing beforehand just where they are located in the file. It is therefore a register of information accompanied by a system for retrieving the data. In order to maintain accurate information in the personnel files of each employee, their records must be updated whenever any changes occur in the employee's skills, education, status or capabilities. The employee's supervisor should pass new information to the personnel department.

A skills inventory gives employees a concrete demonstration that the organization recognizes skills and will call on them when needed. The information contained on the inventory will be divided into seven groups:[73]

1. Personal history data; age, sex, marital status, number of dependents, draft and military reserve status and prior military service.

2. Basic skills information including a history of formal education, degrees earned, previous job experience and training, facility with foreign languages, hobbies and other areas of special interest.

3. Special qualifications, experience such as foreign travel or residence, patents, publications, honors and other types of recognition; membership in professional or other occupationally significant organizations and any record of special assignments completed; participation in civic or community service work.

4. Salary and occupational progression history. This would include his present and past salary as well as a history of the positions which he has occupied and the rates of advancement in his career. Because of its confidential nature this part of an employee's profile should be kept separate and sent only to those authorized to examine it.

5. Organizational data such as pension and retirement fund accumulations, beneficiary assignments, life insurance information, disability insurance electives, bonuses received, stock plan purchases, stock options granted and exercised, incentive plan payments, payroll savings bond purchases and any other financial arrangements between the employee and the organization.

[73] Ibid.

290

6. Performance appraisal data from past evaluations and to the present; reports from any psychological tests taken together with test scores; significant health information.

7. Job location preferences as well as any other special interests which the employee might have that could have a bearing on his employment and occupational utilization. For example, at some time an employee might have expressed a desire to a supervisor to be trained for another job if the opportunity arose. Under a computerized system any data on an employee with a particular skill factor could be retrieved more readily for further evaluation.

Although much of the information mentioned above would be on an employee's application form, in the case of long-term employees the information supplied at the time of entry becomes outdated and inaccurate as time passes.

A skills inventory cross reference would also be necessary so that a list of candidates with a specific skill could be isolated for selection of the best choice. For example, a cross reference inventory on all employees who read, write and speak French and Spanish might reveal eight or ten employees with those skills. Thus, flexibility in utilizing those with pre-scribed skill can be achieved.

A catalogue of skill categories, much the same as a library catalogue card file system, should be prepared. Under each skill category would be a card with the name of each employee with that skill. As the need for someone with the particular skill arises, the selection of names is available for consideration.

External Relations

Industrial Relations

Yoder[74] differentiates between the terms "personnel administration," "personnel management," "labor relations" and "industrial relations" in terms of historical, semantic usage and function. For example, the earliest departments were called "personnel;" they emphasized management relationships with individual employees. As labor unions developed, managers had to negotiate and administer labor contracts. Specialized assistance was provided to them by "labor relations directors" and often personnel and labor relations staffs were combined to form a more comprehensive "industrial relations" department.

Of the titles in current practice, the most common is the oldest -- "personnel administration" or "personnel management." For organizations that deal largely with collective bargaining, the "labor relations" title has become almost standard. Departments that combine responsibilities for both individual and group relationships are commonly described as "industrial relation."

----

[74] Dale Yoder, op. cit., p. 11.

Historically, the process of management as the classic economist Adam Smith saw it in the 18th century was one of combining resources -- the "factors of production," land, labor and capital -- to accomplish the goals of the organization. Managers procure, process and sell, finding and employing resources, developing goods and services and seeking markets for their output. The major subprocesses are defined as planning, organizing, staffing, directing and controlling.

"Manpower management is an essential in each of these functions. Every manager who plans, staffs, organizes, directs and controls necessarily accomplishes these functions through people and applies them to people. His responsibilities include planning for people; organizing them; staffing with people and directing them; gaining the commitment, interest and effort of people and applying controls to them." "Manpower management is thus a pervasive responsibility, inseparable from management. It is not the whole of management, but it is a major subsystem in the total management system."[75]

In order to protect its own interests and to achieve goals beyond what it might otherwise obtain from management, labor too has developed its own philosophy and in many fields has organized into unions so that by the weight of their numbers, the members have a chance of equalizing the power of the company or organization. Yet it is imperative that there be a mutual respect between these often opposing forces of labor and management, so that common goals and interests can be attained.

Unionization in the health services industry has grown significantly in the past two decades and this has accounted in large measure, for the rapidly increasing costs of hospital care. The data in Table VI - 6 demonstrates this fact. Skillful management of the industrial relations is vital to the continued success of any organization. Maintaining open communication channels between employees, supervisors and higher management is essential so that real and imaginary problems and grievances can be aired quickly and fairly before the problem grows out of proportion.

Employees of an organization are also members of many other groups both within and without the organization itself. Friendships are formed between people outside of their own department and social activities are engaged in which they create subtle influences among the participant's. The ever-present "grapevine" gossip, the cliques, the influence peddlers are busy during coffee-breaks, lunch recess or while driving together in car-pools. Effective industrial relations policies should be able to cope with the misconceptions of these people by reference to well-established practices and satisfactory relations with the majority of employees.

Unionism has had a long and stormy history in the U. S. culminating in the establishment of laws guaranteeing rights and privileges to both labor and management to pursue their particular interests with protection under the law. This is a highly specialized area of manpower management best left to the professional labor relations expert.[76] Inept handling of unionized labor

---

[75]Ibid.

[76]For a brief, excellent survey complete with many helpful practical hints for handling problems of labor relations, especially with unions, see Wilbert E. Scheer, Personnel Director's Handbook, op. cit., pp. 735-787.

demands can be a serious matter for an organization causing disruption to its business and threats to its existence.

Professional Relations

The most prominent and powerful professional society with which a H.M.O. may become involved is undoubtedly the American Medical Association which reports that it represents 64.1 per cent or 214,053 out of a national total of 334,028 registered physicians in the U. S. as at December 31, 1970.[77] There are dozens of other organizations with which contact and/or membership will be recommended for either the H.M.O. or an individual H.M.O. executive (See Table V - 8 for such a listing.)

Thus, the American Hospital Association is an important organization with which the management of a hospital should maintain liason. The controller will need to keep contact with his American Institute of Certified Public Accountants or the Hospital Financial Management Association while the hospital administrator will maintain membership in either the American College of Hospital Administrators or the Association of University Programs in Hospital Administration or the Hospital Management Systems Society.

TABLE V - 8[78]

SELECTED LIST OF ORGANIZATIONS & PROFESSIONAL ASSOCIATIONS
OF INTEREST TO WORKERS IN HEALTH SERVICE RELATED JOBS

American College of Hospital
 Administrators
840 North Lake Shore Drive
Chicago, Illinois 60611

Assoc. of University Programs
 in Hospital Administration
1642 East 56th Street
Chicago, Illinois 60637

American Medical Association
535 North Dearborn Street
Chicago, Illinois 60610

Hospital Management Systems Society
840 North Lake Shore Drive
Chicago, Illinois 60611

Data Processing Management Assoc.
505 Busse Highway
Park Ridge, Illinois 60618

Systems and Procedures Assoc.
 of America
7890 Brookside Drive
Cleveland, Ohio 44138

American Registry of
Medical Assistants and
Medical Secretaries
P.O. Box 601
Enid, Oklahoma 73701

American Society for
Personnel Administration
52 East Bridge Street
Berea, Ohio 44017

Public Personnel Assoc.
1313 East 60th Street
Chicago, Illinois 60637

American Personnel and
Guidance Association
1605 New Hampshire Ave. NW
Washington, D. C. 20009

American Society for
Hospital Personnel
Directors
840 North Lake Shore Dr.
Chicago, Illinois 60611

---

[77]American Medical News, August 9, 1971, p. 12.
[78]See Table V - 8 of this study for a selected list of some of these organizations and associations.

TABLE V - 8 (continued)

National Assoc. of Accountants
505 Park Avenue
New York, N.Y. 10022

American Institute of Certified
  Public Accountants
666 Fifth Avenue
New York, N.Y. 10019

Hospital Financial Management
  Association
840 North Lake Shore Drive
Chicago, Illinois 60611

American Association of Hospital
  Accountants
840 North Lake Shore Drive
Chicago, Illinois 60611

American Society for
Training & Development
313 Price Place
P.O. Box 5307
Madison, Wis. 53707

American Society of Directors
of Volunteer Services
American Hospital Assoc.
840 North Lake Shore Drive
Chicago, Illinois 60611

American Society of Anesthesiology
515 Busse Highway
Park Ridge, Ill. 60068

American Assoc. of Nurse
Anesthetists
Suite 3010, Prudential Plaza
Chicago, Ill. 60601

American Nurses' Assoc.
10 Columbus Circle
New York, N.Y. 10019

National League for Nursing
10 Columbus Circle
New York, N.Y. 10019

American Society for Hospital
Central Service Personnel
840 North Lake Shore Drive,
Chicago, Ill. 60611

American Society for
Hospital P.R. Directors
840 North Lake Shore Dr.
Chicago, Illinois 60611

American Assoc. of Hospital
Purchasing Agents
840 North Lake Shore Drive
Chicago, Illinois 60611

National Assoc. of Hospital
Purchasing Agents
840 North Lake Shore Dr.
Chicago, Illinois 60611

American Society for Laboratory
Animal Science
P.O. Box 10
Joliet, Ill. 60434

American Society of Biological
Chemists
9650 Wisconsin Ave. N.W.
Washington, D. C. 20014

American Society of Medical
Technologists
Suite 25, Herrman Prof. Bldg.
Houston, Texas 77025

American Society for Hospital
Engineers
840 North Lake Shore Drive
Chicago, Ill. 60611

American Society of Radiologic
Technologists
645 North Michigan Ave.
Chicago, Ill. 60611

American Orthotics and
Prosthetics Assoc.
919 18th Street, N. W.
Washington, D. C. 20006

American Assoc. of Inhalation
Therapists
332 South Michigan Ave.
Chicago, Ill. 60604

TABLE V - 8 (continued)

American Board of Pathology
University of Michigan
Dept. of Pathology
1335 East Catherine Street
Ann Arbor, Mich. 48104

American Society of Clinical
Pathologists
445 North Lake Shore Drive
Chicago, Ill. 60611

American Pharmaceutical Assoc.
2215 Constitution Ave. N. W.
Washington, D. C. 20037

American Society of Hospital
Pharmacists
4630 Montgomery Ave.
Washington, D. C. 20014

Public Relations Society
of America, Inc.
845 Third Avenue
New York, N.Y. 10022

There are similarly numerous organizations for hospital personnel administrators, purchasing agents, biological chemists and technicians and many others covering almost every professional and technical position.[79] In some instances the H.M.O. will sponsor and subsidize the fees for entry into these associations, but in many others, the individual will join on his own account. Thus AMA membership will be a matter of personal choice by the physicians, whereas membership in the American Hospital Association will be borne by the H.M.O. for the Medical Center Administrators.

The advantages of maintaining membership in such societies are generally well known to those in the professions for which the societies have been formed, as they have become a regular part of everyday working life. Keeping up with the mainstream of events within a profession on a widespread basis is probably the most important reason for joining and the exchange of views and opinions with fellow-members at meetings and conventions, as well as the periodic publications the associations print are also important factors. As a general policy, participation in these groups is to be encouraged.

Separations

Termination

Termination of an employee's service with an organization is costly both in the emotional and financial sense. The organization has an investment in employees who have been a part of it, and for whatever reason the employee's services are to be discontinued, both parties usually lose something from the action.

A policy, preferably in written form and published in the organization manual for the guidance of supervisors, should be used for terminations. When an employee is separated from the payroll, whether because the job has been eliminated, or the employee himself has clearly demonstrated that he cannot perform the job satisfactorily, the specifics should not be left to chance, or worse yet, left to individual whim.

---

[79] U. S. Dept. of Labor, Job Descriptions, op. cit.

Voluntary Termination[80]

When the employee takes the initiative and resigns because he may be unhappy with the job, or because he may have a better opportunity elsewhere or for any other reason, it is customary to expect the courtesy of a notice, usually two weeks prior to his leaving. It is usual to include in the terminal pay all the time worked since his last pay period, until the date of separation, plus pay for any earned vacation still unused.

Involuntary Termination[81]

This may arise out of action initiated by the organization which usually follows a warning or two to an unsatisfactory performer, possibly even after a probationary period has elapsed without visible improvement. When such a discharge is given it is considered proper although not required legally, to give the employee with at least one year's service a two-week notice or two-weeks' pay in lieu of notice. Most usually, the organization prefers to be rid of such a potential troublemaker, by paying him the two-weeks' salary in lieu of notice, rather than have him unproductively waiting out his time.

In the case of an employee with less than a year's service, the same policy might allow one week's pay in lieu of notice.

Though many organizations have well established and well documented hiring procedures, their termination procedures, (especially firing) are quite primitive and clumsy, Scheer[82] notes five main reasons for discharging an employee:

1. for cause, such as dishonesty;

2. continuous disobeyance of necessary orders;

3. personality conflicts;

4. inability to perform--incompetence;

5. worse than lack of skill -- lack of will

Dismissal seems to be appropriate in cases where the employee:[83]

1. lacks initiative or concentration;

2. has outside interests which interfere;

3. makes too many errors;

---

[80]W. E. Scheer, op. cit., p. 220.

[81]Ibid.

[82]Ibid. p. 224.

[83]Ibid., pp. 224-5.

4.   becomes hopelessly confused with unfamiliar terminology;

5.   is slow and creates serious bottlenecks;

6.   develops questionable behavior;

7.   has a poor memory;

8.   is a malcontent and makes disparaging remarks against management;

9.   has inadequate skill for the job;

10. is undependable;

11. cannot cope with a reasonable volume of work;

12. borrows money frequently from other employees;

13. is a disturbing influence;

14. has chronic tardiness;

15. becomes involved in a personality conflict.

It is the prerogative of the supervisor to report unsatisfactory performance or behavior to the attention of the department manager who may give a warning to the employee putting him on notice that a repetition of the offense or lack of improvement in the work will lead to dismissal.

The ultimate responsibility for discharge must remain with the departmental manager and it is always a distasteful experience, for heartless separation is a reflection on the organization whose reputation is on trial at such times. For undesirable separations a further distinction is made;[84] separations are classified as "avoidable" or "unavoidable." Avoidable separations may have arisen through misunderstanding between the quitting employee, his supervisor, his fellow employees or the organization itself. Better job opportunities, better pay scales, working conditions and transportation facilities may be other reasons why valuable employees leave. Staff turnover is costly and the impact on the organization of too rapid a turnover indicates a fault in its industrial relations. Exit Interviews can help in finding explanations for the employee's separation. They may disclose a significant pattern and suggest revisions in organizational manpower management. Some employers prefer post-separation questionnaires,[85] mailed to those who have left. It is thought that these elicit more candid, thoughtful responses, but the evidence is not conclusive because the response to the questionnaires has been very small. Another school of thought feels that the exit interview should be conducted by personnel department representative just prior to the employee's departure. Here again, emotions may cloud the issues

---

[84]Dale S. Yoder, op. cit., p. 277.

[85]Ibid.

and the interviewer's interpretation may be inaccurate. The idea of an exit interview is a valid one in terms of trying to improve human relations on the job, but in practice it falls far short of the ideal.

The exit interview when conducted in the personnel office should cover these points:[86]

1. Try to uncover the real story behind the termination.

2. Locate trouble spots that contribute to staff turnover.

3. Assure the terminating employee of his rights -- pensions, insurance, and any other benefits.

4. Distribute the Unemployment Compensation brochure as required by law.

5. Go over final paycheck and other settlement compensation (pay for unused vacation, separation pay, pay in lieu of notice, refund of employee savings account funds, etc.)

6. Make a necessary record of the circumstances surrounding the termination to satisfy government regulations and union agreements, where applicable.

7. To part as friends.

Retirement

A job gives status to a person, a meaning and satisfaction to life and a feeling of contribution to the general welfare to the community. A major source of concern for the worker is about economic security and the possibility of dependency in old age. Population life-span has increased considerably during the 20th century, but it has also increased the problems of those who have reached the customary retirement age of 65 years. To some, it is freedom from a lifetime of work, to others a dreaded point of no return.

Retirement requires a serious adjustment to one's life-style and few are ever well prepared for it. Employee retirement is one of the more recent personnel functions to be included in organizational personnel programs. Provision for retirement traditionally was viewed as being the private concern and responsibility of each employee who in days gone by returned to the old family farm of his youth or to the small country town of his birth.

Changing patterns in U. S. life-style and rapid urbanization have blocked these possibilities, for few people retiring now lived on a farm in their youth. Pension funds and social security programs to supplement them give a measure of financial relief to those in retirement. Still, it is important for an organization to assist their employees on the way into retirement so that they can become better able to help themselves. Many larger organizations have retirement programs designed to do this by

---

[86]
W. E. Scheer, op. cit., p. 229.

counseling on health problems of older people, use of leisure time and recreation; community resources for older people; housing and living arrangements; revenue producing hobbies and activities; family adjustment problems and, for those who are able and wish to, counseling or participation in volunteer community service projects.

After retirement most ex-employees like to maintain some ties with their old organization. Keeping them on the mailing list for the house organ, the annual report and other publications helps them keep those ties fresh. Some organizations present their retiring employees with a lifetime membership identification card with their photo on it in a laminated plastic finish. This testifies to long service and as a link in the affiliation between retiree and organization.[87]

During the preparation for retirement, booklets describing important facts and features of retirement are distributed during a seminar-type of program. Films, speakers and printed material also form part of the schedule. Important information as follows is passed on to the retiring employees:

Eligibility for Social Security upon retirement with a thorough explanation of how to compute and calculate benefits.

Complete explanation of pension benefits including taxation.

The pro's and con's of investment and explanation of investment "jargon" and opportunities.

The physical aspects of aging, including basic nutritional needs and an explanation of common symptoms to check regularly.

Mental health in later life, noting changes in attitudes which occur during retirement and explaining senility.

Leisure time activities turned into profit-making ventures, and free services available to retired persons.

Housing: Retirement hotels, apartment buildings, and communities; the pro's and con's of relocating.[88]

Even with all the assistance and preparation given to the retiring employee, the hard reality eventually reaches him and it is up to him to try to adjust to it.

_____

[87]Ibid. p. 229.

[88]
W. E. Scheer, op. cit., p.714.

Layoff

In time of economic stress for a company, organization or industry the most immediate reaction that occurs is layoff, the release of significant numbers of employees from the payroll so as to lighten the load by curbing the expenses. Payroll costs are a major expense to most organizations and flexibility in the management of manpower is essential to the life of the organization.

Beach[89] defines a layoff as "an indefinite separation from the payroll due to factors beyond the employee's control." Loss of sales, raw material shortages, seasonal fluctuation in the market, production delays due to strikes in supplier industries or transportation or technological displacement are frequent reasons for layoffs. The period of the duration of the layoff can seldom be predetermined because frequently the causes for the layoff are beyond the control of the employer also. Some temporary layoffs actually become permanent separations especially when the employee successfully obtains another job. Clear distinction should be made between the layoff which is a condition that neither the employer nor the employee usually desire, and a discharge which is a permanent separation brought about by the poor performance or violation of company rules of conduct.

Depending upon company policy and union-employer contract provisions, laid-off workers retain certain rights with their employer. Sometimes seniority rights continue to accumulate for a certain period of time; they may have certain recall rights and time spent on layoff may count towards vacation; pension and sickness benefits. Often the organization hopes that the laid-off workers will maintain their affiliation with it rather than sever relations permanently.[90] Recruiting and training new "green" help when conditions return to normal is costly and time consuming. Unfortunately, the longer the layoff lasts, the less likely it will be for the laid-off workers to return.

Layoff,nonunion[91]

In nonunion situations, the organization usually has more flexibility in determining who will be laid off on the basis of many factors. Among these are ability, age, length of service, number of dependents, financial obligations and health. Job performance and ability are usually given the greatest weight, followed next by length of service. The other factors reflect management's concern with what might be hardship cases if the individual is laid off.

Layoff of organized employees (union)[92]

Layoff procedures have always been of utmost concern to unions and the practices and procedures involved with unions are both complex and varied. The ultimate aim is for the union to maintain its strength and position in the organization and to protect its members jobs as far as possible. It tries hard to insure equitable and impartial treatment among

---

[89]Dale S. Beach, op. cit., pp. 360-361.

[90]Ibid.

[91]Ibid.

[92]Ibid.

individuals based on seniority rights, to prevent dividing influences within the group, and to maintain reemployment rights for those laid off.

Reduction in working hours, prohibition on subcontract work outside the organization where feasible, release of temporary and probationary employees and a ban on overtime are some of the demands made in order to forestall layoffs.

A frank discussion of the situation should be held between management and employees to explain the absolute need for retrenchment in the hope of gaining the sympathy and support of the work-force.

Bulletin-board notices on the method of recall, rights and privileges while on layoff, benefits under unemployment insurance and all other pertinent information on insurance programs, medical scheme payments and so forth, should be posted for all employees to read.

Manpower Control Systems

Manpower Budgets

As an aid to manpower planning a budget system should be instituted.[93] Each department manager will prepare a manpower budget detailing the work to be covered in his department and the personnel required to perform this work. Comparison of the personnel requirements between related departments would show whether fair estimates were being made. For example, if the pharmacy dispensary were staffed by two people handling 1,000 prescriptions per month during the current year, showed in their budget estimates for the next year a requirement for an additional pharmacist to handle an increase expected to reach 1,500 prescriptions per month, it would be necessary to check the anticipated growth in subscribers and patient visits from the estimates provided for the same period by the marketing department and the regional medical groups to see if that estimate could be supported by them. In this way it is possible to check and balance the requirements of the various sections, and prevent "empire building" by a too ambitious department head.

For the most part the limiting factor in the supply of personnel will be the availability of funds allocated to manpower requirements. The financial management of the H.M.O. working with the President will prepare a budget in which a high proportion will be earmarked for labor costs. Each department will then be allocated a portion of the total labor cost in proportion to its needs and when the department managers are presented with these facts, they will then be able to determine whether they have financial "room" for additions to their staff. In cases where additional staff is needed, but not provided for financially, a special application to the controller will be necessary.

Employee Ratios

Statistics are available from the American Hospital Association, the American Pharmaceutical Association or the American Society of Hospital

---

[93] See Chapter VII for Financial Operating Plan.

Pharmacists on the number of prescriptions generally handled by a hospital pharmacist per month so that comparisons can be made with the national or regional figure and the experience of the H.M.O. Similarly, the experience of the Kaiser-Permanente Medical Groups shows that the ratio of one physician per 1,000 to 1,100 subscribers gives adequate coverage as reported elsewhere in this study. Studies made of the numerous varied statistics available can be useful as guidelines in comparing the work of the H.M.O.

The desire of the department managers to maintain efficient working units without attempting to build "empires" will be instrumental in maintaining sane employee ratios. Comparison with other groups and Health Maintenance Organizations of comparable size will help keep the ratios in perspective.

Cost Factors

The most significant advance made in health care delivery has been costs. Since 1960, the Department of Labor estimates that hospital room rates have risen by 155.6 per cent[94] as against 31.1 per cent for all consumer prices; physicians' fees have increased 57.7 per cent while other medical costs have increased 52.5 per cent.[95] Unfortunately, the advance has been adverse for the consuming public whose income has not kept apace with the rising health costs. Thus, protection is afforded those who became subscribers to a prepaid group practice health plan of the H.M.O. type. Over 65 per cent of all health care costs are labor costs[96] because of the nature of the services provided and careful attention to labor costs is vital to the survival of a health maintenance organization. Greater emphasis on preventive medicine and ambulatory rather than hospitalized care whenever possible are key factors in holding down major expenses in providing service to subscribers.

In comparing the H.M.O. Plan Inc's manpower utilization rates with those experienced by similar plans in other areas, and evaluating the cost per subscriber, it will be possible to determine whether the most effective value is being obtained from the manpower employed. If, for example, the H.M.O. system handles 4,000 patient visits per month for a total cost of $420,000, while another organization handles 4,800 patient visits per month for a total cost of $410,000, then it must be assumed that H.M.O.'s cost controls, employee ratios or subscriber utilization rates are less satisfactory. As the H.M.O. experience grows, these ratios will be observed and compared so that systems designed to give better control will be pursued.

CONCLUDING REMARKS

Growth of Group Practice

"Group practice is inevitable and will become the family health care center of the future" predicted American Medical Association President,

---

[94]"Aid for Blue Cross in Nixon's Plan," Business Week, Feb. 27, 1971, pp. 94-96.

[95]"Presidential Prescription for Health," Time Magazine, March 1, 1971, pp. 11-12.

[96]American Medical News, March 1, 1971.

Dr. Walter C. Bornemeier.[97] Such a statement from the President of the major
official organization of the medical profession in the U. S. presumes the
recognition and tacit consent, long withheld by the profession, to deliver
health care to the public through such groups. It is curious to note that
the 1970-1971 President of the AMA did not consider manpower, particularly
licensed physicians, at this time to be the biggest deterrent, especially
in view of the past vehement opposition by the AMA to group practice.

However, while the formation of group practices has grown over the
past 25 years, the major portion of medical services is still provided on a
fee-for-service basis by solo or two and three partner practices. "Young
doctors, especially those entering practice from now on, will opt for group
practice," predicted AMA President Bornemeier in his final report to the
House of Delegates in Atlantic City at the AMA's Annual Convention.[98]

At the 24th National Conference on Rural Health in Atlanta, early
in 1971, Dr. Bornemeier stated that solo practitioners will not be able to
afford the necessary sophisticated equipment, nor can they hope to acquire
the vast range of new skills to practice alone, "therefore, people will
drive past the local doctor's office and on into the county seat for
important illnesses. "Who wants to be a doctor for unimportant illnesses?"
"Another consideration is that practice alone, away from consultation, away
from staff meetings, away from doctor talk with doctors who face similar
problems, just gets too lonesome."[99] The answer for rural and suburban areas
is to establish group practices in the population centers with satellite
clinics in surrounding areas.

The question is raised as to why a licensed physician, after having
spent eight years in academic training plus one to three years in hospital
internship and residency, would want to join a prepaid group practice plan
rather than set up his own fee-for-service practice, as an independent
entrepreneur. Traditionally, until rather recent times, by far the largest
majority of graduating physicians chose the private practice method of earning their livelihood. The American Medical Association until the past eight
or ten years fought strenuously against the principle of prepaid group
practice and tried with all its very considerable power to prevent doctors
engaged in such practice from enjoying the rights and privileges at hospitals,
that were then enjoyed by private practitioners. The AMA certainly tried to
make prepaid group practice doctors like second-class citizens.

But the climate of social conscience is changing and gradually,
very gradually, there is growing acceptance for prepaid group practice and
even the AMA has reversed its formerly adamant position. While still a
majority of graduating physicians choose to go into private practice, a not
insignificant minority has been deciding to enter public medical practice and
prepaid group practice.

---

[97] American Medical News, April 15, 1971, p. 1.

[98] American Medical News, June 28, 1971.

[99] American Medical News, op. cit.

During a personal interview with a medical school senior student, due to graduate within the next year, this author learned that lectures were given the students on the various options open to them in the pursuit of their careers and there was no longer the traditional derogation of or bias against prepaid group practice. Students whose families had paid for all of their training generally felt obligated to enter private practice to justify their family's long years of support. Others whose families could not extend that support to set them up in practice, felt that joining a prepaid group practice presented the best opportunity for them to commence their career.

The younger doctor graduating in the past three or four years, has followed the example of his age-group colleagues in the other professions, notably the law, in pursuing social-conscience activity more willingly than his Establishment father or older brother. The new doctors are apparently willing to break out of the mold which has shaped their predecessors and have even declared their independence from the American Medical Association. Fortune Magazine in its January 1970 issue, devoted largely to the crisis in American medicine, stated that delegates of the Student American Medical Association declared their independence when at their convention they passed resolutions critical of the fee-for-service concept of medical care, and endorsed greater participation in group practice schemes. The S.A.M.A. has attracted 24,000 members out of a total national medical school enrollment of 37,500 students.

The following reasons are given why doctors might prefer working for subscriber prepaid group practice plans rather than as private fee-for-service doctors:[100]

1. a guaranteed income is assured immediately whereas a doctor setting up a new practice may select a location which will not be successful for quite a long time.

2. H.M.O. medical groups assure regular hours of work, thus permitting the doctor a regulated family life which is not always possible in private practice.

3. guaranteed vacations which are not always possible under private practice conditions, especially in the early years of a practice's development.

4. professional leave for study purposes is encouraged and subsidized.

5. no administrative-clerical duties to worry about; (no bookkeeping, simpler tax statements, no bad debts.)

6. group interchange of ideas; cross consultation available quickly and easily; better equipment and facilities available for prompt testing of patients.

---

[100]Interview with F. C. Smith Jr. Administrator, HIP Kings Highway Medical Group, Brooklyn, N.Y., June 21, 1971.

7. no heavy expenditures of personal funds, no finance charges for equipping and maintaining an office.

8. in the event of illness or other forced absence from work, income continues without worrying about loss of patients.

9. fringe benefits package, including provision for retirement.

During the past ten years or so, vast progress has been made in medical research, development of technological aids in both diagnosis and treatment, and extension of hospital and health insurance plans including Medicare and Medicaid, together with the expansion of the awareness by the population in health matters. The affluence of the 1960's with higher per capita income have made health services a particularly rapid growth sector of the economy. As a result, serious shortages of health services personnel have arisen and despite intensified training programs, the shortages, relative to need, remain.

> Approximately 3.7 million persons are now engaged in health services, 2.4 million of whom are employed in hospitals. Projections for 1975 indicate that jobs in health services will increase to 5.5 million, 3.4 million of which will be in hospitals. Accordingly in 1975, hospital employment of health service personnel will have increased an estimated 40 per cent over the current level of employment. This increase will be reflected in every hospital health service occupation, ranging from an estimated five per cent increase in pharmacists to an estimated 50 per cent increase in attendants and nurses.[101]

Here lies a golden opportunity to inspire and encourage the young, intelligent people to train for service in those areas. The H.M.O. should endeavor to maintain strong ties to the nearest medical school, nursing schools and relevant departments of nearby colleges so that a reserve pool of trained people can be drawn from as required. Laboratory technicians, accountants, administrators are usually college trained people, and by maintaining good relationships with the college, recruiting of potentially valuable personnel can be simplified.

The strength of the organization-to-be will come not from elaborate concrete and glass structures, nor from complex computerized systems, but from the selection and development of its human resources of competent, dedicated men and women who will give the organization the vitality and character to make it work for the benefit of the community it is pledged to serve. The challenge of the present is to prepare for the future; it is hoped that the facts presented in this manpower plan will assist in that task.

---

[101] U. S. Dept. of Labor, Job Descriptions, op. cit., p. xiv preface.

APPENDIX A

SPECIMEN PARTNERSHIP AGREEMENT BETWEEN PARTICIPATING
PHYSICIAN-PARTNERS IN A REGIONAL MEDICAL GROUP

XYZ MEDICAL GROUP

AFFILIATED WITH THE HEALTH MAINTENANCE ORGANIZATION, INC.

PARTNERSHIP AGREEMENT

December 7, 1971

TABLE OF CONTENTS

AMENDED PARTNERSHIP AGREEMENT

        Agreement made as of June 1, 1971 by and between Dr. A., Dr. B.,
Dr. C., Dr. D., Dr. E., Dr. F., Dr. G., Dr. H., Dr. I., Dr. J., Dr. K.,
Dr. L., Dr. M., Dr. N., Dr. O., Dr. P., Dr. Q., and such additional persons
as may from time to time be admitted as partners pursuant to the provisions
hereof (all hereinafter referred to as the "Partners") as follows:

                        WITNESSETH:

        WHEREAS, each of the above named parties is a licensed physician
and surgeon, duly admitted to the practice of medicine in the State of New
York, and

        WHEREAS, the parties hereto are now co-partners practicing medicine
under the firm name and style of XYZ MEDICAL GROUP, pursuant to a certain
partnership agreement dated December 1, 1970, and,

        WHEREAS, the parties hereto desire to amend said partnership agree-
ment and continue to be partners in the practice of medicine under the firm
name and style of XYZ MEDICAL GROUP, hereinafter sometimes referred to as
the "Partnership."

        NOW, therefore, the parties hereto agree that said partnership
agreement is hereby amended in its entirety to read as follows:

                        ARTICLE I

                NAME, OFFICE AND CONTINUATION

Section 1. The parties hereto agree to become and continue to be partners
in the practice of medicine under the firm name and style of XXX REGIONAL
MEDICAL GROUP.

Section 2. The office of the Partnership should be maintained in the Town
of ABC, County of DEF, State of N.Y.

Section 3. The Partnership shall continue until the partners shall determine
that the partnership agreement shall be terminated in accordance with
ARTICLE XIX hereof.

Section 4. The resignation, death or expulsion of any partner shall terminate
the partnership only with respect to the person so resigned, dead or expelled,
and the Partnership shall otherwise continue without the necessity of executing any new agreement among the remaining partners; nor shall the addition
of any person as a new partner affect the continuity of the Partnership.

ARTICLE II

PURPOSE

The purpose of the Partnership heretofore formed and existing among the above named persons shall continue to be for the purpose of rendering group medical, surgical and allied care and services pursuant to arrangements between the Partnership and the Health Maintenance Organization (hereinafter referred to as H.M.O.) or any successor thereof, any similar organization, and other organizations or individuals, and shall continue until terminated as provided herein.

ARTICLE III

DUTIES OF PARTNERS

Section 1. Each partner shall render professional medical and surgical services for such persons insured under H.M.O. contracts and policies as may be enrolled with the Group in accordance with the terms of the Group's agreement with H.M.O. or similar organizations, and also to render such other professional medical and surgical services as may be necessary to discharge the Group's obligations under any other arrangements entered into by the Group.

Section 2. Insofar as their partnership duties do not require the partners to devote their time and services exclusively to the Partnership, the partners shall be free to engage in and carry on their individual medical practices as long as the same does not conflict with the services required to be rendered pursuant to this agreement, and the income derived and the expenses incurred in connection with such individual medical practices shall be solely the assets and obligations of such individual partners except as may be otherwise provided by agreement with the Group.

Section 3. Each partner shall devote such time to the care of Group patients at such places as may be necessary or as may be required by Group policies or needs as determined by the Medical Director subject to the disapproval of the Executive Committee.

Section 4. The partner shall have the use of the Partnership premises, equipment, facilities, supplies and hired personnel for nongroup patients subject to the provisions of this agreement and such regulations and conditions as the Group may fix.

Section 5. Each partner shall prepare such reports of his professional services and on such forms and at such times as may be determined by the Medical Director subject to the disapproval of the Executive Committee.

Section 6. Each partner shall devote such time to attendance at Group and committee meetings as the Group or appropriate committee may require for the interest of the Group.

Section 7. No partner shall engage in any conduct that is injurious to the good order, peace, reputation or interest of H.M.O. or the Group, or derogatory to its dignity or the morale of the members of the Group, or inconsistent with the purposes of H.M.O. or the Group.

Section 8. Each partner shall comply with all the rules and regulations of the Group, and such further rules and regulations of H.M.O. or other organizations with which the Group has entered into arrangements which impose duties and obligations upon the Partnership and/or the members thereof. When new contracts or arrangements are made by the Group with H.M.O. or others, this paragraph shall be deemed to refer to the current contract or arrangements.

Section 9. All partners shall have one vote on all questions and matters and votes that may come up before the Partnership.

Section 10. Each partner, at his own cost and expense shall carry malpractice insurance, public liability insurance, automobile liability insurance and such other insurance as may be required by the Partnership in such amounts, with such company and in such forms as are satisfactory to the Partnership for the protection of the Group and H.M.O. except for such coverage as the Partnership may agree to assume at its own cost and expense.

ARTICLE IV

RESPONSIBILITY OF PARTNERS

Section 1. The parties agree that none of the partners shall, without the previous consent in writing of all the other parties to this agreement:

    (a) Employ any monies, property or effects belonging to the Partnership, or engage the credit thereof, or contract any debt or account thereof, except in the due and regular course of business and as authorized by this agreement and upon account of and for the benefit of the Partnership.

    (b) Mortgage, assign or charge or otherwise encumber their interest in the Partnership or in the property or profits thereof or in any manner or form whatsoever dispose of his share of, or interest in the Partnership.

    (c) Compound, settle, release or discharge any debt due to the Partnership without receiving the full amount thereof, except as may otherwise be authorized by the Executive Committee.

    (d) Do or knowingly suffer any act or thing whereby the property or effects of the Partnership thereof, may be attached or taken in execution.

Section 2. The parties further agree that none of them will, directly or indirectly, use the Partnership name for the accommodation of any person, firm, association or corporation or make or endorse or draw or sign any note, check, bill of exchange, bond or undertaking, or any paper or other evidence of indebtedness that purports to obligate the Partnership in any way, for the benefit of another.

310

Section 3. Each partner shall punctually pay, satisfy and discharge all his present and future private debts, obligations, liabilities and engagements and indemnify and save free and harmless all other partners, and the property and effects of the Partnership, therefrom and from all actions, proceedings, damages and expenses of any and every kind on account thereof.

Section 4. All partners agree that the Partnership or the partners individually shall indemnify a partner or partners who shall have incurred an individual liability for a regular or specially authorized Partnership obligation or liability.

ARTICLE V

MEDICAL OFFICES

Section 1. The partnership shall establish and maintain a Group Center and sub-centers and branches. All the medical and surgical instruments, pharmaceutical products and medicines, furniture, fixtures and other equipment acquired by the Partnership shall be and remain Partnership property, and shall be kept at said offices except as otherwise directed by the Executive Committee. Group records, etc., which the Group shall have acquired shall remain the property of the Group unless other disposition is made by the Group.

Section 2. Each partner shall make available to the Partnership in furtherance of its Group practice his private office and equipment, if any, but the Group shall have no possessory rights thereto. A partner may not maintain his office in a location that is incompatible with the partner's practice in the Group.

ARTICLE VI

MEDICAL DIRECTOR

Section 1. There shall be a Medical Director. The Medical Director shall be elected by a majority of the votes cast at a membership meeting. Nominations for Medical Director shall be made at the partnership meeting preceding the meeting at which the election is held. Candidates must be partners and must accept in person or in writing within three days after nomination. The balloting for the election of Medical Director shall be by secret ballot. Ballots together with written notice of the election meeting shall be mailed to all partners. The ballots may be cast in secret at the meeting or by mailing same in a sealed envelope to a person previously designated by the Executive Committee no less than three days prior to the date of election. Mailed ballots shall be produced at the election meeting and the ballot of a partner shall be opened and counted if he is not present at the meeting. The election for Medical Director shall be held during the last month of the term of the incumbent Medical Director. If no candidate receives a majority of the votes cast, a run-off election shall be held between the two candidates with the highest number of votes, at the next Partnership meeting. The Medical Director shall serve for two years and until his successor is elected.

Section 2. Except as otherwise directed by the Partnership, the functions of
the Medical Director shall be:

(a) To preside over all meetings of the Partnership and of the
Executive Committee.

(b) To represent the Partnership at meetings of medical groups
or elsewhere.

(c) To serve as the chief administrator of the Partnership.

(d) To serve as an ex-officio member of all committees.

(e) To assign the duties of the physicians including the partners
and to arrange the schedule of their office hours as required, subject to
the disapproval of the Executive Committee.

(f) To employ personnel including an Administrator for the Partnership and to fix their hours, duties and compensation, subject to the disapproval of the Executive Committee.

(g) To purchase supplies and equipment. Items over $500.00 shall
be subject to prior approval of the Executive Committee.

(h) To be responsible for the professional direction of and
general supervision of the quality of medical care in the Group.

(i) To be responsible for interviewing prospective contract
physicians and partners.

(j) To be responsible for the general supervision of the continuing
education of physicians in the Group.

(k) To act as the Executive officer the Partnership and perform
such duties in the interest of the Partnership which are not delegated
specifically herein, to the Executive Committee or the Partnership.

(l) To select and change the partners who serve on committees
established by the Executive Committee.

(m) To be responsible for the preparation of the agendas of the
Executive Committee and the Partnership meetings.

(n) To be responsible for the calling of all meetings of the
Executive Committee and of the Partnership in accordance with the provisions
herein.

(o) To perform such other functions as may be delegated to him by
the Partnership or by the Executive Committee.

Section 3. The compensation of the Medical Director for the performance of
his respective duties in connection with his office shall be determined by
the Partnership upon recommendation of the Executive Committee.

ARTICLE VII

EXECUTIVE COMMITTEE

Section 1. There is hereby established an Executive Committee. The Executive Committee shall be composed of six partners in addition to the Medical Director who shall be chairman and a member of the Executive Committee by virtue of his position as Medical Director. The members of the Executive Board shall be elected by a plurality vote of the Partnership at a meeting for a two year term and until their successor is elected. No partner shall be eligible to be a member of the Executive Committee for more than two consecutive terms. Elections as aforesaid shall be held at the Partnership meeting preceding the expiration of the terms of the current members of the Executive Committee.

Section 2. The functions of the Executive Committee shall be:

(a) To supervise the expenditure of any funds and to incur obligations on behalf of the Partnership and, in the performance of such duties, to authorize the execution of contracts and other types of evidence of obligations or indebtedness. However, the consent of the Partnership shall be required whenever the expenditure or obligation per item exceeds $500.00 except if the obligation or contract is the result of collective bargaining with a labor organization representing employees of the Partnership.

(b) To make rules and regulations for the conduct of the affairs of the Partnership.

(c) To designate partners who, in addition to the Medical Director, shall be empowered to sign checks on behalf of the Partnership, withdrawals to be made only by the signature and authorization of two authorized partners.

(d) To elect a Secretary from among the members of the Executive Committee each year to serve for a one year term.

(e) To establish various committees to assist in the conduct and operation of the Partnership.

(f) To determine the amount of drawings to be paid to the partners in accordance with the provisions contained herein subject to the approval of the Partnership.

(g) To provide for the maintenance of proper books and records of account for the Partnership and in this connection to retain the services of a Certified Public Accountant who shall audit the books and render reports to the Partnership at regular intervals and make such other financial reports as may be necessary from time to time.

(h) To perform such other and further duties and responsibilities as may be expressly provided by this agreement or may be delegated to it by the Partnership.

Section 3.

(a) Any vacancy in any office or on the Executive Committee created by resignation, retirement, death or by vote of the Partnership as herein provided shall be filled by the Partnership for the unexpired term.

(b) All decisions of the Executive Committee shall be made by majority vote of a quorum which, in turn, shall consist of a majority of the members of the Executive Committee.

(c) The renumeration and expense allowance of the Executive Committee shall be fixed by a vote of the partners.

(d) The Executive Committee shall keep regular minutes of all its proceedings and the original of each set shall be signed by the Secretary.

ARTICLE VIII

PARTNERSHIP MEETINGS

Section 1. Regular meetings of the Partnership shall be held monthly, except during July and August, at the Group Center or at such other times or places as it may designate. Written notice by mail shall be given to each partner by the Medical Director at least seven days prior to each meeting. Notice of the nomination and election of a Medical Director or the election of members of the Executive Committee shall be contained in the written notice of the meeting whenever such action is scheduled.

Section 2. Special meetings of the Partnership may be called by the Medical Director, the Executive Committee or one-fifth of the members of the Partnership upon three business days' notice by telephone, confirmed by letter not mailed later than three business days before the meeting date.

Section 3. The partners at a regular or special meeting shall be the supreme governing body of the Group with authority to overrule and supersede all decisions and actions of any office or committee of the Group and initiate decisions and actions of its own except as may otherwise be provided by this agreement.

Section 4. Ten partners shall constitute a quorum at a regular or special meeting of the Partnership, except as provided in Article XII, Section 1. Determinations shall be made by a majority vote except where otherwise specified either in the Partnership agreement or in by-laws, if any. When the percentage required results in a fraction (e.g. 2/3 of 14), if the fraction be less than $\frac{1}{2}$, it is to be disregarded; if it is $\frac{1}{2}$ or more, it is to be regarded as a whole number.

Section 5. Unless otherwise indicated in this Partnership agreement, wherever the consent or approval of a certain number or percentage of partners is required to bind all the partners, it shall be considered to mean the number and percentage of the partners present at a meeting.

Section 6. When a quorum is not present at any regular or special meeting, the acts of the meeting must be approved at the next meeting of the Group at which a quorum is present.

Section 7. The Secretary shall keep minutes of all meetings of the Partnership and sign the original minutes.

Section 8. All motions, resolutions, rules and/or regulations heretofore duly adopted by the Partnership shall continue to remain in full force and effect and shall be binding on all present and future partners unless in conflict with the provisions of this agreement or repealed, amended or superseded by further action of the Partnership.

ARTICLE IX

PARTNERSHIP ACCOUNTS, CONTRACTS AND INVESTMENTS

Section 1. All accounts of the Partnership shall be kept in one or more banking institutions selected by the Executive Committee, and withdrawals therefrom shall be made only by check, signed by two authorized partners. All disbursements of the Partnership in excess of $100.00 shall be paid by check.

Section 2. All contracts and obligations binding on the Partnership shall be signed and executed by the Medical Director and at least one other member of the Executive Committee after approval by the Partnership, except as otherwise provided or directed in specific instances by the Partnership.

Section 3. Such funds of the Partnership as the Partnership deems to be in excess of ordinary Partnership requirements may be invested in such manner as the Partnership may authorize.

ARTICLE X

PARTNERSHIP PROPERTY AND EARNINGS

Section 1. All fees and income received by the Partnership for services rendered or to be rendered on behalf of the Partnership, shall be Partnership property, except such fees as the individual partners are permitted to charge and retain in accordance with Group agreement or as may be required by law.

Section 2. Attached hereto and made a part hereof is a schedule designated "Participation Schedule" effective December 1, 1966, in which are set forth the names of the partners, the basic shares of participation of each partner, the longevity shares of each partner and the amount of capital paid in or due by each partner.

Section 3. In addition to the basic shares of participation in the partnership, a 12 share partner shall acquire longevity shares as follows: 5 years - ½ share; 10 years - 1 share; 15 years - 2 shares; and 20 years - 3 shares. Partners with more or less than 12 shares with the years of service set forth

315

above shall acquire longevity shares in the percentage proportion that their share holdings relate to 12 shares.

In the event that the partners basic shares are reduced for any reason, same shall not affect his longevity shares.

The date from which service is computed for longevity shares shall be the date of the commencement of partnership or associate partnership status under this or prior partnership agreements, but shall not include any period of time when a physician was associated with the Partnership in any capacity other than as a partner or associate partner.

Section 4. The participations of the individual partners in the net profits of the Partnership shall be by shares as set forth in the attached "Participation Schedule." The earnings of a share shall be determined by dividing the sum of the participating shares, basic and longevity, of all the partners into the net profits of the Partnership earned by the Partnership in a given fiscal period. The result shall equal the earnings of one share for such fiscal period. Provided, however, that in no event shall a full time physician as the term is defined in the contract with H.M.O. and the Partnership, receive less per annum than the specified earnings in said contract for such full time physician and such additional amount, if any, that the Partnership may determine.

Section 5. Changes in the basic shares of any of the partners may be made by the Partnership at any time by a majority vote of the partners. The Executive Committee shall review the basic share holdings at any time and recommend to the Partnership changes in such basic share holdings whenever it deems it advisable. In the event a change in the basic units of a partner is made, the amount of the capital paid or due by said partner should be increased or decreased as the case may be to correspond with the change in the basic units.

Section 6. The "Participating Schedule" shall be revised any time changes are made in the Partnership or in any other matter set forth in the "Participating Schedule" giving effect to such changes and shall be prepared and signed by the Medical Director of the Partnership and when so signed shall from its effective date supersede the prior "Participating Schedule" and become a part of this agreement as though physically attached hereto.

Section 7. The contributions and drawings of the partners shall be in the same percentage proportion as the sharing of profits and losses, after considering longevity shares and the requirements of full time physicians and shall be in such sums as they may from time to time mutually agree upon. Such contributions shall be without interest.

Section 8. The parties hereto agree that drawings will be paid monthly, in amounts to be determined by the Executive Committee, against the estimated total earnings of the shares held by each partner.

Section 9. There shall be an annual financial report distributed to the partners.

ARTICLE XI

WITHDRAWAL OF PARTNERS

Section 1. If any partner shall desire to withdraw from the Partnership, he shall send written notice thereof to the Medical Director at the principal office of the Partnership at least 90 days (or sooner, if the Executive Committee and the withdrawing partner shall so agree) prior to the date he desires his withdrawal to become effective.

Upon the expiration of such period, his withdrawal shall become effective. Thereupon, his share of the Partnership net assets shall be computed on the basis of his capital accounts as reported in the last accounting report of the Partnership as modified by any changes between the date of that report and the end of the month in which the withdrawal became effective. Any monies that said partner owes against his capital account or equity shall be automatically deducted from his share of the capital account. A withdrawing partner shall be paid his share of the net assets, if any, in quarterly installments during a two year period after the effective date of withdrawal. In case of dissolution of the Partnership, any amounts due a withdrawn partner shall be paid at the same time and in the same proportion as the partners. No interest on any partner's share shall be payable for the period between the effective date of withdrawal and the date of payment.

Section 2. Any partner who withdraws from the Partnership prior to attaining the age of 60 years and prior to being a partner for at least ten years shall receive only 90 per cent of his share of the Partnership assets as set forth in Section 1 of this Article. However, if a partner retires after a minimum of 15 years as a partner there shall be no percentage reduction as provided above regardless of age.

Section 3. Upon the death, retirement or expulsion of any partner, he shall be deemed to have withdrawn from the Partnership effective the last day of the month in which such event occurred and his share of the Partnership net assets shall be computed and paid as provided in Section 1, without any percentage reduction as provided in Section 2 hereof.

Section 4. A partner who has reached the age of 65 years shall be retired at the end of the fiscal year in which he attained the age of 65. A partner may continue as such for a period of no more than two years after reaching his retirement date only when requested to do so upon motion adopted by a 2/3 vote of the Partnership at a regular or special meeting provided he assents to so continue. The Partnership may continue to extend the retirement date of a partner for two year periods in the aforesaid manner.

Section 5. No allowance is to be made for good will of Partnership on severence of partner or partners, nor shall they have any interest in the name of the Partnership.

ARTICLE XII

DISCIPLINE OF PARTNERS

Section 1. Any partner may be expelled from the Partnership or otherwise
disciplined for cause. Charges against a partner seeking his expulsion may
be filed by any other partner with the Medical Director. The Medical
Director may also file charges against a partner. The Medical Director shall
promptly cause a copy of the charges together with notice of hearing before
the Executive Committee, to be served upon the accused and the accuser by
certified mail at least seven days before the hearing.

Both the accuser and the accused may be present at the hearing on
the charges before the Executive Committee, be represented by counsel, and
have the opportunity to be heard. The Executive Committee may likewise
employ an attorney to guide and counsel it at the hearing. Both the accuser
and the accused may present evidence and examine and cross-examine witnesses.
Upon the conclusion of the hearing, the Executive Committee shall consider
the evidence and make a recommendation to the partnership by majority vote
of those attending the hearing.

The Partnership shall act on the recommendation and afford both
the accuser and the accused the opportunity to speak on the recommendation
before voting. If 3/4 of the partners present at the meeting vote to expel
the accused partner, he shall stand expelled from the Partnership seven days
after notice of the expulsion action of the partners has been mailed to him.
Upon expulsion he shall be entitled to his share of the Partnership net
assets which shall be computed and paid as provided in Article XI, Section 1.
If the Executive Committee recommends a form of discipline other than expulsion which may include without limitation, removal or suspension from office,
a reduction of Partnership shares or a fine, such a recommendation shall
require a 2/3 vote of the partners present for adoption. A quorum for a
Partnership meeting at which disciplinary action against a partner shall be
considered, shall consist of 3/4 of all the partners and written notice of
such meeting shall be sent by mail to each partner at least seven days before
the meeting.

Section 2. Proof of bankruptcy, insolvency, or assignment for benefit of
creditors by any partner or the entry of judgment against him remaining
unsatisfied for five days or more may result in immediate expulsion from
this Partnership without the necessity of any charges being preferred.

Section 3. Any physician separated from the Group does hereby agree to continue the treatment of ill patients under his care until reasonable opportunity
has been afforded for the transfer of the patient to another physician in
the Group. Any obstetrician separated from the Group hereby agrees to continue treatment of maternity patients under his care (at the request of the
Medical Director), for a period of six weeks postpartum where such patient,
at the time of his severance is in her last two months of pregnancy.

ARTICLE XIII

VACATIONS, DISABILITY PAYMENTS AND OTHER BENEFITS

Section 1. Vacation schedules may be established and leaves of absence may be granted to any partner by the Executive Committee on such terms and conditions as may seem to it desirable and consistent with H.M.O. requirements.

Section 2. Upon the consent and approval of a majority of the partners, the Group may provide for annuities, pensions or retirement funds or for various types of insurance including but not limited to life, accident, health and death benefit insurance, covering each of the partners, out of the Partnership funds. The Group may also arrange sick leave and disability payments for partners and the extent and duration thereof upon the consent and approval of a majority of the partners.

Section 3. If any partner shall enter the military service of the United States, he shall from the date when he ceased to perform the work for the Partnership receive as his share of the surplus the same sum that he would receive as a partner pursuant to this agreement, less the cost to the Partnership of hiring on a temporary contract basis a satisfactory substitute. He shall, however, remain a partner and upon his release from military duty shall thereafter continue to perform his duties as a partner. Said re-entry into partnership duties shall be by arrangements with the Executive Committee to terminate the services of the substitute.

ARTICLE XIV

NEW PARTNERS

Section 1. A new partner may be admitted to the Partnership only upon the recommendation of the Executive Committee and the consent of three fourths of all the partners.

Section 2. Each new partner shall sign the original counterpart of this agreement, as amended, at the time of his admission and after signing he shall be a party to this agreement with the same force and effect as if he had been one of the original parties to this agreement.

Section 3. The incoming partner shall ratify in writing all acts of the Partnership, adopting them as his own. He shall also ratify in writing any other agreements then existing between the Partnership, H.M.O. and/or other person, firm, group or association, and shall consent to be bound thereby without execution of any new agreement.

Section 4. Except as the Partnership may otherwise provide, each new partner shall contribute a sum of money to the Partnership capital to be credited to his capital account in an amount to be determined by the Partnership and on such terms as the Partnership may decide.

319

Section 5. No partner may become a partner in any other medical group
unless permission is granted by the Group in writing. Such permission may
be granted only by a vote of 2/3 of all present at a regular or special
meeting of the Partnership.

ARTICLE XV

DISCRIMINATION BARRED

The parties agree that no person shall be barred or refused admission to the Partnership as a partner or an employee of the Partnership solely
due to his race, color, creed, country of origin and further, that no person
seeking medical or surgical attention from the Partnership shall in any way
be barred or be refused the same or discriminated against in any way solely
because of the race, color, creed or country of origin.

ARTICLE XVI

OUTGOING PARTNERS

Section 1. Outgoing partners shall deliver all reports, records and data
pertaining to Group patients under his care and all other Partnership property
which may be in his possession to the Medical Director prior to the effective
date of his withdrawal, which reports, records, data and property shall at
all times remain the property of the Partnership.

Section 2. Failure to deliver all reports, records, data and property
belonging or pertaining to the Partnership, H.M.O. or to the enrollees and
patients of the Group shall result in deferment of any financial settlement
with said outgoing partners until all such reports, etc. shall have been
delivered to the Group.

Section 3. Outgoing partners shall not solicit patients of the Partnership
and the Partnership shall be entitled to notify patients formerly under the
care of such outgoing partners that the latter are no longer connected with
the Partnership.

ARTICLE XVII

ARBITRATION

If at any time during the existence of this Partnership or after
the dissolution thereof, any question, disagreement, or difference shall
arise between the partners or any of them, concerning the Partnership, its
affairs, transactions, business or accounts, or the meaning or interpretation
of this agreement, or the rights, duties or obligations of the partners
under the terms of this agreement, such question,disagreement or difference
shall be submitted to the arbitration of three disinterested persons, one to
be appointed by each of the parties to the dispute or disagreement, and the
third to be chosen by the two so appointed. Upon the failure of the

arbitrators selected by the parties to agree upon a third arbitrator within ten days after the designation of both, either party may request the American Arbitration Association to appoint the third arbitrator in accordance with its rules then pertaining. If either party to the dispute neglects to appoint an arbitrator within ten days after service upon him or them of notice to appoint an arbitrator, then the arbitrator appointed by the party so giving notice shall proceed to hear and determine the matters in difference between the parties. The award or decision made by the arbitrator or arbitrators shall be final and conclusive as to the parties to this agreement, their executors, administrators and assignees.

ARTICLE XVIII

MISCELLANEOUS

Section 1. Except as may otherwise be provided,whenever notice is required to be given or is given pursuant or relative to this Partnership agreement, whether by a partner to the Partnership or by one partner to another or by the Partnership to a partner, the same shall be made in writing and be addressed to the sendee at his last known address as it appears on the books of the Partnership.

Section 2. The parties agree that the failure of the Partnership or any one or more of the parties, to insist in any one or more instances, upon a strict performance of the Partnership or of the rules and regulations thereto shall not be construed as a waiver or a relinquishment for the future of such term, condition, covenant or provision but the same shall continue and remain in full force and effect.

Section 3. This Partnership agreement shall be governed by and construed in accordance with the laws of the State of New York.

Section 4. The parties agree that this Partnership agreement shall be binding upon and inure to the benefit of the parties hereto and all subsequently duly admitted new partners, their respective heirs, executors, administrators, legal representatives and assigns.

ARTICLE XIX

TERMINATION AND AMENDMENT OF AGREEMENT

Section 1. This agreement may be terminated by the affirmative vote of 3/4 of all the partners at a special meeting called for that purpose. Such termination shall become effective upon such date as may be fixed by such a vote provided, however that the Partnership has completed, or been released from, any contractual obligation to the fulfillment of which its continued existence and operation may be requisite.

Section 2. Upon the voluntary termination or other dissolution of the Partnership:

(a)   A financial statement should be prepared and rendered by a Certified Public Accountant reflecting a balance sheet, a profit and loss statement, a statement of the account of each partner and any other matters which the Partnership may then deem requisite.

(b)   The Partnership shall be dissolved, all debts and obligations paid, the books shall be closed, the interest of each partner determined and the assets of the Partnership distributed in proportion to such interest.

Section 3.   The Executive Committee shall serve as a liquidation committee, unless a majority of the partners decide to elect a special liquidating committee.

Section 4.   The parties further agree that such voluntary or other dissolution of the Partnership shall be made and conducted in accordance with the provisions of the Partnership Law of the State of New York.   However, all Partnership expenses and expenditures shall be paid and the distribution of profits and losses in such proceeding shall be made pursuant to the provisions respectively relating thereto, as set forth elsewhere in the Partnership agreement.

Section 5.   The parties likewise agree to execute and deliver any and all instruments necessary or incidental to such dissolution and the completion of the business of the Partnership.

Section 6.   This agreement may also be amended, altered or modified by affirmative vote of 2/3 of all the partners at a regular meeting or a special meeting provided notice of such proposed amendment, alteration or modification has been given 1) at a previous Partnership meeting or 2) by mail sent to each partner at least seven days before the meeting, at which the amendment, alteration or modification is put to a vote, or by an agreement in writing signed by 2/3 of the partners.   Any such amendment, alteration, or modification shall be effective and binding upon all of the partners, irrespective of their consent thereto.

APPENDIX B

SPECIMEN AGREEMENT BETWEEN LICENSED PHYSICIAN,
(NON-PARTNER) EMPLOYEE AND A H.M.O. REGIONAL
MEDICAL GROUP

AGREEMENT made June 5th, 1971 between XYZ MEDICAL GROUP, a co-partnership (hereinafter referred to as the "Group"), and JOHN DOE, M. D. (hereinafter referred to as "Dr. Doe").

WHEREAS, the Group has been organized to and does render medical services to subscribers of the HEALTH MAINTENANCE ORGANIZATION, (commonly known as and hereinafter referred to as "H.M.O."), pursuant to an agreement with said H.M.O.; and

WHEREAS, the parties mutually desire that Dr. Doe become associated with the Group as a family physician rendering medical care and treatment to patients assigned to him by the Group on an associated but nonpartnership basis;

NOW, THEREFORE, in consideration of the premises and the mutual covenants herein set forth, it is covenanted and agreed as follows:

1. <u>Medical Services</u>: Dr. Doe shall render such medical care and treatment and perform such procedures singly or in consultation as may be required upon such patients as may be assigned to him by the Group during his tour of duty.

2. <u>Tour of Duty</u>: Dr. Doe's tour of duty shall consist of such hours and days as may be determined by the Group after consultation with Dr. Doe, but in no event shall be less than 27 hours per week. It is further understood that the aforesaid tour of duty shall be conducted only at the premises of the Group or such other place as the Group may designate.

3. <u>Professional Standards</u>: Dr. Doe agrees that he will render services of the highest professional standards conscientiously and expeditiously to the satisfaction of the Executive Committee of the Group. In the event that a majority of the Executive Committee shall determine that Dr. Doe has failed or refused to comply with this provision of this Section, the Agreement may be terminated by the Group without further notice or a hearing of any type or nature, notwithstanding Section 14 and anything herein to the contrary.

4. <u>Compensation</u>: For all services rendered by Dr. Doe, the Group shall pay him the sum of $2,083.33 monthly. The aforesaid amount shall be the total and complete compensation to be paid by the Group to Dr. Doe, for his above described services, notwithstanding any bonus, rebate or allowance granted or provided by H.M.O. to the Group or to a physician pursuant to the terms of said H.M.O. "full time" program.

5. <u>Vacations</u>: Dr. Doe shall be entitled to four (4) weeks' vacation after each year of service during which time his compensation will be paid in full. The period of vacation shall be mutually agreed upon between Dr. Doe and the Group.

6. Insurance: Dr. Doe shall secure and maintain for the full term of this agreement the following insurance coverage to protect the Group as well as himself from liability at his own cost and expense in an amount satisfactory to the Group:

> (a) personal injury and property damage automobile insurance;
>
> (b) general personal liability insurance;
>
> (c) malpractice insurance (medical).

The required insurance policies shall be made available to the Group for its inspection at any time upon request.

7. Status: The Group agrees to consider Dr. Doe as a partner, two years after the date of this Agreement, provided this Agreement is in force and affect at that time.

8. Working Facilities: The Group agrees to furnish Dr. Doe with office facilities and such other facilities suitable to the performance of services at the Group premises, and Dr. Doe agrees not to maintain an office and not to provide medical services outside of the Group premises, except with the consent of the Group. Any compensation or fees received directly by Dr. Doe from patients not assigned to him by the Group shall be transferred and delivered to the Group in accordance with the provisions of the aforesaid H.M.O. "full time" program.

9. Expenses: It is understood and agreed that Dr. Doe is not to incur or authorize any expenses on behalf of the Group without the written consent of the Group's Medical Director and/or its Executive Committee.

10. Disability: If Dr. Doe is unable to perform his services as herein provided by reason of illness or incapacity for a period of more than one week, the compensation otherwise payable to him shall terminate. Notwithstanding anything herein to the contrary, the Group may terminate this Agreement at any time if Dr. Doe shall be unable to perform his duties as herein provided, for whatever cause, for a continuing period of more than one month and all obligations of the Group herein shall cease upon such termination.

11. Termination: Either party may terminate this Agreement without cause at any time upon at least three (3) months' written notice by one to the other. In such event, Dr. Doe shall continue to render his services and shall be paid his regular compensation up to the date of termination.

12. H.M.O.: Notwithstanding anything herein contained to the contrary, the Group may terminate this Agreement whenever it no longer is in written contractual relations with the H.M.O.

13. Restrictive Covenant: It is understood and agreed that for a period of one (1) year from the termination of this Agreement, Dr. Doe will not associate in any manner whatsoever with any other Medical Group in the county area, in contractual relations with H.M.O.

14. Arbitration: Any controversy or claim arising out of, or relating to this Agreement or the breach thereof, shall be settled by arbitration by an arbitrator mutually selected by the parties within 48 hours after demand by one party against the other for arbitration. Upon failure of the parties to select an arbitrator within the period herein specified, the arbitrator shall be selected by the American Arbitration Association in accordance with its rules then obtaining. The award of the arbitrator shall be final and binding upon the parties.

15. Notices: Any notice required or permitted to be given under this Agreement shall be sufficient if in writing and if sent by registered or certified mail by one party to the offices of the other party.

16. Entire Agreement: This instrument contains the entire agreement of the parties. It may not be changed orally, but only by an agreement in writing signed by the party against whom enforcement of any waiver, change, modification, extension or discharge is sought.

17. Assignment: This Agreement may not be assigned, transferred or conveyed by either party without the written consent of the other.

18. Effective Date: This Agreement shall become effective June 5, 1971.

IN WITNESS WHEREOF, the parties have executed this Agreement on June 5th, 1971.

       XYZ MEDICAL GROUP

BY:_____   _____
        Medical Director   John Doe, M.D.

APPENDIX C

SPECIMEN AGREEMENT BETWEEN EXECUTIVE

EMPLOYEE AND AN ORGANIZATION

Specimen Agreement Between Executive
Employee and an Organization

AGREEMENT dated January 1, 1970, between H.M.O. Plan hereinafter called the
Employer, and Joseph P. Doe, hereinafter called the Employee.

1. Employment. The Employer hereby employs the Employee and the Employee
hereby accepts employment upon the terms and conditions hereinafter set
forth.

2. Term. Subject to the provisions for termination as hereinafter provided,
the term of this agreement shall begin on January 1, 1970, and shall terminate on December 31, 1972, with the right on the part of the Employer to
extend this agreement for an additional period of three years upon written
notice to the Employee given not less than four months prior to December 31,
1972.

3. Compensation. For all services rendered by the Employee under this
Agreement, the Employer shall pay the Employee a salary of $15,000 a year,
payable in equal monthly installments at the end of each month.

4. Duties. The Employee is engaged as office manager of the Employer, to
supervise and direct credit, personnel, public relations, and servicing.
The precise services of the Employee may be extended or curtailed, from time
to time, at the direction of the Employer. If the Employee is elected or
appointed a director or an officer of the Employer during the term of this
Agreement, the Employee will serve in such capacity or capacities without
further compensation; but nothing herein shall be construed as requiring the
Employer, or anybody else, to cause the election or appointment of the
Employee as such director or officer.

5. Extent of Services. The Employee shall devote his entire time, attention,
and energies to the business of the Employer, and shall not during the term
of this Agreement be engaged in any other business activity whether or not
such business activity is pursued for gain, profit, or other pecuniary
advantage; but this shall not be construed as preventing the Employee from
investing his assets in such form or manner as will not require any services
on the part of the Employee in the operation of the affairs of the companies
in which such investments are made.

6. Working Facilities. The Employee shall be furnished with a private office,
stenographic help, and such other facilities and services, suitable to his
position and adequate for the performance of his duties.

7. Disclosure of Information. The Employee recognizes and acknowledges that
the list of the Employer's customers, as it may exist from time to time, is
a valuable, special, and unique asset of the Employer's business. The
Employee will not, during or after the term of his employment, disclose the
list of the Employer's customers or any part thereof to any person, firm,
corporation, association, or other entity for any reason or purpose whatsoever.
In the event of a breach or threatened breach by the Employee of the provisions of this paragraph, the Employer shall be entitled to an injunction
restraining the Employee from disclosing, in whole or in part, the list of

the Employer's customers, or from rendering any services to any person, firm, corporation, association, or other entity to whom such list, in whole or in part, has been disclosed or is threatened to be disclosed. Nothing herein shall be construed as prohibiting the Employer from pursuing any other remedies available to the Employer for such breach or threatened breach, including the recovery of damages from the Employee.

8. <u>Expenses</u>. The Employee is authorized to incur reasonable expenses for promoting the business of the Employer, including expenses for entertainment, travel, and similar items. The Employer will reimburse the Employee for all such expenses upon the presentation by the Employee, from time to time, of an itemized account of such expenditures.

9. <u>Vacations</u>. The Employee shall be entitled each year to a vacation of three weeks, during which time his compensation shall be paid in full. Each vacation shall be taken by the Employee over a consecutive period beginning on or after July 1 and ending on or before September 30.

10. <u>Disability</u>. If the Employee is unable to perform his services by reason of illness or incapacity for a period of more than two weeks, the compensation otherwise payable to him during the continued period of such illness or incapacity shall be reduced by 50 per cent. The Employee's full compensation shall be reinstated upon his return to employment and the discharge of his full duties hereunder. Notwithstanding anything herein to the contrary, the Employer may terminate this agreement at any time after the Employee shall be absent from his employment, for whatever cause, for a continuous period of more than three months, and all obligations of the Employer hereunder shall cease upon such termination.

11. <u>Termination Without Cause</u>. Without cause, the Employer may terminate this agreement at any time upon 30 days' written notice to the Employee. In such event, the Employee, if requested by the Employer, shall continue to render his services, and shall be paid his regular compensation up to the date of termination and, in addition, there shall be paid to the Employee on the date of termination a severance allowance of $2,000 (less all amounts required to be withheld and deducted). Without cause, the Employee may terminate this agreement upon 60 days' written notice to the Employer. In such event, the Employee shall continue to render his services and shall be paid his regular compensation up to the date of termination, but no severance allowance shall be paid to him.

12. <u>Termination Upon Sale of Business</u>. Notwithstanding anything herein contained to the contrary, the Employer may terminate this agreement upon ten days' notice to the Employee upon the happening of any of the following events: (a) the sale by the Employer of substantially all of its assets to a single purchaser or to a group of associated purchasers; (b) the sale, exchange, or other disposition, in one transaction, of two-thirds of the out-standing corporate shares of the Employer; (c) a bona fide decision by the Employer to terminate its business and liquidate its assets; or (d) the merger or consolidation of the Employer in a transaction in which the share-holders of the Employer receive less than 50 per cent of the outstanding voting shares of the new or continuing corporation.

13. Death During Employment. If the Employee dies during the term of this employment, the Employer shall pay to the estate of the Employee the compensation which would otherwise be payable to the Employee up to the end of the month in which his death occurs. In addition, the Employer shall pay $5,000, within 60 days after the death of the Employee, to the widow of the Employee, or if he is not then survived by his widow to the Employee's surviving children in equal shares, or if there are no such surviving children to the estate of the Employee.

14. Restrictive Covenant. For a period of five years after the termination of this agreement, the Employee will not, within a radius of 300 miles from the present place of business of the Employer, directly or indirectly, own, manage, operate control, be employed by, participate in, or be connected in any manner with the ownership management, operation, or control of any business similar to the type of business conducted by the Employer at the time of the termination of this agreement.

15. Arbitration. Any controversy or claim arising out of, or relating to this agreement, or the breach thereof, shall be settled by arbitration in the city of Chicago in accordance with the rules then obtaining of the American Arbitration Association, and judgment upon the award rendered may be entered in any court having jurisdiction thereof.

16. Notices. Any notice required or permitted to be given under this agreement shall be sufficient if in writing, and if sent by registered mail to his residence in the case of the Employee, or to its principal office in the case of the Employer.

17. Waiver of Breach. The waiver by the Employer of a breach of any provision of this agreement by the Employee shall not operate or be construed as a waiver of any subsequent breach by the Employee.

18. Assignment. The rights and obligations of the Employer under this agreement shall inure to the benefit of and shall be binding upon the successors and assigns of the Employer.

19. Entire Agreement. This instrument contains the entire agreement of the parties. It may not be changed orally but only by an agreement in writing signed by the party against whom enforcement of any waiver, change, modification, extension, or discharge is sought.

In witness whereof the parties have executed this agreement on December 31, 1969.

Corporate Seal   H.M.O. Plan, Inc.
Attest
                                                   by.......................
                                                      Chairman of Trustees
....
        Secretary   ....
                                                      Joseph P. Doe

BIBLIOGRAPHY

Books

Beach, Dale S. Personnel: The Management of People at Work. New York: MacMillan, 2nd ed., 1970.

Chruden, H. J. & Sherman, A. W. Jr. Personnel Management. Cincinnati: South West Publ. 3rd ed., 1968.

Clark, Wallace. The Gantt Chart: Working Tool of Management. London: Pitman Publ. 3rd Ed., 1952.

Davis Keith. Human Relations at Work. New York: McGraw-Hill, 2nd ed., 1962.

Drucker, Peter. The Practice of Management. New York: Harper & Row, 1954.

Greenberg, Selig. The Quality of Mercy. New York: Athaneum Press, 1971.

Holden, Fish & Smith. Top Management Organization & Control. New York: McGraw-Hill, 1951.

Kime, Robert E. Health: A Consumer's Dilemma. California: Wadsworth, 1970.

Newman, W. H. & Summer, C. E. Jr. The Process of Management: Concepts, Behavior and Practice. Englewood Cliffs, N.J.: Prentice-Hall, 1961.

Patten, T. H. Jr. Manpower Planning and the Development of Human Resources. New York: Wiley Interscience, 1970.

Reynolds, L. G. Labor Economics and Labor Relations, Englewood Cliffs, N.J.: Prentice-Hall, 2nd ed., 1954.

Rutstein, David, M.D. The Coming Revolution in Medicine. Cambridge, Mass.: M.I.T. Press, 1967.

Scheer, Wilbert E. Personnel Director's Handbook. Dartnell Publ. 2nd ed., 1970.

Schorr, Daniel. Don't Get Sick In America. Tennessee: Aurora, 1970.

Siegel, Laurence. Industrial Psychology. Homewood, Ill.: Irwin, 1962.

Smalley, H. E. & Freeman, J. R. Hospital Industrial Engineering. New York: Reinhold Publ. 1966.

Steiner, George A. Top Management Planning. New York: MacMillan, 1969.

Tracy, Wm. R. Evaluating Training & Development Systems. New York: American Management Assoc. Inc., 1968.

U. S. Dept. of Labor, Manpower Administration. <u>Job De scriptions and</u>
<u>Organizational Analysis for Hospitals and Related Health Services</u>.
U. S. Supt. of Documents, Revised, June 1971.

Yoder, Dale. <u>Personnel Management and Industrial Relations</u>. Englewood
Cliffs, N.J.: Prentice-Hall, 6th ed., 1970.

Articles

"Aid for Blue Cross in Nixon's Plan," <u>Business Week</u>, Feb. 27, 1971.

<u>American Medical News</u>, Various articles, editorials, news items in this
weekly newspaper of the American Medical Association.

Bennis, W. G. "Revisionist Theory of Leadership," <u>Harvard Business Review</u>,
Jan.-Feb. 1961, p. 150.

"The Crisis in American Medicine," <u>Fortune Magazine</u>, Jan. 1970.

Forsyth, G. C. & Thomas, D. G. "Models for Financially Health Hospitals,"
<u>Harvard Business Review</u>, July-Aug. 1971, Vol. 49, No. 4, pp. 106-7.

Garfield, Sidney R. M.D. "The Delivery of Medical Care," <u>Scientific</u>
<u>American</u>, April 1970, Vol. 222, No. 4.

Greenberg, I. G. & Rodburg, M. L. "The Role of Prepaid Group Practice in
Relieving the Medical Care Crisis," <u>Harvard Law Review</u>, Feb. 1971,
Vol. 84, No. 4.

Larson, L. W. et al. "Report of the Commission on Medical Care," <u>Journal of</u>
<u>the American Medical Association</u>, Special Edition, Jan. 17, 1959.

<u>Medical Economics Magazine</u>. Various issues, background information;
November 1970 through November 1971.

<u>Medical Group News</u>. Editorial, July 1970.

Sackler, A. M. Dr. "The Health Manpower Crisis," <u>Medical and Hospital</u>
<u>Tribune</u>, May 17, 1971.

Smith, R. A. Dr. "A Strategy for Health Manpower," <u>Journal of American</u>
<u>Medical Association</u>, Sept. 6, 1971.

<u>Wall Street Journal</u>. Various issues during 1971 on background topics.

Williams, Greer. "Kaiser: What is it? How does it Work? Why does it Work?"
<u>Modern Hospital Magazine</u>, Feb. 1971.

Reports

<u>American Hospital Association</u>. "Guide Issue of Hospitals," Journal of
American Hospital Assoc., August 1971.

<u>Carnegie Commission on Higher Education</u>. "Higher Education and the Nation's
Health," New York: McGraw-Hill, 1970.

332

Health & Hospital Planning Council of Southern New York, Inc. "Hospitals and
     Related Facilities in Southern New York," 1970 edition.

Health Insurance Plan of Greater New York: Annual Report, 1970.

Health Insurance Plan of Greater New York, "Information for Physicians
     Interested in Joining a Prepaid Group Partnership Practice with
     HIP Affiliation," Feb. 1971.

State of New York, "Report from the Governor's Steering Committee on Social
     Problems on Health and Hospital Services and Costs," Joseph C.
     Wilson, Chairman, April 1971.

U. S. Dept. of Health Education & Welfare, Public Health Service, "Report
     on Medical Care for the American People," October 1932, reprinted
     1970.

Yedida, Avram, "Planning and Implementation of Community Health Foundation
     of Cleveland, Ohio," U. S. Dept. of Health, Education & Welfare,
     Case study, Public Health Service.

CHAPTER VI

FINANCIAL INFORMATION AND CONTROL PROCEDURES

Harry Maccarrone

INTRODUCTION

The purpose of this chapter is to develop a financial information
and control system which will aid the managment in coordinating, monitoring,
controlling, and evaluating the on-going financial operations of the Health
Maintenance Organization.

To achieve this purpose it becomes necessary "to collect, sort,
and organize information on the progress of activities."[1] A well designed
and functioning financial information system could be expected to have the
following benefits:

1. Cost reduction opportunities and the need for increased
    expenditures can be identified. These will aid in the
    determination of realistic operating budgets.

2. It can provide the tools for controlling operations within
    budgeted limits.

3. Sufficient data could be generated to enable

    (a) Rendering reports to governing bodies and

    (b) Providing a basis for the allocating common expenses
         when computing operating costs of each organizational
         component.

    (c) It can provide a basis for the calculation of average
         income and costs per unit of service rendered

---

[1] Peat, Marwick, Mitchell & Co., Health Systems Management, Report to
Community Health Service, (Washington, D. C.: U. S. Department of Health
Education, and Welfare, June 1970), p. 60.

(d) It can provide information for the preparation of the multitude of reports to governmental agencies, insurance carriers, and other interested parties.[2]

Elements of a Financial Information and Control System

The major elements of the information and control plan are:

1. The Chart of Accounts

2. Payroll Accounting subsystem

3. Purchases and Stores Inventory subsystem

4. Miscellaneous Expense Accounting

5. Revenue subsystem

6. Budgeting procedures

7. Financial and Statistical Reports

The interrelationship of these seven elements is shown schematically in Figure VI - 1.

Basic H.M.O. Organization

A basic organization chart for the H.M.O. is shown in Figure VI - 2. The organization contains four components

1. The H.M.O. Foundation, Inc.

2. The H.M.O. Medical Center (Hospital)

3. The H.M.O. Services, Inc.

4. The Regional Medical Groups

It is contemplated that the financial organization will reside within the H.M.O. Services, Inc. entirely but it will provide accounting services for all H.M.O. components.[3]

Accounting Organization

To operate the H.M.O.'s Finance Department effectively, it is necessary to have a logical organization with clearly defined job responsibilities. The organization of the Accounting Department is shown in Figure VI - 3. It consists of several subsepartments (a) Business Office

---

[2]Uniform Chart of Accounts for Hospitals, (Chicago, Ill.: American Hospital Association, 1966).

[3]Further details of these components can be found in Chapter II, "The Organization Plan for the H.M.O."

FIGURE VI - 1

ELEMENTS OF THE HMO INFORMATION AND CONTROL PLAN

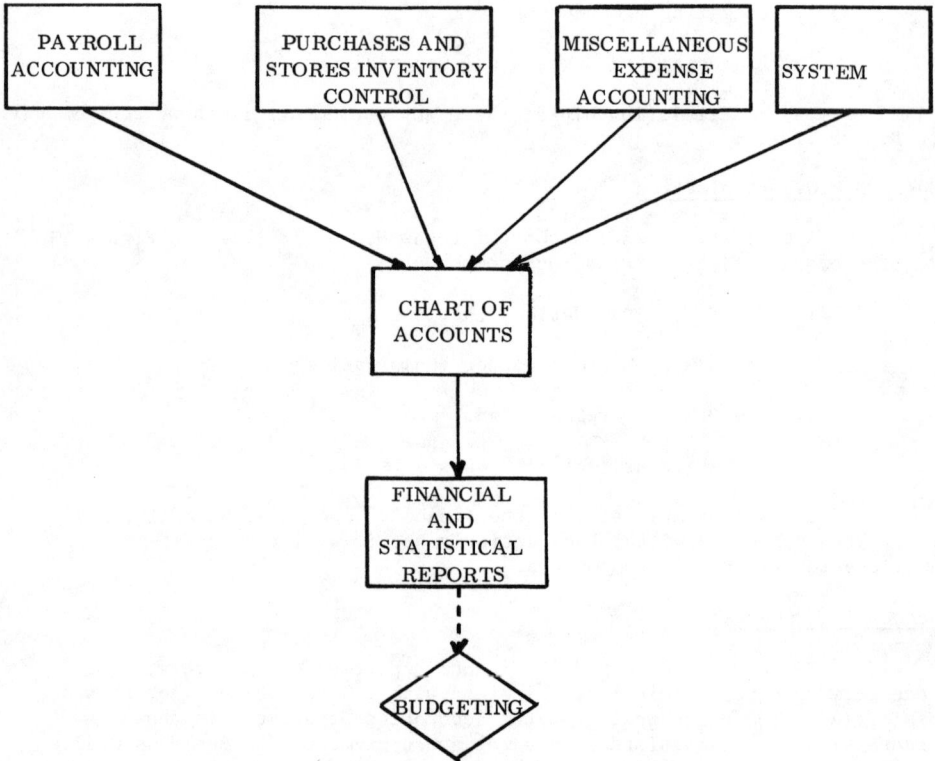


```
┌──────────────┐  ┌──────────────────┐  ┌──────────────┐  ┌──────────────┐
│   PAYROLL    │  │  PURCHASES AND   │  │MISCELLANEOUS │  │              │
│  ACCOUNTING  │  │STORES INVENTORY  │  │   EXPENSE    │  │    SYSTEM    │
│              │  │    CONTROL       │  │  ACCOUNTING  │  │              │
└──────────────┘  └──────────────────┘  └──────────────┘  └──────────────┘
            ╲            │              ╱          ╱
             ╲           │             ╱          ╱
              ╲          ▼            ▼          ╱
            ┌──────────────────────────────────┐
            │          CHART OF                 │
            │          ACCOUNTS                 │
            └──────────────────────────────────┘
                         │
                         ▼
              ┌─────────────────────┐
              │     FINANCIAL       │
              │        AND          │
              │    STATISTICAL      │
              │     REPORTS         │
              └─────────────────────┘
                         ┊
                         ▼
                    ╱─────────╲
                   ╱           ╲
                  ⟨ BUDGETING   ⟩
                   ╲           ╱
                    ╲─────────╱
```

FIGURE VI - 2

HEALTH MAINTENANCE ORGANIZATION CHART

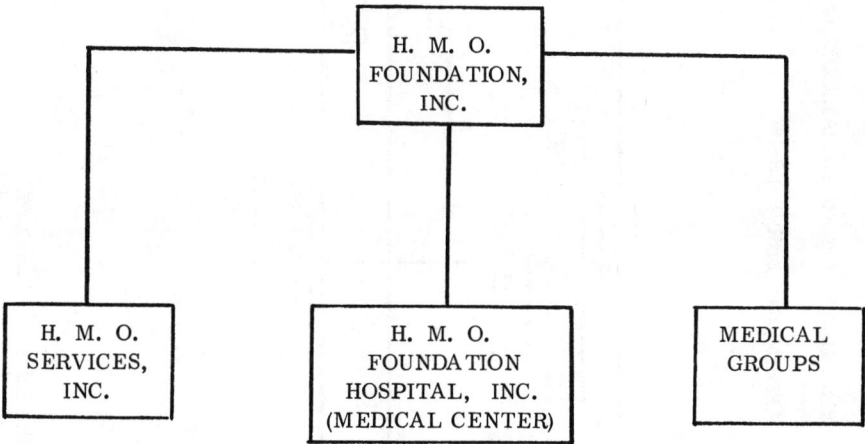

```
                        ┌─────────────────┐
                        │    H. M. O.     │
                        │   FOUNDATION,   │
                        │      INC.       │
                        └─────────────────┘
        ┌────────────────────────┼────────────────────────┐
        │                        │                        │
┌───────────────┐    ┌───────────────────────┐    ┌───────────────┐
│   H. M. O.    │    │       H. M. O.        │    │   MEDICAL     │
│   SERVICES,   │    │      FOUNDATION       │    │   GROUPS      │
│     INC.      │    │   HOSPITAL,  INC.     │    │               │
└───────────────┘    │   (MEDICAL CENTER)    │    └───────────────┘
                     └───────────────────────┘
```

Source: The Kaiser-Permanente Medical Care Program

FIGURE VI - 3

ORGANIZATION CHART FOR FINANCIAL CONTROL

WITHIN HMO SERVICES INC.

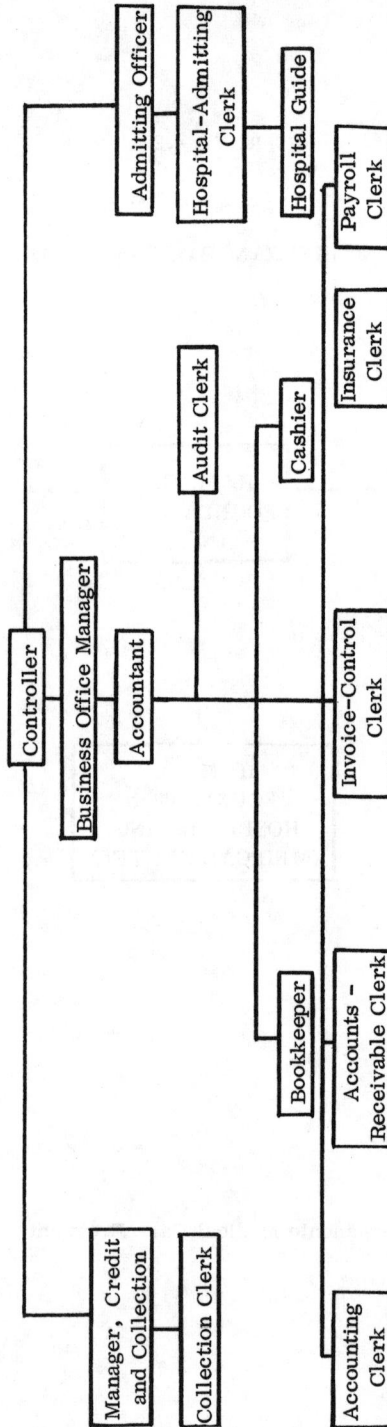

338

Source: Job Descriptions for Hospitals and Organizational Analyses for Hospitals and Related Health Care Services, U.S. Dept. of Labor.

(b) Admitting Office and (c) Credit and Collection Office. Each of these offices have personnel for carrying out their major functions. The department will be headed by a Controller.

The Controller

The Controller's responsibilities are summarized as follows:

1. To direct and coordinate H.M.O. activities concerned with financial administration, general accounting, membership business services, and financial and statistical reporting.

2. To devise and install new or modified accounting systems to provide complete and accurate records of the H.M.O.'s assets, liabilities, and financial transactions.

3. To plan methods for insuring timely receipt of membership fees and payments on patient accounts.

4. To compile information about new equipment, such as cost and labor saving features.

5. To supervise subordinates in the preparation of the H.M.O.'s budgets based on past, current, and anticipated revenues and expenditures.

6. To direct the preparation of financial and operating reports for planning effective administration of the H.M.O.'s activities by management.

7. To prepare detailed analyses of financial statements to reflect variances in income and expenditures from budgeted amounts.

8. To make recommendations to the H.M.O.'s administration concerning means of reducing operating costs and increasing memberships and revenues, based on knowledge of market trends, financial reports, and industry operating procedures.

9. To participate in discussions with the finance committee concerning such matters as the purchase of equipment and construction of new facilities.

10. To compute and record depreciation on buildings and equipment.

11. To arrange for audits of the H.M.O. accounts.

12. To review insurance policies to ascertain that coverage is adequate.

13. To supervise the preparation of cost reimbursement
    reports to Government Agencies (Medicare, Medicaid)
    and private third party agencies.[4]

CHART OF ACCOUNTS

The system has as its foundation a detailed chart of accounts that
permits the routine accumulation of financial information in classifications
most useful to management for planning and control purposes. Appendix I at
the end of this chapter contains the detailed chart of accounts. The chart
of accounts, summarized in Table VI - 1, is based on the recommendation of
the American Hospital Association (AHA) and it is adapted to the special
requirements of the H.M.O.[5,6]

As the scope and operations of the H.M.O. change, new accounts may
be needed and others deleted. Current revisions of the AHA chart of accounts
manual can be used as guides for making changes. The clerical procedures
that are influenced by these changes must then be updated.[7]

The chart of accounts uses a five digit code, for example 100.01.
Account numbers three digits to the left of the decimal point identify primary
or control account classifications; numbers two digits to the right identify
secondary account classifications. Thus, account number 100.01 refers to
cash assets (100) at the Long Island Trust Co. Bank (.01).[8]

All asset, liability, and principal or balance accounts are recorded
in balance sheet accounts. Asset accounts are numbered 100-199; liability
accounts 200-218. The difference accounts (assets - liabilities) are listed
as the principal or balance accounts numbered 219-299.[9]

---

[4] Job Descriptions for Hospitals and Related Organizational Analyses for
Hospitals and Related Health Care Services, U. S. Department of Labor,
Manpower Administration, revised edition 1971, U. S. Superintendent of
Labor, pp. 92-93. Job descriptions for other positions can also be found
in this document.

[5] Uniform Chart of Accounts for Hospitals, op. cit., p. 25.

[6] The three organizations (H.M.O. Foundation, Inc., H.M.O. Foundation Hospital,
Inc., and H.M.O. Services Inc.) will use the same chart of accounts to
facilitate consolidation of financial statements.

[7] Uniform Chart of Accounts for Hospitals, op. cit.

[8] Ibid.

[9] Ibid., pp. 62-90.

TABLE VI - 1

CHART OF ACCOUNTS SUMMARY

	Primary Classification		Secondary Classification
Balance Sheet Accounts			
Assets	100-200	XXX	
Liabilities	200-218	XXX	
Principal and Balance	219-299	XXX	
Secondary Account Classifications			.XX
Income and Expense Accounts			
Patient Service Revenue	300-499	XXX	
Deductions from Revenue	500-529	XXX	
Other Revenue (including Memberships)	530-599	XXX	
Patient Expense Centers	600-799	XXX	
General Operating Centers	800-999	XXX	
Revenue			
Inpatient Members	.01		.XX
Inpatient Nonmembers	.02		.XX
Inpatient Medicare	.03		.XX
Outpatient Members	.11		.XX
Outpatient Nonmembers	.12		.XX
Outpatient Medicare	.13		.XX
Expenses			
Salaries, Wages and Fringe Benefits	.01-.19		.XX
Professional and Outside Services	.20-.29		.XX
Supplies	.30-.39		.XX
Interest and Insurance	.40-.49		.XX
Depreciation	.50-.59		.XX
Utilities	.60-.69		.XX
Miscellaneous	.70-.79		.XX
Expense Credits	.80-.89		.XX

Note: Details in Appendix I at end of chapter.

Source: Adapted from Uniform Chart of Accounts for Hospitals,
(Chicago, Ill.: American Hospital Association, 1966).

341

Each primary balance sheet account has subclassifications. For example, the subclassifications of inventory maintained by the H.M.O. Services, Inc. include:

113.00   General Storeroom

113.01   Dietary Supplies

113.02   Pharmacy   10

Revenue Accounts

All member or nonmember revenue is recorded in member or nonmember revenue center accounts which are used to accumulate "revenue" for services performed by the H.M.O. These accounts are set up in the same manner as "fee for service" revenue accounts of a hospital. Services performed by H.M.O. Foundation, Inc., H.M.O. Foundation Hospital Inc., and H.M.O. Services, Inc. should be reflected in their respective accounting records.

Revenue accounts also have a three-digit primary account number and a two-digit secondary account number. For example, the revenue account that is used to accumulate the basic hospital charge in the Operating Room for a member patient is 360.01. This charge is recorded on the H.M.O. Foundation Hospital, Inc. accounting records.

```
                                 360         0        1

    Operating Room----------------------┘        ┊        ┊

    Inpatient-------------------------------------┘        ┊

    Member------------------------------------------------┘ 11
```

All differences between the revenues recorded and the actual receivables are recorded in the deductions from revenue accounts. Revenue accounts are credited for the full value of services rendered to patients at the H.M.O.'s established rates, regardless of the amounts the H.M.O. actually expects to collect for such services. The deductions from revenue accounts are used to record the offsets to revenue earned by H.M.O., but are amounts members or nonmembers, themselves, will not actually pay. These deductions from revenue accounts have a primary classification number in the 500 through 529 and contain contractual adjustments for:

1.   H.M.O. memberships

2.   Medicare

3.   Other (including Blue Cross, HIP, etc.)   12

---

10 Ibid.

11 Ibid., pp. 91-95.

12 Ibid., pp. 94-96.

All other revenues not included as patient service revenue are recorded in other revenue accounts of the respective H.M.O. component generating the revenue. These revenues are accumulated in the primary account classifications 530 through 599. The secondary classifications can later be established to provide additional subclassifications as other revenue accounts are needed.

For example, other revenues generated by the H.M.O. Services, Inc. may include:

     551   Cafeteria Sales--H.M.O.

     552   Barber Shop Sales

     561   Vending Machines

     566 Laundry Service

     568 Medical Record Transcript Fees [13]

Expense Center Accounts

All direct expenses incurred in providing patient services by each H.M.O. component are recorded in the respective patient expense center accounts. All expenses must be recorded in both a primary account number and a secondary expense classification. The patient expense center accounts have initial primary account series of "600" and "700." These numbers correspond to those accounts in the "300" and "400" series which indicate comparable revenue accounts. The second and third digits of the patient expense center accounts are identical to the second and third digits of the corresponding revenue accounts.[14] For example, the revenue account used to accumulate the basic hospital charge in the Operating Room is 360. The corresponding Operating Room expenses are accumulated in primary account 660.[15]

Indirect service expense center accounts are in the "800" and "900" series. The expenses recorded in these accounts result from indirect service or "nonrevenue producing" centers of the respective H.M.O. component. These cost centers include Housekeeping, Dietary, Laundry, Maintenance, etc.[16]

All direct H.M.O. (hospital, clinic, etc.) costs are recorded by expense account. No expense accounts can be used without a corresponding expense center account. The secondary account classifications provide a means of identifying expense within each cost center. The first digit of the secondary classification identifies the type of expense and the second digit provides additional classifications within the expense type.[17]

---

[13]Ibid., pp. 96-99.

[14]Ibid., pp. 103-16.

[15]Ibid.

[16]Ibid., pp. 101-03.

[17]Ibid.

Secondary Classifications

First Digit	Description
0 & 1	Salaries, Wages and Employee Benefits
2	Professional and Outside Services
3	Supplies
4	Interest and Insurance
5	Depreciation
6	Utilities
7	Miscellaneous
8	Expense Credits [18]

A full account number for regular salaries for employees working in the Operating Room would be 660.<u>01</u>.

Regional Medical Group Expenses

All Regional Medical Group expense accounts have a primary classification of 757. This account is used to record all[19] direct expenses associated with the Regional Medical Groups for which H.M.O. components will not be reimbursed. These expenses include:

1. Salary payments to Doctors operating the Regional Medical Groups.

2. Drugs and supplies requisitions by the Regional Medical Groups for H.M.O. members.[20]

Inter-Organizational Expenses

The inter-organizational accounts ("Due to"/"Due from") have primary classifications 147 through 150. Whenever a chargeable service is performed by one H.M.O. component on behalf of another, the inter-organizational accounts are used to record the receivable/payable that has been created on the respective H.M.O. component's account records. For example, assume the H.M.O. Foundation Hospital, Inc. requests medical supplies from Central Storage and Warehouse maintained by H.M.O. Services, Inc. and H.M.O. Services, Inc. will record a receivable "due from" H.M.O. Foundation Hospital, Inc.

---

[18]Ibid.

[19]The appointment service function is recorded in expense account 986 by the H.M.O. Service, Inc. The appointment service expense is not a chargeable expense to the Regional Medical Groups.

[20]The salary arrangements with the medical doctors operating the Regional Medical Groups are discussed in Chapter VI "The Manpower Plan."

(inter-organizational account 148) and reduce inventory (inventory account 113). The H.M.O. Foundation Hospital, Inc. will record the transaction as "due to" H.M.O. Services, Inc. (inter-organizational account 149) and record the expense in the appropriate cost center.

PAYROLL ACCOUNTING

The payroll accounting system is designed to do the following:

1. Accumulate the direct payroll expense by the incurring cost center.

2. Calculate the accumulated payroll related fringe benefits.

3. Determine the month-end labor and labor related accruals.[21]

The flow chart in Figure VII - 4 shows the relationships of the payroll subsystems described in this section.

Labor Reporting

Some nursing personnel may work interchangeably in patient and ancillary cost centers. To properly record nursing time, the nurse's time sheet in Table VI - 2 should be completed and reconciled to the time cards on a daily basis by nursing personnel assigned to two or more cost centers. The time sheets indicate by cost center the actual hours worked each day. This makes it possible to manually compute the nursing expense by cost center.

The following procedure should be used by the payroll clerk to accumulate the nursing expense biweekly.[22]

1. Total the hours worked in each cost center on each nurse's time sheet.

2. Total the daily employee compensation hours by each cost center and reconcile these totals to the total hour column.

3. Determine the percentage of total hours spent by the employee in each cost center by dividing the cost center total hours by total hours. Post this amount to the employee time sheet "percentage" line.

---

[21]Accounting Manual for Long-term Care Institutions, (Chicago, Ill.: American Hospital Association, 1968), p. 77.

[22]It is assumed that there will be biweekly payroll.

FIGURE VI - 4 (Continued)

PAYROLL FLOW CHART
WITHIN HMO SERVICES, INC.

ACCOUNTING

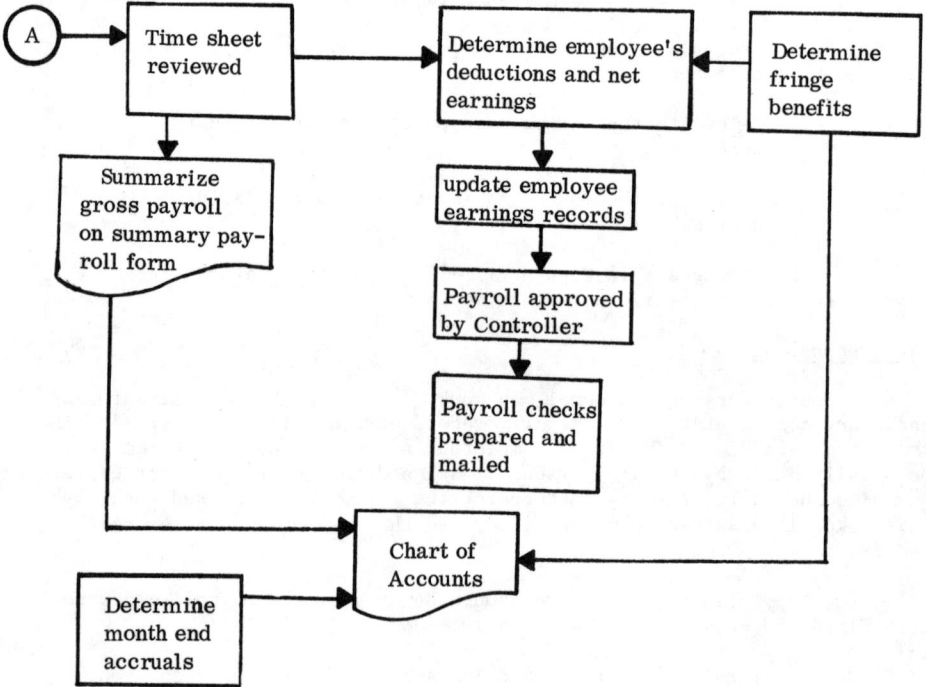

PAYROLL FLOW CHART
WITHIN HMO SERVICES, INC.

COST CENTER   DEPARTMENT HEAD

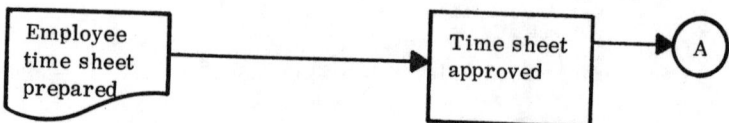

TABLE VI - 2

Payroll Report For Nurses Working In Two Or More Cost Centers

Employee_____   Position_____

From_____To_____   Ward_____

Date	Time In	Time Out	Total Hours	General Practise	Hospital 1st Floor	Medical & Surgical	Hospital 2nd Floor	Medical & Surgical	Hospital 3rd Floor	Pediatrics	ICU	Obstetrics	Newborn	Operating and Recovery Room	Labor and Delivery Room	Emergency Room	Other				
1																					
2																					
3																					
4																					
5																					
6																					
7																					
8																					
9																					
10																					
11																					
12																					
13																					
14																					
15																					
16																					
17																					
18																					
19																					
20																					
21																					
22																					
23																					
24																					
25																					
26																					
27																					
28																					
29																					
30																					
31																					
Total Hours																					
%																					
Gross Pay																					

Employee _____   Date _____

Source: Adapted from various Long Island Hospital payroll forms.

TABLE VI - 3
H. M. O.

NURSING SERVICE

SUMMARY PAYROLL REPORT

FROM _____ TO _____

Employee	Gross Pay	G. P.	M & S 1st Fl.	M & S 2nd Fl.	M & S 3rd Fl.	Ped.	ICU	O. B.	Newborn	O. & R.	Emergency	Other				
Totals																

Source: Adapted from various Long Island Hospital payroll forms.

4. Post the total amount earned in the "Gross Pay" box and allocate it to the appropriate cost center. Reconcile the cost center totals to gross pay.

5. Record each employee's payroll allocation by cost center on the summary sheet (See Table VII - 3).

6. Total the payroll amounts by cost center making sure the combined totals of the cost centers equals the total of the "Gross Pay" column.[23]

Forms shown in Tables VI - 2 and VI - 3 can be adapted for use for other departments' employees who work in two or more cost centers.

Fringe Benefits

Fringe benefits consist of payroll related payments including the employer's portion of Social Security, Workmen's Compensation, and Employee H.M.O. Coverage. These amounts must be accounted for regularly. This can be accomplished by having the payroll department allocate the fringe benefits to the cost centers and allocating benefits for employees working in two or more cost centers proportionately. For example, if an employee worked 75 per cent of his time in Pediatrics (account 630) and 25 per cent in Newborn Nurseries (account 640), the employee's fringe benefits would be charged proportionately between the two cost centers.[24]

Payroll and Payroll Related Accruals

The H.M.O. employees are paid on a biweekly basis, whereas most accounting departments are on a calendar month. If the account period and the payroll period do not end on the same day, employees will have worked several days for which they have not yet been paid. These amounts plus related fringe benefits are recognized by the use of accrual entries.

Payroll accruals should be made during the month-end closing by the Accounting Department as follows:

1. Divide the total payroll paid during the last payroll period in all cost centers by the work days in that payroll.

2. Multiply the amount obtained in step 1 by the number of workdays worked but not yet paid.

---

[23] P. Taylor and B. O. Nelson, Management Accounting for Hospitals, (Philadelphia, Pa.: W. B. Saunders Co. 1964), pp. 286-299.

[24] Ibid.

3. Prepare a journal entry to record the amount accrued at the end of the month.

4. Reverse the month-end journal entry at the beginning of the next month by journal entry.[25]

For example, assume the last pay period in October ended October 25. The next pay period would end November 8 (14 days later). Salaries and wages earned from October 26 through October 31 should be reflected as an October expense. Thus, 6/14 of the last payroll can be used to set up the month-end accrual by:

1. Debiting the various department salaries and wages in the same proportion as the last payroll.

2. Crediting payroll deductions account.

3. Crediting salaries and wages payable.[26]

Fringe benefit accruals include liabilities arising from specific payroll related benefits. To calculate the fringe benefit accrual for each cost center, total payroll accrued should be multiplied by the appropriate percentage factor for each of the following fringe benefits:

1. FICA

2. Workmen's Compensation

3. Employee H.M.O. Coverage

4. Other fringe benefits

To record these accruals, a journal entry listing each component is prepared. This entry must also be reversed in the following month. For example, if the percentage factor for FICA is 5.2 per cent of gross payroll, 5.2 per cent of the gross payroll accrual would represent the FICA month-end accrual. A journal entry would be made:

1. Debiting FICA expense to the various cost centers in same proportion as the payroll accrual.

2. Crediting the FICA payable account.

PURCHASING AND STORES INVENTORY CONTROL

Approximately 25 per cent of a hospital's expenses originate from purchases.[27] Weak controls over the purchasing procedures can be extremely

---

[25]Accounting Manual for Long-term Care Institutions, op. cit., p. 78.

[26]Ibid.

[27]P. Taylor and B. O. Nelson, op. cit., p. 261.

costly; good controls can result in significant savings.

The purchasing and stores inventory control phases of the H.M.O. accounting system are intended to do the following:

1. Provide control over purchasing and receiving.

2. Provide quantitative inventory control.

3. Accumulate materials, supplies, and other expenses by the incurring cost centers as the related documents are received in the Accounting Department.

4. Determine the monthly accounts payable balance.

The system consists of the following parts:

1. Purchasing and receiving of goods.

2. Physical distribution of stores and nonstore items.

3. Cost allocation of goods to the appropriate cost centers.

Purchasing and Receiving

The control and accounting of material purchases begin with the purchasing and receiving function. The following procedures should be followed by the purchasing and receiving department of the H.M.O. Services, Inc.:

1. Use a purchase requisition for all purchase requests except for certain food purchases where an open purchase order may be used for vendors with whom business is done on a day-to-day basis.[28]

2. Require a three part purchase order.[29]

3. Code purchase orders by cost center and H.M.O. component.

4. Use a two part receiving report.

5. Send vendor invoices to the accounts payable department in the Accounting Department.

---

[28] For details regarding purchase requisition forms see Taylor and Nelson, p. 262.

[29] For details regarding purchase order forms see Taylor and Nelson, p. 263.

FIGURE VI - 5

PURCHASING AND RECEIVING FLOW CHART
WITHIN HMO SERVICES, INC.

DEPARTMENT HEAD

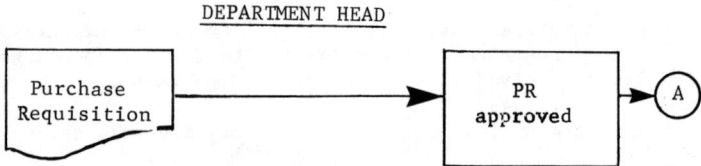

FIGURE VI - 5 (continued)

PURCHASING AND RECEIVING FLOW CHART
WITHIN HMO SERVICES, INC.

PURCHASING AND RECEIVING

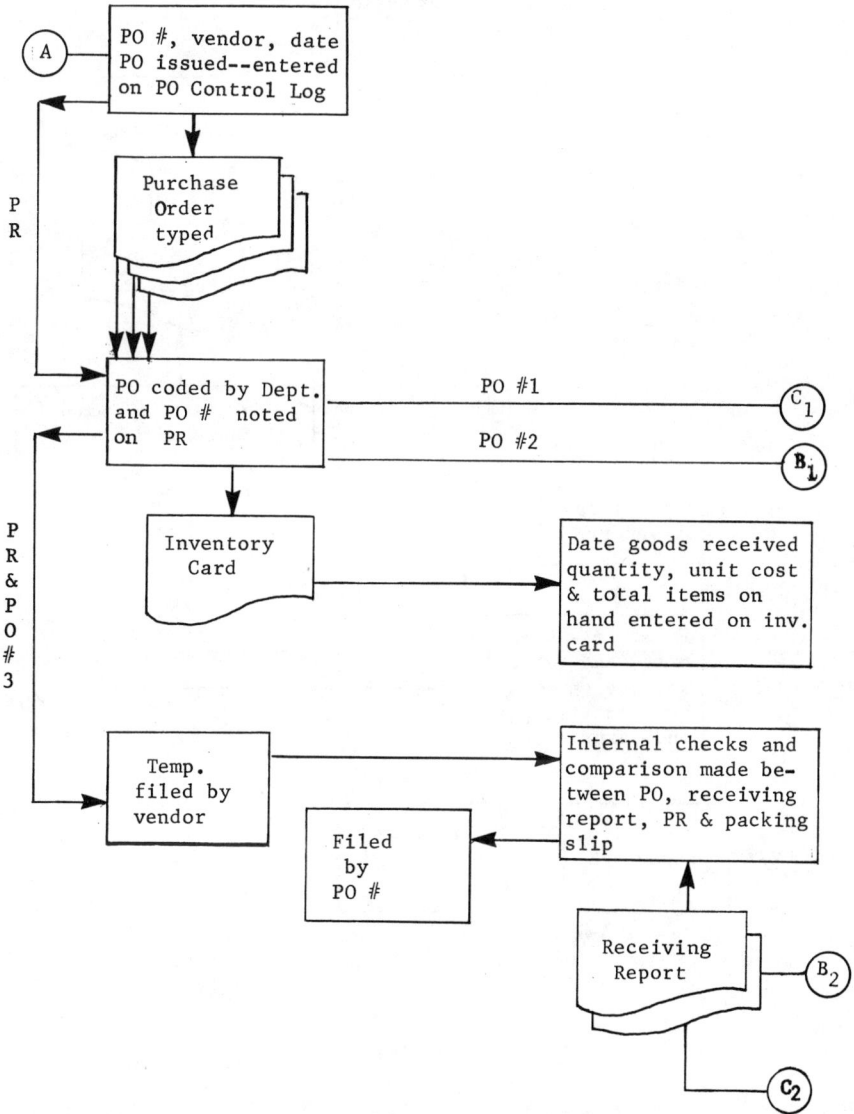

FIGURE VI - 5 (continued)

PURCHASING AND RECEIVING FLOW CHART
WITHIN HMO SERVICES, INC.

ACCOUNTING

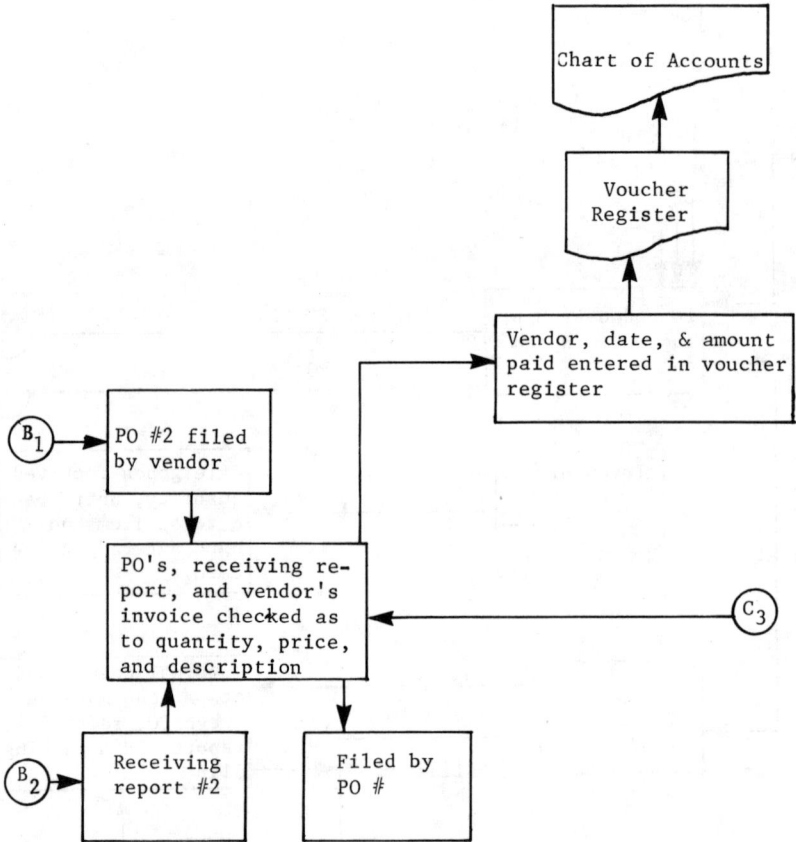

FIGURE VI - 5 (continued)

PURCHASING AND RECEIVING FLOW CHART
WITHIN HMO SERVICES, INC.

<u>VENDOR</u>

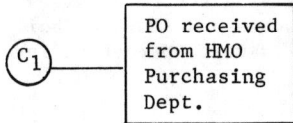

PO received
from HMO
Purchasing
Dept.

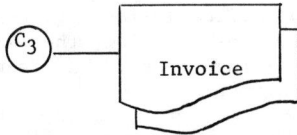

Invoice

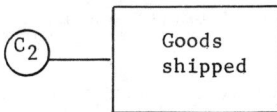

Goods
shipped

6. Receiving all merchandise ordered by the
   Purchasing and Receiving Department, which
   inspects the goods and forwards receiving
   reports to the Accounting Department.[30,31,32]

        See Figure VI - 5 for the Purchasing and Receiving Flow Chart
illustrating the above procedures.

        These procedures result in the following:

1. Segregation of duties among the ordering,
   physical control of the purchases, recording
   of the accounts payable, and receipt of the
   vendor's invoice.

2. Assignment of responsibility to one department for the receipt of merchandise in good
   condition.

        The purchasing and receiving system provides for all goods to be
received in the Centralized Warehouse and Storage Facilities of the H.M.O.
Services, Inc. At this point, a quantity perpetual inventory is used to aid
in accounting for these items.[33]

        Stock items are held in storerooms. A stock requisition form should
be used to draw stock. When the storeroom receives a requisition from a cost
center, it will issue the goods and make the necessary entry in the perpetual
inventory records.

        Nonstock items are materials and supplies not usually held in the
storeroom inventory, but ordered specifically for a requesting cost center.
When a nonstock item is received by the storeroom, the purchase order should
be pulled and matched with the receiving report. The documents should then
be forwarded to the Accounting Department.

Cost Distribution

        The cost distribution system serves as a means for assigning pur-
chase material costs to the proper cost center and H.M.O. component. Two
methods to do this are:

1. Assign costs to the requisitioning cost center
   as goods are requisitioned from inventory.

2. Assign costs to the purchasing cost center as
   invoices are received.

_____

[30]For details regarding receiving report forms see Taylor and Nelson, p. 264.

[31]P. Taylor and B. O. Nelson, op. cit., pp. 261-265.

[32]Developed in discussions with John T. Norton, C. P. A.

[33]For details regarding perpetual inventory system see Taylor and Nelson,
   pp. 267-275.

356

The second method is preferrable for the H.M.O. because it requires less time and it is simpler.

When the Accounting Department receives an invoice and matches it to the purchase order, it knows to which cost center and H.M.O. component the expenses should be charged. In instances where two or more cost centers are involved, a suitable basis should be established for the allocation.

Allocation of nonstores items is relatively simple. For example, legal service invoices should be charged to the legal expense account (900.22), telephone bills to the telephone expense account (900.68).

See Figure VI - 5 for the Purchasing and Receiving Flow Chart illustrating the relationship between the purchasing, receiving, inventory, and accounts payable systems.

OTHER EXPENSE ACCOUNTING

Certain expenses incurred by cost centers are charged to one center by another center. Although no actual cash payments are made by the cost center receiving the material or service. Examples of these book transactions include depreciation and internal maintenance.

Depreciation

Depreciation is the recovery of prepaid fixed asset cost charged to a specific accounting period.[34] Depreciation is a valid operating expense and is recognized as such by the reimbursement regulation of the Health Insurance For the Aged Act, Title XVIII.[35]

Accurate depreciation records are the prerequisite to an effective property control system, which will permit the Controller to:

1. Select the optimum depreciation for third party reimbursement and cash flow.

2. Substantiate third party reimbursement reports for audit purposes.

3. Obtain adequate physical control.

4. Properly allocate depreciation to departments.

---

[34] James A. Cashin and Garland C.Owens, Auditing, (New York, N.Y.: The Roland Press Company, 1963), p. 345.

[35] Audit Program for Hospitals Under the Health Insurance for the Aged Act Title XVIII, U. S. Department of Health, Education and Welfare.

5. Evaluate the adequacy of property insurance.

6. Develop capital budgets for funding requirements.

Recovery of Depreciation Charges

The present Medicare regulations, as described in the Social Security Administration's publication, HIM-15, Provider Reimbursement Manual, provide a health care institution with various methods for calculating allowable depreciation. Each method requires certain backup data to substantiate the reasonableness of the depreciation expense. Through installation of a reliable property control system, the H.M.O. will be able to ensure proper reimbursement. Several key factors regarding the Medicare regulations should be noted:

1. Either straight line or accelerated depreciation may be used.

2. The same method does not have to be used for each asset.

3. The method of depreciation on each asset may be changed only once following the initial selection.[36]

In order to take full advantage of these options, depreciation on land improvements, buildings and fixtures, and other depreciable property must be identifiable and properly recorded on the H.M.O.'s accounting records. The Medicare regulations also state that the depreciation must be based on the historical cost or the fair market value at the time of donation for donated assets. To ensure proper reimbursement for depreciation, H.M.O.'s records must show for each asset: the acquisition date, the original cost and the useful life.[37]

Physical Control

The following are the physical control requirements of the H.M.O.:

1. All operating fixed assets must be included, including gifts and donations.

2. All assets in the following categories must be included:

   a. Land improvements

   b. Buildings

   c. Building fixtures and fixed equipment

   d. Major movable equipment

---

[36] Herman Miles Somors, Medicare and the Hospitals, (Washington, D.C.: Brookings Institution, 1967), pp. 171-74.

[37] Ibid., pp. 171-75.

3. Assets must be clearly identifiable in the property control records as to the location, the account, the classification, the department cost center, and the H.M.O. component.

4. Capitalization policies must be defined and updating procedures for the property control records documented.

5. Property control records must be readily verifiable for internal audit and management purposes.[38,39]

These procedures will provide the H.M.O. with the information needed to insure that:

1. All assets have been included in the depreciation computation.

2. Depreciation is being charged to the proper cost center and H.M.O. component.

3. The existence and location of each asset can be readily verified through observation.

4. The appropriate information has been included for insurance purposes.[40]

Internal Maintenance

All outside maintenance and repairs to specific equipment should be charged to the incurring H.M.O. component's cost center through the accounts payable system. Internal maintenance jobs that have a total labor content of one or more hours or a total material cost of $25.00 or more should be charged to the requesting H.M.O. component cost center.[41]

Materials and supplies requisitioned for a specific repair should be charged directly to the cost center receiving the repair by noting the department's code number on the purchase order. General material and supplies usage should be estimated by the Maintenance Department and priced at the requisition unit price. See Table VI - 4 for a sample H.M.O. repair requisition form.

[38]Hospital Audit Guide, AICPA, Re-exposure Draft, January 22, 1971.

[39]Benjamin Newman, Accounting Theory, A CPA Review, (New York, N.Y.: Wiley Press, 1967), pp. 577-78.

[40]Ibid., p. 578.

[41]This is an arbitrary cutoff, for purposes of illustration.

TABLE VI - 4

HMO

REPAIR REQUISITION

REPAIR REQUISITION

HMO COMPONENT_____   COST CENTER_____

DATE_____   DEPT. HEAD_____

DESCRIPTION:

APPROVED BY_____

The labor cost for each maintenance requisition shoud be computed by the Accounting Department. The number of hours worked should be multiplied by the average hourly rate of the Maintenance Department. Cost requisitions should then be accumulated by the Accounting Department and charged to the department requesting the repair.

REVENUE SYSTEM

The H.M.O. accounting system is designed with an emphasis on expense accumulation. However, the system must also deal with the special requirements of revenue accumulation for H.M.O. members, nonmembers, and Medicare patients. The H.M.O. Revenue System includes the following:

1. Revenue is assigned to the period in which it is earned.

2. Revenue is recognized at established rates for all patient services, even though many of the charges will later be discounted (for Medicare, nonmembers) or not billed at all (members).

3. Revenue is segregated by the revenue center producing the revenue.

4. Revenue is recorded by Member, Nonmember, and Medicare classifications.

5. Revenue statistics that reflect the activity levels of the revenue producing cost centers are generated.

Membership Revenues

Membership revenues are the fees prepaid by H.M.O. subscribers for medical services. Since H.M.O. fees involve a prepayment, membership revenues must be recorded through a deferred revenue or unearned revenue account (revenue account 217.50 on the H.M.O. Foundation, Inc. accounting records). Monthly, as income is earned, the deferred revenue account is reduced and earned revenue recognized (revenue account 570).[42]

It is important for H.M.O. management to know what medical facilities are being used by members. The above revenue recognition procedure does not provide this information. Therefore, the revenue system must be further modified to segregate and accumulate the various medical service charges to H.M.O. members.

When a member receives a service, the "revenue" is recorded in the appropriate revenue center coded "Members" on the accounting records of the

---

[42]
Developed in discussion with John T. Norton, C. P. A.

H.M.O. organization performing the service. This is the same procedure followed for "Nonmembers" or "Medicare" patients. However, if this "revenue",
is not collectible; no account receivable is set up. Instead, the contractual
adjustment allowance account is charged (account 510). For example, if a
subscriber has an operation which is covered by his H.M.O. membership, the
established H.M.O. charge for the service would be recorded in Medical and
Surgical-Member revenue account 310.01. Since the subscriber would not have
to pay for the service, the contractual allowance account 510 would be charged
rather than accounts receivable account.

The advantages for this procedure are that it:

1. Permits management to know through financial
   statements what medical facilities are being
   used.

2. Shows management which revenue centers are
   not being run efficiently when compared to
   corresponding cost centers.

3. Is necessary for Medicare and Blue Cross
   reimbursement computations.

4. Is helpful in pricing membership fees at
   "break-even" levels.

Census Taking

The census is an accounting of all inpatients at the H.M.O. The
census shows the names and number of patients at each nursing station which
is the basis for accumulating patient charges for daily hospital services.

The following procedures should be followed when taking the census:

1. Nurses should complete the room census at
   midnight.

2. In the morning the nursing station should
   submit the census to the Medical Records
   Department.

3. The Medical Records Department should
   prepare the Daily Census Report each
   morning by utilizing the previous day's
   Census Report as a worksheet, and updating
   it for admissions and discharges.[43]

4. The Medical Records Department should
   forward the completed Daily Census Report
   to the Accounting Department in the morning.

---

[43] For details regarding census reports see Taylor and Nelson, pp. 177-78.

5. The Accounting Department should use the Daily Census Report as the source to post the daily patient service charges to the patient billing ledgers.[44]

6. A copy of the Census Report should be filed in the Accounting Department as a permanent record.[45,46]

Patient Charges

Patient charges (other than hospital services) originate in other departments which provide ancillary services and supplies. Ancillary services may include specialized professional services performed for patients by one or more of the following departments:

1. General Practice

2. Operating and Recovery Rooms

3. Labor and Delivery

4. Laboratory

5. Emergency

6. Radiology

7. Physical Therapy

8. Pharmacy

9. Central Supply

The following procedures should be followed in processing the charge slips issued by these departments:

1. Each of the above departments should complete daily charge slips at the time the service is provided to the patient. See Table VII - 5 for a sample H.M.O. CHARGE SLIP.

2. The charge slips should be completed in their entirety with the exception of the pricing of the service. This should now be the responsibility of the Accounting Department.

---

[44] For details regarding patient billing ledgers see Taylor and Nelson, p. 189.

[45] P. Taylor and B. O. Nelson, pp. 175-78.

[46] Developed in discussions with John T. Norton, C. P. A.

363

TABLE VI - 5

HMO

CHARGE SLIP

HMO
CHARGE SLIP

HMO COMPONENT_____

DEPARTMENT_____

PATIENT NAME_____   Patient No._____

DESCRIPTION OF SERVICE_____

_____

_____

TOTAL COST $_____   Approved by_____

                                    No. 0000001

364

5.   Procedures should be established to be
     certain that price books are kept up-to-
     date in all departments.

Patient Discharge Procedure

The following procedures should be followed when discharging
patients:

1.   Physician

     The attending physician should write "HOME" on
     the patient's chart when the patient is ready
     to be discharged.

2.   Nurse

     The nurse should check the last charge slip
     issued to be sure that all medication given
     to the patient has been recorded. A dis-
     charge notice should then be sent to the
     Accounting Department and the cashier.
     See Table VI - 6 for H.M.O. DISCHARGE NOTICE.

3.   Accounting Department

     Upon notification of discharge, the Accounting
     Department should:

     a.   Locate the patient's billing ledger.

     b.   Review the unrecorded charge slips for
          applicable charges to be added to the
          patient's account.

     c.   Determine H.M.O. Coverage and reduce
          patient's account accordingly.

     d.   Record Blue Cross, HIP, and other
          insurance credits.

     e.   Determine amount due from patient.

4.   Cashier

     Before the patient is discharged, the cashier should:

     a.   Obtain the patient's billing ledger from
          the Accounting Department.

     b.   Ask the patient or responsible party to
          pay the patient's portion of the estimated
          bill not covered by the H.M.O. prepayment
          contract. If the patient cannot pay his
          portion of his estimated bill, ask him to
          pay for his take-home drugs and have him
          sign a promissory note for the balance.

TABLE VI - 6

HMO

DISCHARGE NOTICE

HMO
DISCHARGE NOTICE

NAME_____   DATE_____

PATIENT NO._____   APPROVED BY_____

LEAVING TIME_____

COMMENT_____

_____

_____

No. 0000001

However, the Pharmacy, Operating Room, Emergency Room, and General Practice are the only exceptions to this procedure. These departments should price the charge slip originating within their respective areas. Further, other charges not included in the H.M.O. Price Book because of their unusual nature should be priced by the originating department.

3. The charge slips should be forwarded to the Accounting Department.[47]

In conjunction with the above, the following procedures should be followed within the Accounting Department regarding patients' accounts:

1. Patient billing ledgers should be filed alphabetically within each type of membership for members and by third party payers for nonmembers. This will facilitate the necessary billing and collection process.

2. All patient charges, both members and nonmembers, should be posted to the patient's billing ledgers daily.[48]

H.M.O. Price Book

Since the H.M.O. will provide medical services for members, the H.M.O. Price Book listing the charges for all medical services is required. The H.M.O. Price Book is the basis for all patient charges. The following procedures should be adhered to regarding the H.M.O. Price Book:

1. Every chargeable service including drugs, laboratory tests, X-Rays, central supply items, or surgical charges should be included with respective prices in the H.M.O. Price Book.

2. The Accounting Department should have the responsibility for maintaining the H.M.O. Price Book.

3. The Accounting Department should be notified of any change (addition, deletion, or price change) by the department supervisor or other responsible individual.

4. Whenever the H.M.O. Price Book is updated, notice of the change should be sent to all personnel who have a copy.

---

[47] P. Taylor and B. O. Nelson, op. cit., pp. 188-96.

[48] Ibid.

c. Issue a receipt for the money received.

d. Return the patient's billing ledger to
the Accounting Department.[49,50]

BUDGETING

The revenues realized and the expenses incurred by H.M.O. as
collected and recorded can also provide information to aid management in
planning and controlling its activities. Budgeting is the principal management tool used to control operations.[51]

Advantages of Budgeting

The budgeting program used for the H.M.O. has several advantages
to management. It:

1. Requires management to think ahead and
review past trends within H.M.O. and
the health care industry.

2. Requires the establishment of goals for
H.M.O. These goals include financial
operational goals as well as health care
delivery goals.

3. Stimulates a cost consciousness among
department heads and other employees.

4. Provides standards against which results
can be compared. These standards are
used for evaluating employee performances
and controlling costs.

5. Provides the necessary information for
corrective action.

6. Enables management to anticipate cash
requirements of operations.[52,53]

Prerequisites to Budgeting

Before an effective budgeting system can be developed, there are
certain prerequisites, including:

---

[49]Ibid., pp. 219-21.

[50]Developed in discussions with John T. Norton, C. P. A.

[51]Accounting Manual for Long-term Care Institutions, op. cit., p. 91.

[52]Ibid.

[53]Systems and Procedures, Ed. Victor Lazarro, (Englewood Cliffs, N.J.:
Prentice Hall, Inc. 1968), pp. 262-63.

368

1. The firm support and acceptance of the budget program by H.M.O. management (including department heads).

2. A sound organizational structure within which responsibilities are clearly defined.

3. A chart of accounts which conforms to the organizational structure. This will guarantee that actual results can be identified with specific individuals or functions.[54]

Other Budgeting Factors

Other factors that may effect the cost of future outlays include:

1. Price level changes which cause costs of most commodities and services to increase or decrease.

2. Technological advances that may: a) render certain commodities or services obsolete, or, b) change the quality of the commodity resulting in an increase or decrease in price.

3. Changes in quantities of commodities purchased: this may effect quantity discounts and change unit costs.

4. Changes in the supply and demand of certain commodities; this may cause an increase or decrease in costs.

5. Legislative action (federal, state, and local), such as the Minimum Wage and Hour law, may effect staffing policies and costs.[55]

H.M.O. can have some control over the above factors.

The Operating Budget

The operating budget is a 12 month projection of the H.M.O.'s profit and loss statement. It includes projections of revenues, deductions from revenues, and expenses.[56]

---

[54]Accounting Manual for Long-term Care Institutions, op. cit., p. 92.

[55]Cost Finding and Rate Setting for Hospitals, (Chicago, Ill.: American Hospital Association, 1968), p. 12.

[56]Accounting Manual for Long-term Care Institutions, loc. cit.

Budgeting Revenues

The budget of revenues starts with a careful review of the mix between anticipated member patients and nonmember patients. Statistical data must be compiled to estimate the amount and types of member and nonmember services. Estimates must also be made to determine chargeable member services that are not covered by their contracts (such as telephone, television, private room, etc.). When this is completed, the budget for revenues can be developed, as follows:

1. Determine total membership fees by taking the total number of members multiplied by their respective membership rates.

2. Determine member revenues not covered by contracts.

3. Determine revenues from nonmembers.

Deductions from Revenues

Deductions from revenues include a) allowances, the differences between gross revenue charges and the amounts received (or to be received) from patients or third party payors for H.M.O. services and, b) provision for uncollectible receivables.[57]

The budget for revenue deductions should be developed by relating past experience adjusted for expected variations to the total budgeted patient service revenue. Variations in the percentage of deductions to gross revenues may be due to changes in patient mix (i.e. relatively fewer contractual patients), changes in reimbursement rates by third party agencies (e.g., Blue Cross), or changes in admission policies.[58]

Percentage of deductions to gross revenues, classified by type of deduction, should be developed. These percentages can then be applied to budget revenues to determine the estimated deductions from revenues.[59]

Budgeting Expenses

Each department is given a worksheet (see Table VI - 7). Historical data is inserted by the accountant or statistician.[60] The department head in conference with the administrator determines the budget figures. The participation by the department head in the development of the budget encourages acceptance and responsibility.[61]

---

[57]Ibid.

[58]Ibid.

[59]Ibid.

[60]After the first year of operation, historical data will be available to H.M.O.; for the first year information should be obtained from health care industry in preparing the expense budget.

[61]Accounting Manual for Long-term Care Institutions, op. cit.,p. 93.

TABLE VI - 7

DEPARTMENTAL EXPENSE BUDGET WORK SHEET

| | Total | Expense Budget by Month | | | | | | | |
		1	2	3	9	10	11	12
Expense Experience								
Last Year:								
Salaries and Wages	$	$	$	$	$	$	$	$
Supplies and Other	$	$	$	$	$	$	$	$
Total Last Year	$	$	$	$	$	$	$	$
This Year:								
Salaries and Wages	$	$	$	$	$	$	$	$
Supplies and Other	$	$	$	$	$	$	$	$
Total This Year	$	$	$	$	$	$	$	$
Expense Budget								
Salaries and Wages:	$	$	$	$	$	$	$	$
Employee Name								
Employee Name								
Employee Name								
Proposed Addition								
Total Salaries and Wages Budget	$	$	$	$	$	$	$	$
Supplies and Other--								
This Year	$	$	$	$	$	$	$	$
Projected Increase in Resident Days (%)	%	%	%	%	%	%	%	%
Increase in Supplies and Other Expense	$	$	$	$	$	$	$	$
Unadjusted Supplies and Other Expense Budget	$	$	$	$	$	$	$	$
Estimated--% Price Increase								
Supplies and Other Expense Budget	$	$	$	$	$	$	$	$
Total Expense Budget for Department	$	$	$	$	$	$	$	$

(4th through 8th month omitted)

Source: Accounting Manual for Long-Term Care Institutions, American Hospital Association (Chicago, Ill., 1968), p.97

371

Completing the Operating Budget

The accountant must compile the budgets from all parties involved into a projected profit and loss statement for the budget period. After an administrative review, the final result is obtained by combining the partial budgets into a master budget.

The Cash Budget

Using the approved master budget which will include both the operating budget and the plant and equipment budget, a cash budget can be developed. Table VI - 8 can be used for this purpose.[62]

Budgeting Cash Receipts

The major portion of cash receipts will be from membership fees. The fees may be due quarterly, semiannually, or annually (depending on payment plan). From this information the cash inflow from membership fees can be determined.

Another significant portion of cash receipts will be collections on patient accounts receivable. A study of collection experience in hospitals and other health care institutions will provide a guide to the budgeting of cash receipts from patients or their sponsors.[63] For example, if hospital experience in the locality shows that 60 per cent of billings usually are collected in the month billed and 40 per cent in the following month. If January billings are $10,000 then it can be estimated that $6,000 will be collected in January and $4,000 in February.[64]

Other items, such as donations and government grants are usually more difficult to budget. Specific dates as to when these items will be collected is often unknown. Therefore, the accountant must use his seasoned judgement in estimating all cash receipts and in anticipating cash shortages so that bank loans can be sought.

Budgeting Cash Disbursements

Budgeting of payment on accounts payables is based upon an analysis of the budgets for plant and equipment, supplies, utilities, and other non-payroll expenses. The accountant should also confirm credit arrangements with suppliers, inventory requirements, and other factors that may effect the timing of cash outlays.[65]

---

[62]Ibid.

[63]After the first year of operations, past collection experience will be a better guide in estimating cash flow from patient receivables.

[64]Accounting Manual for Long-term Care Institutions, loc. cit.

[65]Ibid., pp. 93-94.

TABLE VI - 8
CASH BUDGET

Cash Budget by Month

	1	2	3	(4th through 8th month omitted)	9	10	11	12
Opening Balance	$	$	$		$	$	$	$
Budgeted Cash Receipts:								
Collections on Accounts Receivable	$	$	$		$	$	$	$
Collections on Membership Fees								
Grants and Contributions								
Investment Income								
Proceeds from Sale of Investments								
Loan from Bank								
Other Receipts	$	$	$		$	$	$	$
Total Cash Receipts	$	$	$		$	$	$	$
Total Cash Available	$	$	$		$	$	$	$
Budgeted Cash Disbursements:								
Payments on Accounts Payable	$	$	$		$	$	$	$
Payment of Salaries and Wages								
Payments of Taxes								
Repayment of Bank Loans								
Payments on Mortgage								
Purchase of Equipment								
Purchase of Investments								
Other Disbursements	$	$	$		$	$	$	$
Total Cash Disbursements	$	$	$		$	$	$	$
Closing Balance	$	$	$		$	$	$	$

Source: Adapted from Accounting Manual for Long-Term Care Institutions, (Chicago, Ill: American Hospital Association, 1968), p. 98.

Budgeting of payment for payroll is based upon the anticipated manpower needs of the H.M.O. Once these needs are estimated, the budget for payroll expenditures can be determined by adding wage and fringe benefit payments plus any increments caused by additions or subtractions to the payroll or wage adjustments.[66]

Budgeting of payment for bank loans and mortgages are relatively simple. After the loans are made, schedules of the amounts and payment dates are supplied by the bank.[67]

Budget and Financial Reports

Budgets should be used along with financial reports to enable management to gain better control over expenses. For example, "this year versus last year" comparison:

	This Year	Last Year
Dietary Expense	$55,000	$52,000

This comparison has some value; but, it does not tell management what the dietary expense should have been for the period. They cannot evaluate the performance of the dietary department from this information alone.[68]

However, if the actual dietary expenses were compared to the budget amount, management could take necessary corrective action to prevent excessive spending in the dietary department.

	This Year	Budgeted
Dietary Expense	$55,000	$45,000 [69]

H.M.O. monthly financial reports with "actual versus budget" comparisons enable an administrator to detect unfavorable trends and to correct them before any serious damage is done.[70]

FINANCIAL AND STATISTICAL REPORTS

One of the principle objectives of the accounting system is to generate accurate and meaningful information about the H.M.O.'s operations for use by the various management levels and for external use.

---

[66] Ibid.

[67] Ibid.

[68] Ibid., pp. 94-95.

[69] Ibid.

[70] Ibid.

Financial Reports

Financial reports summarize the overall financial position and performance of the H.M.O. These reports are prepared on a daily, monthly, quarterly, and annual basis.

The most important financial reports are the statement of operations statement of income and expense, or an income statement.[71]

Table VI - 9 contains the recommended format for the H.M.O.'s statement of operations. It is designed to reflect totals of the basic categories of revenues and expenses for the current month, and the year to date, in comparison with the budgeted amounts. Actual revenues and expenses are accumulated from the following accounts in the general ledger:

1. Patient Service Revenue   300-499

2. Deductions from Revenue Centers   500-529

3. Other Revenues   530-599

4. Patient Expense Centers   600-799

5. General Operating Centers   800-899

The Balance Sheet reflects the financial position of the H.M.O. at a specific point in time in terms of assets, liabilities, and capital or fund balances. Table VI - 10 contains the recommended format for the H.M.O's Balance Sheet which contains summaries of various asset and liability accounts. It should be prepared on a monthly basis. See Figure VI - 6 for Accounting Cycle Summary which shows how the Balance Sheet and Operating Statements are generated from the accounting system.[72]

The controller of the H.M.O. should be aware of the cash position of the H.M.O. on a daily basis. This is necessary to determine whether planned expenditures can be made or whether the H.M.O. should obtain some additional short term borrowings to meet current cash needs.

The Cash Flow Statement report provides a summation of cash received for the day (which should equal the amount of cash receipts recorded in the cash receipts journals), the cash disbursements for the day (which equal the amount of cash disbursements recorded in the cash disbursements journals), and the prior day's closing cash balance. Thus, the Cash Flow Statement provide a handy summary of cash, inflows, outflows and balances.

The daily Cash Flow Statement is also used as the source for preparing the monthly Cash Flow Statement which summarizes the cash activity for the month and year to date. See Table VI - 11.

---

[71]Ibid., pp. 99-100.

[72]Ibid., p. 101.

TABLE VI - 9

STATEMENT OF OPERATIONS
FROM_____TO_____

	Current Month Actual Budgeted	Year to Date Actual Budgeted
Revenue:		
Inpatient		
Outpatient		
Total Patient Service Revenue		
Deductions from Patient Service Revenue		
Other Revenue		
Total Revenue		
Expenses:		
Nursing services		
Other professional services		
General services		
Fiscal services		
Administrative services		
Depreciation		
Miscellaneous		
Total Expenses		
Net Income (Loss)		

Source: Adapted from Hospital Audit Guide, AICPA Re-exposure Draft,
January 22, 1971, p. 55.

TABLE VI - 10

BALANCE SHEET
(DATE)

	Current Month	Prior Year

Current Assets:
  Cash
  Receivables
    Membership Fees
    Inpatient
    Outpatient
  Allowance for Uncollectible Accounts
  Other Receivables
  Inventories
  Prepaid Expenses

        Total Current Assets

Fixed Assets
Accumulated Depreciation

        Total Fixed Assets

        Total Assets

Current Liabilities:
    Accounts Payable
    Accrued Salary Expenses
    Other Current Liabilities

        Total Current Liabilities

Long Term Debt:
    Notes payable

        Total Long Term Debt

        Fund Balance

Source: Adapted from Hospital Audit Guide, AICPA Re-exposure Draft,
January 22, 1971, p. 53.

FIGURE VI - 6

ACCOUNTING CYCLE SUMMARY

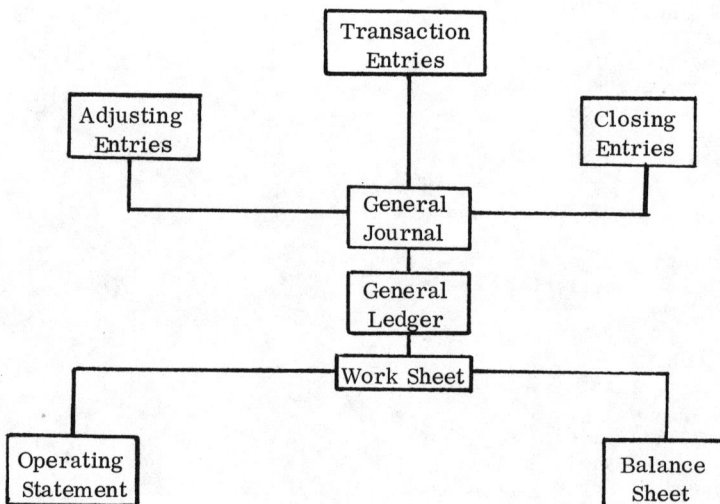

Source: Accounting Manual for Long-Term Care Institutions, American Hospital Association (Chicago, Ill., 1968), p. 24.

TABLE VI - 11

CASH FLOW STATEMENT

FROM_____TO____

	Daily $	Month to date $	Year to date $
Balance at beginning of period			
Add Cash Receipts:			
Collection of Membership fees			
Collection on Accounts Receivable			
Cash Transactions			
Other (specify)			
Deduct Cash Disbursements:			
Payroll			
Operating Expenditures			
Capital Expenditures			
Other (specify)			
Balance at end of period	$	$	$

Management Reports

Management reports are used by the H.M.O. cost center supervisors to control the direct costs for which they are responsible. In addition, these reports are used by the H.M.O. administration to evaluate individual cost center supervisor's performance. The information available in management reports is used to:

1. Make pricing decisions.

2. Study proposed or existing services.

3. Evaluate any H.M.O. policy having financial implications.

The direct costs incurred by each cost center should be accumulated on a monthly basis. The H.M.O. Accounting Department should produce a full cost allocation to determine the financial viability of each H.M.O. cost center that generates patient revenue. Table VI - 12 contains the format of the statements used for this purpose.[73]

Profit per Unit of Service Statement

The Profit per Unit of Service Statement compares the revenue and the fully allocated costs of certain revenue producing services provided by the H.M.O. This information should be used at least quarterly to evaluate the H.M.O.'s current price structure. The Profit per Unit of Service is derived by dividing the fully allocated cost of a cost center by the units of service that occurred during that period.[74]

The Profit per Unit of Service will vary because of levels of occupancy, levels of service, and the mix of services performed during the period. Occupancy or utilization levels are a major factor in profit per unit of service data.[75]

Other Management Reports

The information generated by the accounting system can also be used for various types of special analysis. Management reports are not limited to the reports described above. The monthly reports are primarily designed to indicate areas for additional analysis.

External Reports

The final reimbursements made to the H.M.O. under the health insurance programs are determined as a result of annual audited cost reports. The

---

[73]P. Taylor and B. O. Nelson, op. cit., p. 17.

[74]Accounting Manual for Long-term Care Institutions, op. cit., pp. 102-03.

[75]See Accounting Manual for Long-term Care Institutions, pp. 102-03, 112, for formats that may be adopted for Unit of Services analyses.

TABLE VI - 12

COST CENTER INCOME STATEMENT
COST CENTER_____
FROM_____ TO_____

	Quarter	Year to date
Revenue:		
Inpatient		
Members		
Nonmembers		
Other		
Outpatient		
Members		
Nonmembers		
Medicare		
Other		
Total Revenues		
Direct Expenses:		
Salaries and Wages		
Employee Benefits		
Professional and Outside Services		
Supplies		
Equipment Depreciation		
Maintenance		
Total Direct Expenses		
Allocated Expenses:		
Administrative		
Plant Maintenance		
Laundry and Linen		
Housekeeping		
Dietary		
Nursing Administration		
Medical Records		
Plant Depreciation		
Interest and Insurance		
Utilities		
Miscellaneous		
Total Allocated Expenses		
Total Expense		
Net Income (Loss)		

accounting system is designed to produce the information necessary for the generation of these health insurance program cost reports. In addition, the accounting system is designed to provide the flexibility to analyze alternatives to determine how to maximize reimbursement.

APPENDIX I

LONG ISLAND HEALTH MAINTENANCE ORGANIZATION

CHARGE OF ACCOUNTS

Assets

OPERATING FUND ASSETS
100.00-110.49 Cash in Banks
    110.01 Long Island Trust Bank
    110.05 Long Island Trust Bank (Equipment Fund)
    110.10 Long Island Trust Bank (Trust Account)
    110.15 Valley National Bank
    110.20 First National City Bank

110.50-110.99 Imprest Cash Funds
    110.50 Petty Cash Fund
    110.60 Cashiers Change Fund
    110.70 Cafeteria Change Fund

112.00-112.09 Accounts and Notes Receivable - Inpatients
    112.01 LIHMO Memberships
    112.03 Medicare
    112.04 Blue Cross
    112.05 Other Insurance
    112.06 Creditors Services
    112.07 Indigent
    112.08 Other

112.10-112.19 Accounts and Notes Receivable - Outpatients
    112.10 LIHMO Members
    112.11 Nonmembers
    112.13 Medicare
    112.14 Blue Cross
    112.15 Other Insurance
    112.16 Creditors Services
    112.17 Indigent
    112.18 Other

112.20-112.89 Other Receivables
    112.61 Staff Physicians
    112.62 Other Employees

113.00-113.99 Inventories
    113.00 General Storeroom
    113.01 Dietary Supplies
    113.02 Pharmacy

114.00-114.99 Prepaid Expenses
    114.00 Insurance

PLANT FUND ASSETS
145.00-145.99 Land, Building & Equipment
145.00-145.09 Land
  145.00 Hospital

145.30-145.39 Buildings
  145.30 Hospital

145.50-145.59 Fixed Equipment
  145.50 Hospital

145.70-145.79 Major Movable Equipment
  145.70 Hospital

146.00-146.99 Accumulated Depreciation
146.30-146.39 Accumulated Depreciation - Buildings
  146.30 Hospital

146.50-146.59 Accumulated Depreciation - Fixed Equipment
  '146.50 Hospital

146.70-146.79 Accumulated Depreciation - Major Movable Equipment
  146.70 Hospital

147.00-150.00 Inter-Organizational Accounts
  147.00 Due From (Due To) H.M.O. Foundation, Inc.
  148.00 Due From (Due To) H.M.O. Foundation Hospital,Inc.
  149.00 Due From (Due To) H.M.O. Services, Inc.
  150.00 Due From (Due To) Regional Medical Groups

Liabilities

OPERATING FUND
217.00-217.19 Accounts Payable and Accrued Payroll
  217.00 Accounts Payable
  217.10 Accrued Payroll

217.20-217.29 Payroll Taxes and Deductions Payable
  217.20 FICA
  217.21 Employee LIHMO Coverage
  217.23 Workmen's Compensation

217.50-217.59 Deferred Income
  217.50 LIHMO Membership
  217.54 Medicare
  217.55 Blue Cross
  217.56 Other

217.70-217.89 Other Current Liabilities

Principal and Balance Accounts
219.00 Accumulated Earnings (Deficit) - LIHMO
219.20 Bond Fund

Revenue

310-359 Daily Patient Services
310.01 Medical and Surgical - Members (1st Floor)
310.02 Medical and Surgical - Nonmembers (1st Floor)
310.03 Medical and Surgical - Medicare (1st Floor)
311.01 Medical and Surgical - Members (2nd Floor)
311.02 Medical and Surgical - Nonmembers (2nd Floor)
311.03 Medical and Surgical - Medicare (2nd Floor)
312.01 Medical and Surgical - Members (3rd Floor)
312.02 Medical and Surgical - Nonmembers (3rd Floor)
312.03 Medical and Surgical - Medicare (3rd Floor)
330.01 Pediatrics - Members
330.02 Pediatrics - Nonmembers
330.03 Pediatrics - Medicare
340.01 Intensive Care - Members
340.02 Intensive Care - Nonmembers
340.03 Intensive Care - Medicare
346.01 Obstetrics - Members
346.02 Obstetrics - Nonmembers
346.03 Obstetrics - Medicare
350.01 Newborn Nurseries - Members
350.02 Newborn Nurseries - Nonmembers
350.03 Newborn Nurseries - Medicare

360 - 389 Other Nursing Services
360.01 Operating and Recovery Rooms - Members (Inpatient)
360.02 Operating and Recovery Rooms - Nonmembers (Inpatient)
360.03 Operating and Recovery Rooms - Medicare (Inpatient)
370.01 Labor and Delivery Rooms - Members (Inpatient)
370.02 Labor and Delivery Rooms - Nonmembers (Inpatient)
370.03 Labor and Delivery Rooms - Medicare (Inpatient)
375.01 Central Supply - Members (Inpatient)
375.02 Central Supply - Nonmembers (Inpatient)
375.03 Central Supply - Medicare (Inpatient)
375.11 Central Supply - Members (Outpatient)
375.12 Central Supply - Nonmembers (Outpatient)
375.12 Central Supply - Medicare (Outpatient)
378.11 Emergency Room - Members (Outpatient)
378.12 Emergency Room - Nonmembers (Outpatient)
378.13 Emergency Room - Medicare (Outpatient)

402 - 499 Ancillary Services
402.01 Laboratory - Members (Inpatient)
402.02 Laboratory - Nonmembers (Inpatient)
402.03 Laboratory - Medicare (Inpatient)
402.11 Laboratory - Members (Outpatient)
402.12 Laboratory - Nonmembers (Outpatient)
402.13 Laboratory - Medicare (Outpatient)
410.01 Blood Bank - Members (Inpatient)
410.02 Blood Bank - Nonmembers (Inpatient)
410.03 Blood Bank - Medicare (Inpatient)
410.11 Blood Bank - Members (Outpatient)
410.12 Blood Bank - Nonmembers (Outpatient)
410.13 Blood Bank - Medicare (Outpatient)

402 - 499 Ancillary Services, Continued
415.01 EKG - Members (Inpatient)
415.02 EKG - Nonmembers (Inpatient)
415.03 EKG - Medicare (Inpatient)
415.11 EKG - Members (Outpatient)
415.12 EKG - Nonmembers (Outpatient)
415.13 EKG - Medicare (Outpatient)
421.01 Radiology - Members (Inpatient)
421.02 Radiology - Nonmembers (Inpatient)
421.03 Radiology - Medicare (Inpatient)
421.11 Radiology - Members (Outpatient)
421.12 Radiology - Nonmembers (Outpatient)
421.13 Radiology - Medicare (Outpatient)
430.01 Pharmacy - Members (Inpatient)
430.02 Pharmacy - Nonmembers (Inpatient)
430.03 Pharmacy - Medicare (Inpatient)
430.11 Pharmacy - Members (Outpatient)
430.12 Pharmacy - Nonmembers (Outpatient)
430.13 Pharmacy - Medicare (Outpatient)
436.01 Inhalation Therapy - Members (Inpatient)
436.02 Inhalation Therapy - Nonmembers (Inpatient)
436.03 Inhalation Therapy - Medicare (Inpatient)
436.11 Inhalation Therapy - Members (Outpatient)
436.12 Inhalation Therapy - Nonmembers (Outpatient)
436.13 Inhalation Therapy - Medicare (Outpatient)
437.01 Physical Therapy - Members (Inpatient)
437.02 Physical Therapy - Nonmembers (Inpatient)
437.03 Physical Therapy - Medicare (Inpatient)
437.11 Physical Therapy - Members (Outpatient)
437.12 Physical Therapy - Nonmembers (Outpatient)
437.13 Physical Therapy - Medicare (Outpatient)
456.11 Physician's Fees - Members (Outpatient)
456.12 Physician's Fees - Nonmembers (Outpatient)
456.13 Physician's Fees - Medicare (Outpatient)

510 - 519 Contractual Adjustments
510 LIHMO Membership
511 Medicare
512 Blue Cross
515 Other

550 - 599 Other Revenues
551 Cafeteria Sales - LIHMO
552 Barber Shop Sales
561 Vending Machines
565 Telephone and Telegraph
566 Laundry Service
568 Medical Record Transcript Fees
569 Other
570 H.M.O. Membership Fees

APPENDIX I (continued)

Patient Expense Centers

600 - 699 Nursing Division
600 Administration and Training
610 Medical and Surgical (1st Floor)
611 Medical and Surgical (2nd Floor)
612 Medical and Surgical (3rd Floor)
630 Pediatrics
640 Intensive Care
646 Obstetrics
650 Newborn Nurseries
660 Operating and Recovery Rooms
670 Labor and Delivery Rooms
675 Central Supplies
678 Emergency Room
679 General Practice

700 - 799 Other Professional Services Division
702 Laboratory
710 Blood Bank
715 EKG
721 Radiology
730 Pharmacy
736 Inhalation Therapy
737 Physical Therapy
756 Physicians Fees
757 Regional Medical Group

800- 999 General Operating Centers
801 Dietary
830 Plant Services
850 Housekeeping
860 Laundry
900 Administration
942 Medical Records
981 Provision for Depreciation - Building
985 Insurance
986 Appointment Services

Secondary Expense Accounts

Salaries and Wages
.01 Regular Salaries
.02 Overtime Premium
.03 Standby and Call Time
.04 Temporary Help
.05 Bonus

Employee Benefits
.11 FICA
.12 Workmen's Compensation
.13 Employee LIHMO Coverage

Professional and Outside Services
   .21 Professional Remuneration
   .22 Legal Fees
   .23 Audit Fees
   .27 Repairs and Maintenance
   .28 Service Contracts
   .29 Other Outside Services

Supplies
   .31 Food
   .32 Blood
   .33 Anesthesia and Oxygen
   .34 Drugs and Pharmaceuticals
   .35 Linens
   .36 Educational and Office
   .37 Maintenance
   .38 Other Supplies - Patient
   .39 Other Supplies - Non-Patient

Interest and Insurance
   .41 Interest
   .42 Insurance

Depreciation
   .51 Equipment

Utilities
   .65 Gas
   .66 Electricity
   .67 Water
   .68 Telephone and Telegraph

Miscellaneous
   .71 Professional Meetings and Travel
   .72 Dues and Subscriptions
   .73 Postage
   .74 Freight
   .75 Equipment Rental
   .76 Bad Debts
   .79 Other

Expense Credits
   .80 Inter-departmental

Source: Adapted from Uniform Chart of Accounts for Hospitals, (Chicago,Ill.:
        American Hospital Association, 1966).

BIBLIOGRAPHY

Accounting Manual for Long Term Care Institutions, Chicago, Illinois:
       American Hospital Association, 1968.

Audit Program for Hospitals Under the Health Insurance for the Aged Act,
       Title XVIII, U. S. Department of Health,Education, and Welfare.

Birand, Ives. System of Medical Records for Clinical and Statistical
       Purposes for Outpatient Clinics, Medical Outposts, and Health
       Centers, Geneva: World Health Association, 1960.

Cashin, James and Owens, Garland C. Auditing, New York, N.Y.: Roland Press
       Company, 1963.

Cost Finding and Rate Setting for Hospitals, Chicago, Illinois: American
       Hospital Association, 1968.

Cost Finding for Hospitals, Chicago, Illinois: American Hospital
       Association, 1957.

Hay, Leon. Budgeting and Cost Analysis for Hospital Management, Second
       Edition, Bloomington, Indiana: Pressler Publications, 1963.

_____. Health is a Community Affair, Report of the National Commission
       on Community Health Services, Cambridge, Mass.: Harvard University
       Press, 1966.

Heiser, Herman C. Budgeting Principles and Practice, New York: The
       Roland Press Company, 1959.

Hospital Audit Guide, AICPA, Re-exposure Draft, January 22, 1971.

Job Descriptions for Hospitals and Organizational Analyses for Hospitals and
       Related Health Care Services, U. S. Superintendent of Labor, 1971.

Lozarro, Victor. Systems and Procedures, Englewood Cliffs,New Jersey:
       Prentice-Hall, Inc. 1968.

_____. Preliminary Report of the Governor's Steering Committee on
       Social Problems on Health and Hospital Services and Costs,
       New York, April 15, 1971.

Medicare Audit Guide, AICPA, New York, N.Y. 1969.

Newman, Benjamin. Accounting Theory, A CPA Review, New York, N.Y.: Wiley
       Press, 1967.

Peat, Marwick, Mitchell & Company, Health Systems Management, Report to
       Community Health Service, Washington, D. C.: U. S. Department
       of Health, Education and Welfare, 1970.

Seawell, Lloyd Vann. Principle of Hospital Accounting, Berwyn, Illinois:
       Physicians Record Company, 1960.

389

Taylor, P. and Nelson, B. O. Management Accounting for Hospitals,
        Philadelphia, Pa.: W. B. Saunders Company, 1964.

Uniform Chart of Accounts, Chicago, Ill.: American Hospital Association,
        1966.

Conferences

Norton, John T. C.P.A. involved with Hospital, Medicare, Medicaid, and other
        Long-term Health Care Institution accounting and procedures.

CHAPTER VII

THE PUBLIC RELATIONS PLAN

James Aubrey Kirklin

LE RAISON D'ETRE

Today, there exists a world of complex relationships with inescapable interdependences between its inhabitants and the institutions they have
created. Several trends are responsible for these growing interdependences[1]
and for the growing need for public relations activities to cope with the
resultant problems. The population explosion, urbanization, rapid advance-
ments in science, automation, rising education levels and accompanying
aspiration levels, the social revolution, and the separation of ownership
and control of business all have come about with such rapidity as to make
acceptance of changes difficult. Eric Hoffer,[2] in his book, The Ordeal of
Change, presents a cogent and lucid picture of the tensions and conflicts
that arise from such changes.

Specialization has also created an additional need for interpretation and dissemination of information about the organization's activities.
Percy Tannenbaum supports this by saying "perhaps it would be best to give
up the idea that the mass media can become reliable disseminators...because
they are not equipped to supply information and their audience is not equipped
to handle it."[3]

Although the goals and functions of today's organizations vary,
they all seek, in their respective ways, to serve their publics. Sallie
Bright believes that "The extent to which any organization will be permitted
to serve the community depends directly on how much people understand and how
they feel about the needs it is attempting to meet, and about the methods it
is using to meet them, and about the quality of its performance. A sound

---

[1] Scott M. Cutlip and Allen H. Center, Effective Public Relations,
(Englewood Cliffs, N.J.: Prentice-Hall, Inc., 1964), p. 54.

[2] Eric Hoffer, The Ordeal of Change, (New York: Harper and Row Publishers,
Inc., 1963).

[3] Percy Tannenbaum, "Communication of Science Information," Science, Vol. 14,
(May 10, 1963).

Public Relations program is directed to these three points, to the end that
people may better be served."[4] In this sense, the Public Relations function
is intended to illuminate the gray area between the organization and its
publics and to aid in building lasting and meaningful relationships.

The concept of Public Relations itself presents a justification for
its existence. Conceptually, Public Relations is both task and policy-
oriented. According to the management concept,[5] Public Relations is public
responsibility, or in-a-word accountability. Advocates of these positions
point out that "Responsible performances on the part of a corporation, governmental agency or nonprofit organization is the foundation of sound Public
Relations."[6] Further, holders of the management viewpoint place the responsibility for public accountability in the laps of corporate directors, board
members and trustees, and not in its staff or line organization. The leadership is responsible for the design of organizational policies, while the
followers are left to implement them.[7]

A particular need for public relations exists in the health field.[8]
The increasing cost of medical care, overcrowded hospitals, understaffing,
long waits in the emergency room, the apparent lack of concern for a patient's
well-being, and the exclusive interest in his ability to pay are just some of
the gripes heard from users of the medical system. When these situations or
conditions do exist, there are no doubt reasons for them. With the proper
employment of a public relations program, the public can be made aware of these
reasons, and the H.M.O., of their public's complaints. The result ought to be
a better understanding of each others' plight and a more harmonious relationship.

The health field is dynamic. New developments in medical care,
techniques for treating chronic illnesses, chemotherapy, patient services,
etc., go a long way toward upgrading the care of the industry's clientele.
Yet, unless these developments are made known, it's like winking at a girl
in a dark room - no one but you knows it. "The getting credit is where the
Public Relations Department can help."[9]

There is also the need to inform the public of changes in the
delivery of medical care; i.e., the way in which people can pay for medical
care or be treated, e.g., preventive medicine or acute episodic care.

---

[4]Sallie Bright, Public Relations Programs, (New York: National Public
Relations Council, Inc., 1970), p. 3.

[5]Scott M. Cutlip, op. cit., p. 6.

[6]Ibid., p. 6.

[7]Harold P. Kurtz, Public Relations for Hospitals, (Springfield, Ill.:
Charles C. Thomas, 1969),p. 3.

[8]Jim Reed, "Basics in Medical Public Relations," Arizona Medicine,
(October 1968), p. 894.

[9]See, e.g., James R. Neely, "Guidelines for Implementation," Hospitals,
(Journal of the American Hospital Association, March 16, 1971), p. 79.

Such is the case of a Health Maintenance Organization new in concept, and different from the **typical** fee-for-service system of medical care. Complete and effective dissemination of information about it is a requisite to its successful implementation. Only when people become aware of its benefits will they begin to seek it out.[10]

The Samaritan Health Service of Phoenix, Arizona, faced a similar situation. The Good Samaritan, Grand Canyon, and Holbrook hospitals had combined to form the Samaritan Health Service. Their objective was to provide complete, qualitative health care, and to inform the public and gain their acceptance of the plan. A condensation of their informative approach is reprinted in Table VII - 1.

TABLE VII - 1

SAMARITAN HEALTH SERVICE
PHOENIX, ARIZONA

Objectives:

The plan was to: 1) present a philosophy of containing costs; 2) make health care more easily accessible to all people; 3) elevate the level of care, accompanying all this with the additional objective of making Samaritan Health Service and its contents a known fact to the people of Arizona through a meaningful public relations effort.

Method:

The method itself depended upon the time-honored basics associated with public relations; news media, coorporate publications, newsletters, explanatory brochures, speakers bureau, annual report, etc. In each instance it was necessary to keep telling a story which was advantageous to Samaritan Health Service, and setting it apart from the single-hospital concept. To give this effort impact, a logo was developed which was carried prominently on all printed matter.

Results:

Acknowledgement and acclamation of the efforts of Samaritan Health Service have been both parochial and universal. In depth, features and articles have appeared in local and national news media. Favorable editorial comments have been garnered in the press and on television.

Conflict, tension and resistance accompany change. The extent to which these factors operate depends upon how well-accepted the concept of an H.M.O. becomes in the public mind. If the public rejects the idea, it becomes necessary to change their minds. A public relations program designed to disseminate information that will have appeal to each of the H.M.O.'s publics will improve the H.M.O.'s chances of being accepted. The public relations

---

[10]See, e.g., Ira G. Greenberg and Michael L. Rodburg, "The Role of Prepaid Group Practice in Relieving the Medical Care Crisis," Harvard Law Review, (February 1971), pp. 927-932.

program must demonstrate to these publics that an H.M.O. can meet their needs more fully than other alternatives.

There are groups who are neither subscribers nor employees of the H.M.O. Into this group fall other health organizations, trade associations, businesses, governments and the community at large. Their reaction to an H.M.O. may be a crucial factor in the H.M.O.'s success because by denegrating the H.M.O., or by encouraging opposition to its existence they can seriously impede the H.M.O.'s acceptance and growth.

Paul de Kruif's[11] excellent study of the origins of the Kaiser-Permanente Plan[12] provides a poignant account of the difficulties generated by opposition groups not directly involved with the plan. De Kruif shows how Kaiser was able to win over his opposition by demonstrating the ways in which the Kaiser Plan could improve upon the existing medical system's approach to episodic care. Through conferences, tours, cost-benefit studies, examples of the success achieved by other groups employing the same approach - in short, by using positive communicative techniques - Kaiser was able to overcome his opposition.

BASIC PUBLIC RELATIONS OBJECTIVES

The basic objective of this P.R. plan is to help insure "...the continuity of the organization and its survival as a health entity."[13] The extent of the P.R. departments success in furthering this objective depends on the importance management attaches to public relations. "If management thinks of the public relations operations in a small way, then it will occupy a small place in the company's scheme of things. If management thinks it is important, then it will occupy a prominent place and its contribution will be great."[14]

A preliminary goal, then, must convince the management of the important part public relations can play.

In his advisory capacity, "the public relations officer analyzes public opinion and counsels line and other staff officers on the public relations aspects of the organization's communications problems...' In the operational role, he handles the organization's communications outside the line function. In mature organizations, the function embraces both."[15]

---

[11]Paul de Kruif, Kaiser Wakes the Doctors, (New York: Harcourt Brace, 1943).

[12]Scott Fleming, "Kaiser Foundation-Permanente Program," Hospitals, Journal of the American Hospital Association, March 16, 1971).

[13]Scott M. Cutlip, op. cit., p. 208.

[14]Ibid.,

[15]Ibid.

The term public implies that the public is a homogeneous group in mind, spirit and opinion. This is not so, "...The public is not one great monolith, but rather a group of segments, often overlapping, and at times, almost completely indefinable."[16] Consequently, before it can begin to effectively deal with public opinion, the public relations department must identify its publics. Some of the publics an H.M.O. will have to deal with are diagramed in Figure VII - 1. The arrangement is hierarchial and denotes that the levels closest to the H.M.O. have the greatest influence upon its operation.

The public relations department, through the use of survey techniques,[17] determines the attitudes and sentiments prevalent in the segments of the H.M.O.'s publics. Awareness of these attitudes and sentiments will aid in designing a program that will help gain acceptance.

The public relations program will identify the specific techniques for achieving its objectives. These techniques include in-house publications and newsletters, personal contact and mass media approaches.[18] Each can be effective in specific situations, and each will have different costs. Since start-up costs for an H.M.O. are great and working capital limited,[19] the public relations program will have to take cost effectiveness into consideration when choosing the techniques.[20]

Throughout its life the H.M.O. will face the problem of response to shifting challenges and priorities. The public relations department constantly monitors the H.M.O.'s operation and environment and their effects upon one another. They will be sensitive to the psychological and physiological needs of its publics; they will anticipate changes in the delivery of medical care, assess economic, social and political changes and their consequences. The public relations department must also be able to evaluate the effectiveness of its own programs in responding to these changing challenges and priorities.

The public relations department is also the nexus of the Marketing and the Finance department's own public relations efforts. Marketing will face the difficult task of recruiting subscribers. To do so, marketing must be able to effectively communicate with nonsubscribers and existing subscribers to convince them of the H.M.O.'s merits. The public relations department coordinates its work with that of the marketing department in writing and designing copy for publication and distribution.

Finance, too, will have to convince the financial community that the H.M.O. is found in concept, is necessary for the public good and is a

---

[16]Harold P. Kurtz, op. cit., p. 12.

[17]Scott M. Cutlip, op. cit., Chapter 7.

[18]Ibid., p. 180.

[19]James R. Neely, op. cit., p. 76.

[20]Interview with Barry Zeeman, H.M.O. Planning Director, L.I. Jewish Medical Center, Lake Success, N.Y., November 1971.

FIGURE VII - 1

The H.M.O.'s Publics. The levels
closest to the H.M.O. have the
greatest influence on its operation.

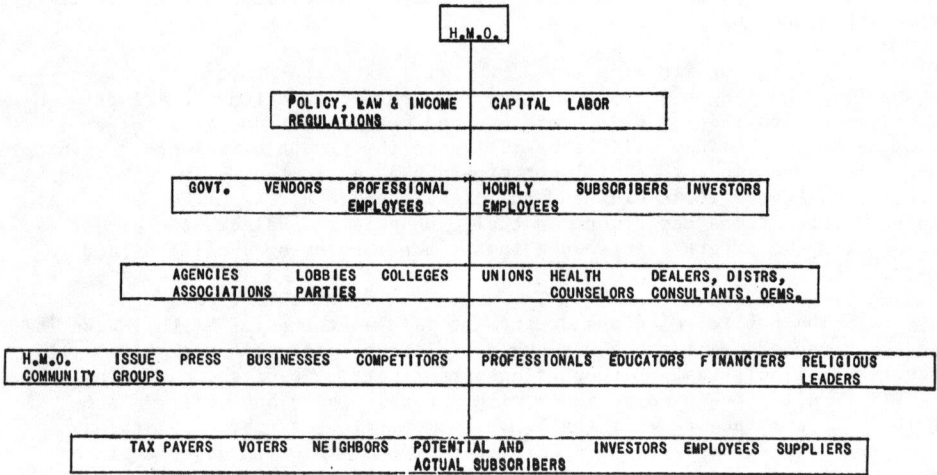

```
                          ┌──────────┐
                          │  H.M.O.  │
                          └──────────┘
          ┌──────────────────────┼──────────────────────┐
          │ POLICY, LAW & INCOME  │  CAPITAL   LABOR      │
          │ REGULATIONS           │                      │
          └──────────────────────┴──────────────────────┘

    ┌──────────────────────────────┼──────────────────────────────┐
    │ GOVT.   VENDORS  PROFESSIONAL │ HOURLY      SUBSCRIBERS  INVESTORS │
    │                 EMPLOYEES     │ EMPLOYEES                     │
    └──────────────────────────────┴──────────────────────────────┘

 ┌───────────────────────────────────┼───────────────────────────────────┐
 │ AGENCIES       LOBBIES   COLLEGES  │ UNIONS  HEALTH       DEALERS, DISTRS, │
 │ ASSOCIATIONS   PARTIES             │         COUNSELORS   CONSULTANTS, OEMS. │
 └───────────────────────────────────┴───────────────────────────────────┘

┌──────────────────────────────────────┼──────────────────────────────────────┐
│ H.M.O.  ISSUE  PRESS  BUSINESSES  COMPETITORS │ PROFESSIONALS  EDUCATORS  FINANCIERS  RELIGIOUS │
│ COMMUNITY GROUPS                       │                                        LEADERS │
└──────────────────────────────────────┴──────────────────────────────────────┘

  ┌──────────────────────────────────────┼──────────────────────────────────────┐
  │ TAX PAYERS   VOTERS   NEIGHBORS  POTENTIAL AND │      INVESTORS  EMPLOYEES  SUPPLIERS │
  │                                 ACTUAL SUBSCRIBERS │                                 │
  └──────────────────────────────────────┴──────────────────────────────────────┘
```

396

good risk. It must do this through a cogent presentation of facts and figures which support its claims. The public relations department can assist the finance department in fact-finding, and in preparing these reports.

Through the joint effort, they will facilitate internal communication, will engender better departmental cooperation, and will prevent duplication of efforts, manpower, materials and supplies.

IDENTIFICATION OF THE H.M.O.'S PUBLICS

The Public Relations program is aimed at reaching various people, groups, or fraternal and trade associations, collectively referred to as the H.M.O.'s publics. Harold P. Kurtz believes that most medical institutions have the following publics:[21]

1. The subscriber public. This represents the H.M.O.'s most important public. Without subscribers, there would be no need for a H.M.O.

2. The visitor and family public. These are members of the subscriber's family or are friends of the patient or his family.

3. The medical staff public. The medical staff consists of the medical personnel employed in curative and diagnostic activities.

4. The employee public. Ancillary help not involved in medical care.

5. The volunteer public. People who donate their time and assistance to health care organizations without remuneration.

6. Geographic public. People living near the H.M.O. who may be affected by such things as parking, construction, land acquisition, noise, etc.

7. Special public. This is a catch-all for the number of splitter groups, organizations or people who do not fit into any of the above categories.

Some of the Special Publics[22] are:

a. religious organizations

b. eleemosynary organizations, e.g., Red Cross, Cancer Society, etc.

---

[21]Harold P. Kurtz, op. cit., pp. 12-13.

[22]Scott M. Cutlip, op. cit.

c. civic organizations, e.g., Kiwanis, Lions, Rotary, etc.

d. political organizations, e.g., American Legion, VFW, League of Women Voters, GOP, Democrats.

e. legislative and governmental organizations, e.g., Mayor's office, Governor, Courts, Senate, Congress.

f. civil service groups, e.g., fire department, police, schools.

g. institutions of higher learning.

h. trade and professional associations, e.g., AMA, AHA, ADA.

i. regulatory agencies, e.g., insurance companies, planning agencies.

j. unions, e.g., AFL-CIO, UAW.

k. medical and nursing students, paramedics.

The Employee Publics[23] are:

Administrative Departments

a. Executive

b. Financial Management

c. General Clerical

d. Personnel

e. Purchasing and Receiving and Stores

f. Public Relations

g. Training

Professional Care Division

a. Central Services

b. Clinical Labs

c. Food Service

d. Medical Library

---

[23] Jack Abeshouse, "Manpower Development," Chapter VI.

e. Medical Records

f. Nursing Service

g. Outpatient

h. Pharmacy

i. Physical Medicine and Rehabilitation

j. Radiology-Nuclear Medicine

k. Social Services

l. Technical Services

Plant Operations and Maintenance

a. Mechanical Services

b. Housekeeping

c. Laundry

Medical Staff Department

H.M.O. Members

a. Interns

b. Residents

c. G.P.'s

d. Specialists

e. Consultants

f. Surgeons

g. Teaching doctors and Researchers

Non-H.M.O. Members

a. Interns

b. Residents

c. Solo-practitioners

d. Prepaid groups

e. Community groups

f. Other hospital staff

    Private
    Community
    State
    Federal

g. Retired M.D.'s

h. Teaching and Research fellows

ATTITUDES TOWARDS H.M.O.'S

A harmonious adjustment between an institution and its publics
requires a free exchange of opinions and information.[24] There are several
segments of the health care industry which are influential in the development
and acceptance of prepaid group practice and H.M.O.'s. These include:

1. The Medical Profession

2. Medical Societies

3. Third-Party Insurers

4. Governments

5. Regulatory Agencies

6. Unions

7. Industrial Groups

8. Universities

9. Consumer Groups

10. Minority Groups

Each of these groups has its special position on the H.M.O. concept.

The Medical Profession

The medical profession is not a monolithic structure[25] and opinion
on prepaid group practice and H.M.O.'s tends to be varied. Physicians tend

---

[24] Scott M. Cutlip, op. cit., p. 108.

[25] See e.g., Richard W. Dodds, "A Framework for Political Mapping of Conflict
in Organized Medicine - Especially Pediatrics," (Reprints of this article
may be obtained by writing to him at 1513 44th St., N.W., Washington, D.C.
20201).

to worry about press coverage, news stories and public statements,[26] and rely upon their medical affiliates to voice their opinions. It is generally only those in the public eye who are free to voice an opinion.

For example, American Medical Association President, Dr. Walter C. Bornemeier, stated, "Group practice is inevitable and will become the family health care center of the Future."[27] He also believes that "...Young doctors, especially those entering practice from now on, will opt for group practice."[28] Dr. Bornemeier, speaking at the Washington, D. C. Medical Society, stated that "...the AMA itself should help young doctors start group practices."[29]

Group practice is increasing. For example, in 1946, there were 404 groups; in 1969, there were 6,372, and the projection for 1975, based on survey trends, is 16,000.[30] This would seem to indicate that more and more physicians are turning to group practice. For those fee-for-service groups already in operation, they "...have indicated unexpected interest in establishing H.M.O.'s, a most desirable source of support for the strategy."[31]

National Medical Societies

The most vocal group so far has been medical students. A _Fortune_ article cites a poll of the Student American Medical Association regarding fee-for-service practice. "At its convention last year delegates passed resolutions critical of the fee-for-service concept of payment for medical care, and endorsed greater participation in group practice.[32] This position is supported again by a survey taken by California Medical Association, Bureau of Research and Planning.[33] In its report, "...forty-five per cent of freshmen, 39 per cent of seniors, and only 27 per cent of residents agreed that the emphasis of the organized medical profession on fee-for-service, solo practice was unrealistic in terms of cost of medical care to the

---

[26] See, e.g., Kurtz, _op. cit._, p. 22.

[27] _AMA News_, April 5, 1971.

[28] _Ibid._,   June 28, 1971.

[29] Stuart Auerbach, "AMA President Pushes Aid for Group Practice," _Washington Post and Times Herald_, 93:24a, (September 10, 1970).

[30] _Medical Group News_, July 1970, (Jack's Paper).

[31] Paul M. Ellwood, Jr., "Concept and Strategy," _Hospitals_, (Journal of the American Hospital Association, March 16, 1971), p. 56.

[32] _____, "Shaking Up the Curriculum," _Fortune_, (January 1970), p. 89.

[33] California Medical Association, Bureau of Research and Planning, Division of Socio-Economics and Research, "Survey on Medical Student Attitudes," _Socio-Economic Report_, Vol. 9, (September 1969), pp. 1-6.

public."[34] Further, "...A very small minority of each group, including six per cent of freshmen, two per cent of seniors, and 11 per cent of residents, agreed that 'solo practice offers greater opportunities for the physician to provide good quality medical care than does group practice'."[35] All of this goes on to support the contention that young doctors will tend to opt for group practice, if given the choice.

The California viewpoints of its component societies regarding the H.M.O. concept. Responding to President Nixon's 1971 National Health Message, the society took the position that "...the H.M.O. concept should be implemented only in carefully selected areas on a pilot basis, with well-publicized evaluation in terms of cost effectiveness, efficiency and quality of patient care, before any special effort is made to implement H.M.O.'s nationally."[36]

The AMA has come out with a similar position. "While AMA has no clear-cut objection to H.M.O.'s," the report said, "their value still needs to be tested and each should be judged on an individual basis. Some potential organizational patterns suggest that a nonmedical organization may exercise control over the provision of medical service..."[37] Even though the AMA has not fully endorsed the H.M.O. concept, to admit that it has no clear-cut objection is a move toward endorsement. Previously, the AMA has been too concerned with government intervention to clearly define[38] its position on H.M.O.'s and prepaid group practice.

Unlike the AMA, the American Osteopathic Association, while endorsing the National Health Insurance proposal, has refused to support any particular plan or methodology for implementing such a plan.[39] Instead, AOA delegates stated that "...this should be handled by the various lawmakers at state and national levels."[40] The AOA's new President, W. S. Horn, D. O., added "...Physicians are in a poor position to make decisions concerning methods of distribution of health care... Physicians are not economists,

---

[34]Ibid., p. 136.

[35]Ibid.

[36]_____, "H.M.O.'s - Past and Present," California Medical Association News, Vol. 16, (May 7, 1971), p. 1.

[37]_____, "Further Testing of H.M.O.'s Urged," American Medical News, 14:7, (July 5, 1971).

[38]Ira G. Greenberg and Michael L. Rodburg, "The Role of Prepaid Group Practice in Relieving the Medical Care Crisis," Harvard Law Review, (February 1971), pp. 954-955.

[39]See, e.g., "AOA House of Delegates OK's National Health Insurance," AOA News Review, 13:1, (September 1970).

[40]Ibid., 13:1.

lawyers, legislators or sociologists, but any drafting of a compulsory national health insurance program must necessarily involve these groups of people."[41]

In turn, the Association of American Physicians and Surgeons has stated strong disapproval of any National Health Insurance program. The AAPS feels that...

> Whereas, all proposals for National Health
> Insurance have the effect of creating the
> false impression that payment for medical
> services by the government will improve the
> quantity and quality of medical care, and
> whereas, the evidence concerning Medicare,
> Medicaid and other programs demonstrate
> government payment does not improve the
> quantity and quality of medical care.
> Therefore, be it resolved that the Assembly
> and House of Delegates of the Association of
> American Physicians and Surgeons, Inc.
> oppose any system of National Health Insurance
> regardless of how devised."[42] /Author's emphasis/

Further, support for a new system of comprehensive health care supported by the government is voiced by the American Hospital Association[43] and the National League of Nursing.[44] At the same time, the AHA warns of the problems of implementation, development, funding and lack of incentives for recruitment of subscribers and providers of health care; the AHA also cautions against dependence on a free market approach to provide needed health care.[45] "The concept's free market approach may leave large geographic areas uncovered by any form of health insurance... The H.M.O. strategy does not encourage providers to relocate in areas that have an inadequate supply of providers."[46]

County and Local Medical Societies

County and Local Medical Societies have played an equally important role in the development of group practices and H.M.O.'s. This is possible

---

[41]Ibid.

[42]_____, "Resolutions Adopted by the Assembly and Delegates of the Association of American Physicians and Surgeons," Association of American Physicians and Surgeons, Inc. (October 1970).

[43]James R. Neely, "Guidelines for Implementation," Hospitals, (Journal of American Hospital Association, March 16, 1971), p. 80.

[44]_____, "NIN Convention Resolutions," Nursing Outlook 19: 393, (June 1971).

[45]James R. Neely, op. cit., p.81.

[46]Ibid.

because "local medical societies are largely autonomous."[47] Thus, despite
its influence, the AMA's neutrality in this regard does not assure that
prepaid group practice will remain unchallenged. "County medical societies
may continue to regard prepaid group practice as an unfair mode of competition,"[48] and while most state societies do not have any official position,[49]
at least one state society has indicated that its general attitude would be
in opposition to this type of medical practice."[50]

   Local societies may oppose group practice in several ways. "First,
they may expel or refuse to admit to the local society physicians participating in such plans."[51] Second, "a physician may be denied hospital privileges...
denial of hospital privileges may prevent a doctor from practicing his
specialty and may impair his ability to practice generally."[52] For a group
whose referral and hospitalization needs are internally met, these difficulties may be ameliorated.[53] Yet, for the new doctor facing an uncertain
future, should he leave the plan, these difficulties may be a deterrent to
his joining. Members may also suffer a loss of professional status and civic
esteem resulting from vociferous vilification by his nonmembers peers.[54]

   Action has been taken to lessen, and when possible, outlaw the use
of these discriminatory practices.[55] Courts have reviewed expulsions, and
when found to be in violation of the society's by-laws or constitution, have
invalidated them on the grounds that..."those constitute a contract between
that member and the association, or in the theory that the member is deprived
of a property right."[56] In the case of denial, these arguments against

---

[47]For support of this view, see AMA Judicial Council Opinions and Reports,
2: '69, (disciplinary action may depend on local attitudes), see also,
Greenberg & Rodburg, "Prepaid Group," p. 956.

[48]See, e.g., Greenberg, "The Decline of the Healing Art," Harper's,
(October 1960), p. 136.

[49]Greenberg & Rodburg, "Prepaid Group," p. 956, (opinion based on survey of
37 societies).

[50]Ibid., p. 956.

[51]Ibid.

[52]Ibid., pp. 956-957.

[53]Ibid.

[54]For support of this view, see William MacColl, "Group Practice and
Prepayment of Medical Care," (Washington: Public Affairs Press, 1966).

[55]Greenberg & Rodburg, "Prepaid Group," p. 957.

[56]See, e.g., "Expulsion and Exclusion from Hospital Practice and Organized
Medical Societies," Rutgers Law Review, #15, (1961), pp. 327, 335.

exclusion have no effect. Courts may review on procedural and substantive fairness on public policy grounds,[57] and, "...those courts potentially could invalidate both expulsions and exclusion."[58] Some states have taken legislative action in passing laws that would prohibit hospital affiliation because of group affiliation.[59] The National Conference on Group Practice has retaliated by requesting that Medicaid, Medicare, and Hill-Burton funds be withdrawn from those hospitals discriminating against group affiliations.[60] Where hospitals receive some state funding, courts have the option of ruling against "black-balling" on the grounds that it constitutes "...an invidious classification, and hence invalid as a denial of equal protection."[61]

Several favorable rulings for group practice plans[62] have lessened the pursuit of county challenges of unethical conduct, and "several local counties have elected to settle out of court."[63] Reversals in opposition are also occurring and there is now "...wide-spread interest by local medical societies in establishing society-sponsored medical care foundations modeled after the San Joaquin or Clackamas County plans."[64] While these reversals may indicate a lessening of opposition to group practice, strong opposition still exists in some areas.[65] And, those not experiencing current opposition, but desiring to expand into new areas, fear opposition there.[66]

---

[57] See, e.g., "American Medical Association: Power, Purpose and Politics in Organized Medicine," Yale Law Journal, #63, (1954), (See Medical Foundation of Bellaire).

[58] Greenberg & Rodburg, op. cit.

[59] See, e.g., N.Y. Public Health Law, Section 206-a, (McKinney supplement, 1970).

[60] Greenberg & Rodburg, op. cit., see also, "Promoting the Group Practice of Medicine," Report of the National Conference on Group Practice, Public Health Service Publication, #1750, (1967), p. 32.

[61] Ibid., p. 957.

[62] See, e.g. AMA v. United States, 317 U. S. 519, 1943; Group Health Cooperative v. King Medical Society, 39 Washington, 2d 586,237 p. 2d. 737, 1951.

[63] Greenberg & Rodburg, "Prepaid Group," p. 958; see also, W. Dearing, "Developments and Accomplishments of Comprehensive Group Practice Payment Programs," Group Health Association of America, Inc., Booklet #16, (1970), (Two Harbors).

[64] Paul M. Ellwood, Jr., op. cit. p. 55; see also, pp. 63-68.

[65] See, e.g., Chase, "The Politics of Medicine," Harper's, (October 1960), pp. 125-26.

[66] Greenberg & Rodburg, op. cit., p. 959.

Lastly, opposition by the AMA[67] and the AAPS[68] to the National Health Insurance Plan indirectly limits group practice and H.M.O. development[69] because included in this proposal, are economic incentives for prepaid group practice and H.M.O. development.[70]

Governmental and Regulatory Agencies

Government - Federal and State - have acted towards group practice in two ways: (1) to facilitate group practice development by making an exception to or by circumventing vaguely-defined legal barriers;[71] (2) state and federal governments have provided financial or planning support, passed enabling legislation, or have submitted medical-care plans of their own design for legislative consideration and funding.[72]

Legal barriers primarily are of two types: one is the corporate practice rule which prohibits a corporation from engaging in a learned profession,[73] the reasoning being that "...the acts of natural persons employed by the corporation are attributable to the corporate person."[74] Incorporation would free those performing the acts from any legal prosecution for malpractice, since the corporation is the entity held legally responsible. This rule was set to protect innocent people from quackery, deception and exploitation, but it has current relevance in preventing a conflict of interest between patient and corporation.[75]

To contend with the corporate practice rule, States have taken various action. "Some states have included in their enabling legislation language which specifically states that an authorized health plan shall not be considered to be engaged in the practice of medicine."[76]

---

[67]Greenberg & Rodburg, Harvard Law Review, op. cit.

[68]Greenberg & Rodburg, "Resolutions Adopted by House of Delegates, April 17, 1971, Association of American Physicians and Surgeons: Chicago, Ill.," Association of American Physicians and Surgeons, Inc. (April 17, 1971).

[69]Greenberg & Rodburg, Harvard Law Review, op. cit.

[70]Ibid.

[71]Interview with Leo Petit, Director of Operations, Providence, R.I.: Rhode Island Group Health Association, (December 1971).

[72]Ibid.

[73]Greenberg & Rodburg, Harvard Law Review, op. cit., p. 960, (see, e.g., Wilcox, Hospitals and the Corporate Practice of Medicine, 45 Cornell Law Quarterly, 432, (1960).

[74]Ibid., pp. 960-961.

[75]See, e.g., Forgotson, Roemer & Newman, "Innovations in the Organization of Health Services: Inhibiting vs. Permissive Regulation," Washington University Law Quarterly, (1967), pp. 400, 413.

[76]Greenberg & Rodburg, Harvard Law Review, op. cit.

New York State, for example, has passed the Non -Profit-Corporation Act, or the Lombardi Law. "The Lombardi Law will enable physician groups to form what would be prototype H.M.O.'s."[77] Further, under Article 44 of the New York Public Health Law, "...The State Health Department encourages new concepts in the delivery of health care under the approval of the Public Health Council of the State of New York is a prerequisite of the consent of the Commissioner of Health."[78]

At the federal level...a number of recent proposals...would remove any lingering doubts as to the rules (Corporate Practice Rule) existant with respect to nonprofit health organizations.[79]

Blue Shield Laws have presented the greatest legal barrier to prepaid group plans, in that they affect the administrative and operational aspects. Blue Shield Laws state that "...

(1) the medical society must approve the article of incorporation

(2) the medical society must be the sole sponsor or have control of the board of directors

(3) the medical society must control the operation of the plan

(4) all physicians who desire must be permitted to participate

(5) a majority of the physicians in the local must participate."[80]

The medical societies were mainly responsible for the enactment of the Blue Shield Law.

Today, there are only 18 states which have Blue Shield statutes which require all health service corporations to incorporate under the Blue

---

[77] Greenberg & Rodburg, "The Nonprofit Medical Corporations Act," Newsletter, Medical Societies' Reference Committee, (1971).

[78] Greenberg & Rodburg, see, e.g., Article 44, Public Health Law, "New York's Approach to Prepaid Comprehensive Group Practice - Considerations for Applicants," New York State Department of Health, (July 1971).

[79] See, e.g., The Proposed Health Security Act, S. 4297 Section 56(a) (4), 116 Congressional Record S 14339 (daily edition, August 27, 1970).

[80] Greenberg & Rodburg, Harvard Law Review, op. cit., p. 963.

Shield Laws.[81] In those states[82] lacking Blue Shield Statutes, or not
requiring conformance to Blue Shield Legislation, there exists other legal
restraints. Local interpretation of these statutes is very subjective, and
the legal climate is in a state of flux. Consequently, "...legal climate can
be ascertained only through direct discussions with those persons responsible
for the interpretation of the statutes."[83]

        Contention with these variances has taken many forms. To permit the
operation of HIP in New York, a legal fiction was created;[84] in Oklahoma,
legal restrictions were ignored;[85] in Colorado, the Attorney General and
Kaiser personnel worked together to insure that the unprofessional rule
provision would not apply.[86] In Massachusetts, the Governor worked with
officials of the Harvard Community Health Plan and Health Inc. to free them
from restrictions of the Blue Shield Laws by permitting them to incorporate
under the Non-Profit Corporations Act;[87] the Governor has promised to take
any steps necessary if that law is found to be insufficient.[88] In New Haven,
Conn., organized labor, in cooperation with Yale University, has prevailed
upon the state legislature to amend the Blue Shield Statute.[89] And in Ohio,
a consumer act was passed to permit the operation of Medical Foundation of
Bellaire, Ohio.[90]

Insurance Regulation

        Regulation of group plans under insurance regulatory statutes is
another major obstruction to their development. Insurance commissioners have

---

[81]Ibid.

[82]See Report of the National Conference on Group Practice, Promoting the
    Group Practice of Medicine, Keynote Address by William H. Stewart, M.D.,
    Surgeon General, U. S. Public Health Service (1967 PHS publication).

[83]Greenberg & Rodburg, Harvard Law Review, op. cit., p. 964.

[84]Ibid., p. 964. (see, A. Kornfield, Memorandum on the Critical Need for
    New Legislation to Encourage the Organization, Promotion and Expansion of
    Prepaid Group Health Care Plans 10 (1970) (Submitted to the New York State
    Legislature).

[85]Ibid.

[86]Ibid.

[87]Ibid., p. 967.

[88]See Press Release, Governor Francis Sargent, Boston, Mass. (April 14, 1970).

[89]Ibid., p. 968.

[90]See, e.g., Wilson, "Health Legislation in Ohio," American Journal of Public
    Health, Vol. 51, (1961).

the authority to "approve the articles of incorporation, set rates, require detailed financial statements, control advertising and solicitation expenses, and determine that funds may be invested only in securities approved for life insurance companies."[91] Insurance commissioners can also require the holding of large reserves, thereby limiting funds for expansion, and they can also set unreasonably low subscription rates.[92]

Courts have been willing to prove laws inapplicable to group plans under the following rationale: (1) group plans contract for service and not for indemnity, and (2) there is no assumption of risk involved.[93] Although broadly stated, the courts are correct in concluding inapplicability of these laws, since the operational differences between group practice and third-party insurance is significantly different.[94]

It has been demonstrated that restrictive law and regulations can be dealt with, and that the attitude of legislators, State officials and members of the courts are favorably inclined towards group practice plans. Yet, to be successful, a first requisite to group development is to assess the legal barriers in an area. For example, Kaiser, the largest prepaid group,[95] first considers, and often with some reservation, the legal climate before moving into an area.[96] "While the organization is willing to deal with administrative agencies on interpretation of the law, it is loathe to engage in any frontal assault on the legislation."[97]

Existing Groups and Hospitals

Existing county and city hospital systems are also favorably viewing prepaid group practice. "A recent survey of the 60 largest public hospital systems revealed that none reject the H.M.O. idea, and many are seriously considering the establishment of such organizations."[98] This is encouraging in that existing hospital systems are uniquely equipped to start up an H.M.O.

---

[91]Ibid., p. 970. (see, e.g., "Group Health Plans: Some Legal and Economic Aspects," Yale Law Journal, No. 53, 1943, pp. 162, 174).

[92]See, MacColl, op. cit.

[93]Greenberg & Rodburg, op. cit., p. 971.

[94]Ibid.

[95]Edmund K. Faltermayer, "Better Care at Less Cost Without Miracles," Fortune, (January 1970), p. 81.

[96]Greenberg & Rodburg, op. cit., p. 975. (see, e.g., Kaiser Foundation Medical Care Program, Annual Report, 1969, at II: Criteria for Expansion).

[97]Ibid.

[98]Paul M. Ellwood, Jr., op. cit.

By contracting with the hospital's own staff, this group will have a commitment to proper organization, utilization and management, lacking in unrelated groups.[99]

Support for H.M.O. development is also coming from a joint undertaking by Kaiser-Permanente and the Health Insurance Plan (HIP) of New York. These two innovators of group practice "...have undertaken a training project for Blue Cross personnel to manage and operate H.M.O.'s."[100] This is a warranted effort, as "...there is an insufficient number of persons with expertise in the organization and management of group practice prepayment plans to support substantial expansion over the next several years."[101] "The problem is most acute in the startupphase,"[102] and the cost for technical assistance is often prohibitive.[103]

Third-Party Insurers

Several large insurance companies have become actively engaged in establishing H.M.O.'s.[104] The extent of their involvement has been in funding these programs through loans or by underwriting their start-up costs. For example, Connecticut General Life Insurance has agreed to underwrite the cost of the Columbia Medical Plan.[105] Other insurance companies have, to a varying degree, agreed to purchase bonds of prepaid group practices or they have granted small loans or grants for demonstration projects. In Seattle, Connecticut Mutual Life Insurance Company made a $9 million mortgage loan to the Group Health Cooperative of Puget Sound;[106] Aetna invested $101,000 in the Harvard Plan;[107] and Metropolitan Life Insurance Company granted $100,000 to Washington University, St. Louis.[108]

Additional support has come in terms of administrative and supportive services. In Rhode Island, Blue Cross has agreed to provide subscriber leads to the Rhode Island Group Health Association.[109] Blue Cross is currently

---

[99]James R. Neely, op. cit., p. 79.

[100]Paul M. Ellwood, op. cit.

[101]Greenberg & Rodburg, op. cit., p. 953.

[102]Ibid.

[103]Ibid.

[104]Ellwood, loc. cit.

[105]Greenberg & Rodburg, op. cit., p. 950. (see, "The Columbia Medical Plan and the East Baltimore Medical Plan," Hospitals, (Journal of the American Hospital Association, March 16, 1971), pp. 69-72.

[106]Ibid., cf. 15.

[107]Ibid., cf. 16.

[108]Ibid., cf. 16.

[109]Interview with Leo Petit. (see Supra, n. 84, p. 25).

working with Long Island Jewish Hospital in its establishment of an H.M.O.
Blue Cross is providing both marketing and planning assistance.[110] Of the 70
Blue Cross Association member plans, some 22 "...have established or are
negotiating affiliations with prepaid group practice plans."[111]

Universities

A growing number of medical schools have begun, or will soon begin,
operation of H.M.O.'s.[112] The organizational form of these plans have been
of three types. The first, is a university-sponsored and designed plan
marketed to the community.[113] The second is a community-established organization having affiliation with a University Medical Center.[114] The last
type is a joint venture between a community and a university.[115] Another
form tried was that of combining an existing clinic, union demand for better
health care, and the Western Reserve University School of Medicine into what
became the Community Health Foundation of Cleveland, Ohio.[116]

The importance of university plans for those wishing to begin their
own is that Community-University plans are mutually supportive. The community
helps to underwrite the cost of the plan,[117] and the latter can perform the
services, teaching and research functions in an actual situation.[118] Of
greater importance is that medical school affiliation provides several
advantages lacking in other organizational forms. For example, "...the alliance promotes physician recruitment by providing teaching outlets and increasing job satisfaction...promotes continuing education..." and exposes medical
students to the prepaid group concept.[119]

Minority Groups

Minority groups, because of their low income, are prime agents of
support for group practice.[120] Low-economic status, poor mobility and poor

---

[110]Interview with Barry Zeeman. (see _Supra_, n. 24, p. 9).

[111]Ellwood, _loc. cit._

[112]_Ibid._

[113]Greenberg & Rodburg, _op. cit._, p. 916.

[114]_Ibid._

[115]_Ibid._

[116]A. Yedidia, "Planning and Implementation of the Community Health
Foundation of Cleveland, Ohio" (Washington, D.C.: U. S. Government
Printing Office, 1968).

[117]Greenberg, & Rodburg, _loc. cit._

[118]_Ibid._

[119]_Ibid._

[120]Lionel F. Swan, "Group Approach to Medical Care," _Nursing Outlook_, Vol. 18,
(January 1970).

health characterize this group.[121] Although, they realize their need for better treatment, their needs have been neglected. The advantages of group practice to them are (1) group practice does not discriminate against the poor, (2) group practice has lower patient costs.[122] These advantages will provide them with equal opportunity for quality medical care and still enable them to afford it.

Active support of prepaid group practice plans has been initiated by the National Medical Association (NMA). The NMA, a predominantly Negro organization,[123] has proposed a method that will meet the needs of minority groups. The NMA established the National Medical Association Foundation (NMAF) to raise money for multi-specialty clinics, extended care facilities and ancillary services.[124] By borrowing 90 per cent of the money needed through secured FHA loans, (the foundation must raise the other ten per cent itself), the NMAF was able to initiate a pilot project in Washington, D.C.[125]

The success of this group to meet its goals seems to be indicative of the positive responses generated by minority groups to better health care. While there may be some problem of financing low-income subscribers, marketing to this group and seeking of their support is warranted. The Federal Government, in its interest in promoting H.M.O.'s, has in the past, subsidized low-income subscription[126] and probably will continue to do so. Additional funds, although severely limited, may also be secured from the Group Health Association of America.[127]

ORGANIZATIONAL ARRANGEMENTS OF
PUBLIC RELATIONS RESOURCES

The Public Relations Department must decide upon its organizational arrangements. How will the P.R. department be involved in promoting the H.M.O.? How will the employees, the medical staff, the administrators, etc. be used in promoting the H.M.O.? A possible arrangement is diagramed in Figure VII - 2.

---

[121] Michael Harrington, The Other America, (New York: MacMillan Co. 1970).

[122] Lionel F. Swan, op. cit., p. 57.

[123] Ibid.

[124] Ibid.

[125] Ibid.

[126] Greenberg & Rodburg, loc. cit.

[127] Ibid., p. 953.

FIGURE VI - 2

H.M.O.

ORGANIZATIONAL ARRANGEMENT

OF ITS PUBLICS

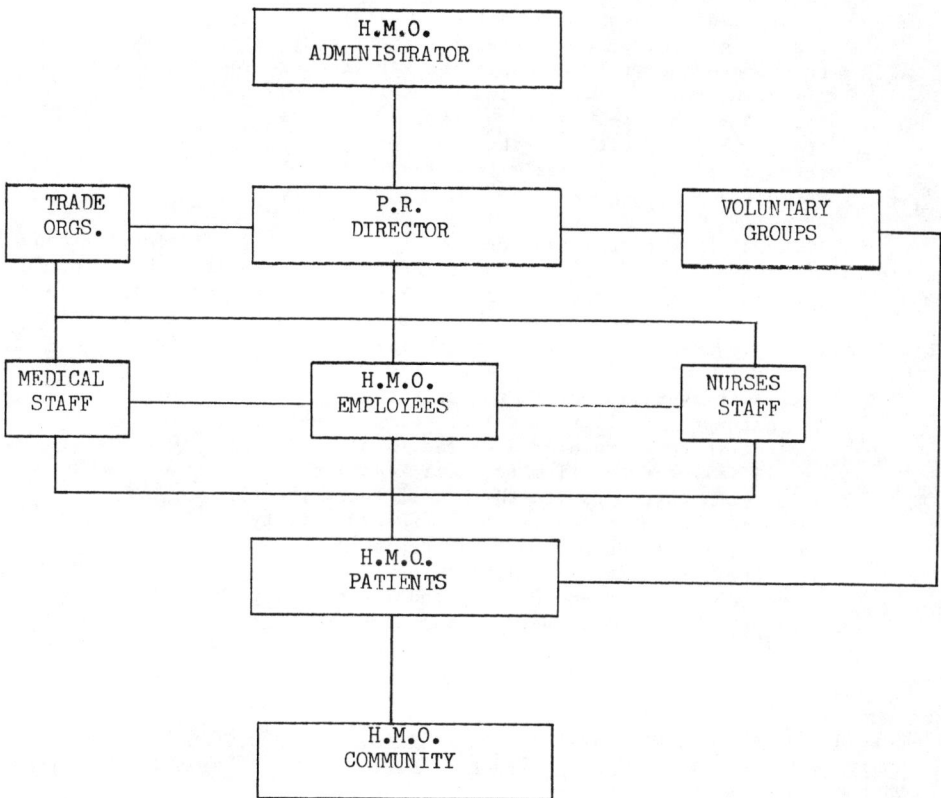

413

Public Relations Director

      If the H.M.O. can afford one, the man of greatest importance in the
P.R. efforts is the full-time director. It is he who will be responsible for
the design and implementation of any public relations efforts. The top
administrator will, of course, have the final say on any major public relations program, but the P. R. director will be its originator.

      There will be two areas of concern for the P. R. Director -
internal and external. External to the organization, public contacts will
be in the form of developing

> ...cooperative relationship(s) with other /H.M.O.'s/
> for exchange of information and services; with
> community agencies to develop understanding of
> /H.M.O./ program and encourage voluntary partici-
> pation; and with professional standards. May
> compile and transmit news articles to press
> regarding /H.M.O./ its activities and functions,
> to promote goodwill, friendliness, and cooperation
> of community. Solicits volunteer services of
> individuals by speaking before various organiza-
> tions. May solicit contributions for /H.M.O./
> through personal contact with citizens in the
> community.[128]

      Internal to the organization, the P. R. Director is primarily con-
cerned with employee and subscriber relations. The degree of involvement in
employee relations may vary within organizations. To whatever extent, the
P. R. department or Director desires the existence of a harmonious relationship between employees on all levels. Of primary interest to him is

> ...(1) an overall concern for the success of
> the enterprise; (2) the attitudes employees
> reflect in their role as ambassadors of good
> or ill will for the firm in their relation-
> ships with customers (in this case, subscribers),
> community and other publics; (3) responsibility
> for creating an environment favorable to the
> personnel, industrial relations function; (4)
> responsibility for encouraging and implementing
> two-way communication between managers and
> men.[129]

---

[128]United States Employment Service: Job Descriptions and Organizational
Analysis for Hospitals and Related Health Services, (Washington, D. C.:
United States Government Printing Office, 1952, pp. 23-24.

[129]Scott M. Cutlip, op. cit., p. 232.

The degree of success will be determined in large part by the effectiveness of internal channels of communication. Because more employee contacts are of a more informal nature than formal, "...he should have at least a certain minimum of accurate and significant information about the institution."[130] Dissemination of this information may be made through department heads, employee meetings, bulletin boards, a house newsletter, the enclosure of a fact sheet in pay envelopes, etc. The important thing is to let employees know about what is happening, be it good news or bad. If one tries to conceal the bad, then rumor may distort it into something worse.

Upward communication is equally important. Employees must be given the opportunity to tell "...(1) what he would like to know about his job, his company and related matters; (2) what he would like management to know about himself and the things that are bothering him."[131] Since it would be impossible for everyone to speak to the H.M.O. Administrator, it is important that the employees' immediate superiors be trained in the area of personal relations so that the employee will feel that his superior is someone he can talk to and get a positive response from.[132]

Other areas of involvement for the Public Relations Director are:[133]

1. The writing of reports, news releases, house publications, etc.

2. The editing of employee publications, employee handbooks, newsletters, and other in-house publications.

3. The securing of agreements with the local press and live media for the placement of news about the organization.

4. The handling of promotion for special events.

5. Frequently, H.M.O. personnel are called upon to speak before various public and civic groups. The P.R. Director can assist these people in writing speeches, or may appear in behalf of the H.M.O. as its spokesman.

---

[130] Alden B. Mills, Hospital Public Relations, (Chicago, Ill.: Physicians' Record Company, 1939), p. 128.

[131] Cutlip, loc. cit.

[132] William F. Whyte, Organizational Behavior: Theory and Application, (Homewood, Ill.: Richard D. Irwin,) p. 315.

[133] Scott M. Cutlip, op. cit., p. 91.

6. Because of his knowledge and experience
   with art and layout, the P. R. Director
   assists in the production of brochures,
   booklets, etc.

7. The P. R. Director is responsible for
   the programming, planning and budgeting
   of the P. R. program.

8. The coordination of efforts between
   advertising and public relations.

The H.M.O. Administrator

In terms of public relations, the role of the H.M.O. administrator
may be a dual one. If a public relations director exists, the H.M.O.
administrator is responsible for determining the scope, place and effectiveness of any public relations attempt.[134]

In the case where no public relations department exists, it then
becomes the responsibility of the H.M.O. administrator to assume, to the
extent of his ability, the aforementioned duties and responsibilities of the
P. R. Director. Those functions he cannot handle will have to be delegated
internally or externally. The latter may require the future hiring of an
outside agency or the seeking of assistance from medical societies that offer
a limited amount of assistance in this area.

Whether or not there exists a formal public relations department,
the H.M.O. administrator will quite often be the official spokesman and
inspirational leader of the organization.[135] He will set the tone and mood
of the organization and strongly influence the prespective his employees will
have towards their place in the organization. He must be cognizant of the
needs of his staff and establish an effective employee relations program that
will be sensitive to these needs, and in turn, develop an employee sensitivity
to patient needs.[136] If employees are abrupt and coarse in their dealings
with patients, this will engender a great deal of patient resentment that
will ultimately blemish the H.M.O.'s reputation and chances for success.

The Medical Profession

In return for its efforts to assure good working relations and
conditions for its physicians, the H.M.O. can rightfully expect its physicians
to reciprocate in assisting the H.M.O.'s.public relations efforts. This can
be done in several ways:

---

[134] Scott M. Cutlip, op. cit., p. 206.

[135] Interview with Leo Petit, (See Supra, n. 88, p. 25).

[136] Interview with Robert K. Kushner, Public Relations Director,
Meadowbrook Hospital, East Meadow, New York, December 1971.

(1) by understanding and supporting the aims
and objectives of the administration; (2) by
cooperating in the /H.M.O.'s/ efforts to
improve its services without, however,
attempting to usurp the powers and duties of
the administration; (3) by upholding the
/H.M.O./ in the eyes of the public, by
suggesting it to wealthy patients as a proper
object of beneficence and by giving actual
assistance as workers when the /H.M.O./
engages in a financial campaign; (4) by
manifesting only kindness and consideration
for patients at all times; (5) by contributing as much as they are able to the advancement of medical science and art; (6) by helping in the educational program for the
interns, residents and junior attending men;
(7) by serving faithfully and to the best of
their ability on the medical board, whenever
chosen; and (8) by observing the highest
medical ethics in all their practice, both
within and without the /H.M.O./[137]

Nurses

The importance of a public-relations-conscious nursing staff is
paramount. Nurses generally comprise half the working staff of a H.M.O.,
and by sheer numbers, have a great impact upon patients.[138] Secondly,
anyone who has ever been a patient will admit that they saw nurses more
often than any other individual. The attitude they carry to the job can
greatly affect the quality of nursing care and ultimately the reputation of
the H.M.O.[139]

Quite often, nurses are rushed and may tend to be abrupt with
patients. In an attempt to have them develop a more gracious attitude towards
patients, one hospital has asked each nurse to see the patient as though he
were a relative.[140] The assumption is that identification will enhance
personalization of service. What is really needed in a nursing staff is a
"social consciousness...so as to preserve in nursing its fine spirit of
service, devotion and self-effacement."[141]

Of equal importance is the treatment visitors receive from nurse
receptionists. For the best situation, the execution of general front-office

---

[137]Ibid., p. 142.

[138]Interview with Robert K. Kushner, (See Supra, n. 158, p. 39).

[139]Harold P. Kurtz, op. cit., p. 28.

[140]Aldon B. Mills, op. cit., p. 132.

[141]Ibid.

policies "...should be entrusted only to people who can make friends of all those whom they meet."[142] If a visitor is mistreated, he will probably tell the patient of this and cause him to think ill of the H.M.O. staff, and may, if the situation is distressing enough, cause anxiety in addition to that caused by his condition.

Additional and valuable free training can also be acquired for the training of telephone operators. Since many people have only telephone contact with the H.M.O., the kind of treatment they receive here is also important. As an assist,the "...telephone company has coaching schools for telephone operators which will assist them to develop a courteous manner over the wire."[143]

H.M.O. Employees

Much of what has been said about nurses' attitudes towards patients applies to ancillary personnel. Those, such as receptionists, orderlies and maids, who come into contact with patients and visitors must be made aware of the psychologic conditions of subscribers.[144] Not unknown to all H.M.O. employees are the mistakes and misfortunes that befall some patients. Relating of these occurrences to a patient may have upsetting consequences but can be avoided through proper sensitivity-training of employees. Patients are generally under a great deal of stress and must be protected from the anxiety that may develop.

Auxiliaries, Guilds and Similar Groups

The presence of these groups in a medical organization can be felt in the added strength they provide. Their importance can range from raising money and creating goodwill to writing of letters and entertaining children. They can act as the eyes and ears of the organization and keep the administration informed through proper channels of communication.[145] These groups can act autonomously but will be receptive to some direction, if provided. Since they are voluntary and are interested in serving the organization, it is paramount that they be kept informed of the organization's needs.

To keep these groups involved, it is necessary that they feel that "...they are actually doing something worthwhile for the H.M.O."[146] The following are some areas of involvement to which these groups have been exposed. The raising of funds for special needs will always be of value. These funds may be used for patient services, new equipment, medical education or civic endowments. Voluntary hospital services are a second important function. Much money, time and a savings in manpower can be realized by the addition of voluntary help. For a complete listing of guidelines and functions performed by voluntary groups, see Appendices II and III of Hospital Public Relations, by Alden B. Mills, Physicians' Record Co., Chicago, Ill.

---

[142]Ibid., p. 134.

[143]Ibid., p. 135.

[144]Ibid., p. 130.

[145]Ibid., p. 143.

[146]Ibid., p. 144.

418

The Rath Organization of Syracuse, N.Y. organized a campaign to inform the taxpayer of the pitfalls of "No-Fault" auto insurance. Table VII - 2 illustrates some of the functions voluntary groups performed. This approach is easily adapted to the needs of nascent H.M.O.'s seeking "public" acceptance, or the recinding of existing prohibitive legislation.

TABLE VII - 2
VOLUNTARY GROUP FUNCTIONS

1) Legislative: - To develop a bill embracing the best features of the /H.M.O./ system which would be in the best interest of the public.

2) Contacts: - To call on business industry, and the /health care field/, obtain new Committee members, and ask support both publicly, in person, and through their own publicity outlets.

3) Speakers Bureau: - To get on the agenda for Fall meetings of various business and fraternal organizations, PTA groups, garden clubs, civic organizations, /health care organizations/, and other community groups throughout the state.

4) Allies: - To call on various other types of organizations to enlist support and coordinate activities.

5) Publicity: - To arrange radio-TV interviews, distribute releases to newspapers, present position statements to editorial writers, holds news conferences.

6) Political Contacts: - To work with candidates as well as incumbents, sharing elements of the campaign with them and asking their support.

7) Union Heads: - To explain to union chiefs the impact of /issue/ on union benefits, and to ask their support.

8) Community Contacts: - To identify and talk with all "special" interests that might be affected by the proposed legislation

Trade Relations

To compete with the large interest groupings, people are organizing into their own interest, trade and professional groups to promote their own self-interests and points of view.[147] Galbraith,[148] in his book American Capitalism, treats extensively the machinations of pressure groups. He contends that power-group formation is an automatic response to the existing power groups of Government and Big Business.

---

[147] Scott M. Cutlip, op. cit., p. 60.

[148] John Kenneth Galbraith, American Capitalism, (Boston, Mass.: Sentry Editions. Imprint of Houghton Mifflin Co., 1956).

Trade associations, in their attempt to assist member contention with opposing groups, have incorporated several services into their operation. Quite often, these services are offered without charge or for a minimal fee. These services may range from the supply of information to legislative representation as a lobbyist.[149] Several associations also have public relations departments which can be employed by H.M.O.'s too small to afford their own.[150] A list of trade associations in the health field may be obtained from part two of the August 1, 1971 issue of Hospitals.[150A]

Each association sponsors a house publication for the dissemination of news and developments in its respective field.[151] Quite often, there is a need for publishable items of interest and these associations will gladly accept articles from members. This will provide trade members with the opportunity to tell the industry what pioneering efforts they are undertaking in the development of new methods and techniques in the field of health care.

Publication of articles and their favorable review is an excellent way for a member to gain professional recognition and acclaim. Publication of impressive undertakings by a staff member brings this to the attention of other members or peers. Their recognition of ability and a progressive manner can lend their vitally-needed support for a nascent organization and can facilitate growth and success by removing doubt as to capability and intent.

The need for information is paramount in any organization dealing with changing public opinion and priorities. Trade organizations can become a prime source of information in this area. Trade associations generally maintain a competent staff of recognized specialists who research the field for answers and issues of community and trade concern. This information is generally available to those who need it. On occasion, consultation and special assistance may be obtained.

SPECIFIC PUBLIC RELATIONS OBJECTIVES

Employee Relations

A specific objective of any public relations program is that of developing good employee relations. Employee relations is the term used to describe the internal relationship between employee and organization. The importance of a good employee relations program can often be found in examples of employee turnover, tardiness, excessive sick leave and prolonged

---

[149]Interview with Shelly Saposnick, Reporter, (New York: Fairchild Publications), (January 1972).

[150]Scott M. Cutlip, op. cit., p. 12.

[150A]"Guide Issue," Hospitals, Journal of the American Hospital Association, Vol. 45, #15, August 1, 1971, pp. 393-416.

[151]Interview with Shelly Saposnick, (See Supra, n. 173, p. 45).

union walkouts.[152] Those firms having a good employee relations program are less likely to be troubled by the above.

Paramount in the development of any employee relations program is the need for a climate of belief.[153] If employees are distrustful or suspicious of management, the likelihood of their accepting any attempt at developing a successful communications program is diminished. This climate of belief is the result of satisfying daily interactions between the employee and his superiors.

Gaining this acceptability, according to Cutlip, is not a complex problem. Rather, he sees it as a three-step process involving "...an expressed interest in the employee's or member's affairs...the actions taken as a result of what is revealed to be necessary in the problems of the employees... (and lastly)...a free and candid flow of information between management and employee."[154] To be effective, the interest must be genuine and humane, the action taken must not be rash or a token effort, and collaborative planning and information exchange must exist on all levels.

The origin for any employee relations plan is at the lowest level of supervision. In most organizations, the lowest level of supervision is that of the supervisor and is "...the basis and framework for any communication program..."[155] In the eyes of some companies, the supervisor is the company management.[156] Proctor and Gamble sees the process of line communication as "...a matter of having sound policies to pass on to employees and of receiving their reactions through man-to-man communication." At P. & G., "...employee communications is viewed as a personnel function, not a mechanical one. It makes each member of supervision wholly responsible for communications in that portion of the operation assigned to him."

The role of the P. R. Director in developing employee relations has been outlined in the previous section. His role is primarily designing, directing and reviewing for effectiveness the employee relations program. The supervisor and the employee counselor are two others having significant involvement with employees.

The involvement of the supervisor is immediate and direct. His role could be likened to that of the Army sargeant in that he is involved with in-line functions and problems.[157] Scott sees the impact of the supervisor in "...creat(ing) the conditions necessary for an efficient and quality-conscious

[152]Interview with Louis Benton, Professor of Management, Hofstra University, Hempstead, N.Y., February 1972.

[153]Scott M. Cutlip, op. cit., p. 223.

[154]Ibid., p. 227.

[155]Ibid.

[156]Wm. G. Werner, "Person to Person," Public Relations Journal, Vol. 12, (April 1956), pp. 3-5.

[157]William G. Scott, Organizational Theory, (Homewood, Ill.: Richard D. Irwin, Inc., 1967), p. 70.

department."[158] Also, the effect of the supervisor on the work climate may
be such as "...to reduce turnover, gain the confidence of employees in
management, sell them on the value and legitimacy of their work, and reduce
gripes, complaints and grievances."[159] According to Whyte, the degree of
success the supervisor has in developing such favorable interpersonnel
sentiments depends on the "...openness of communication between superiors
and subordinates..."[160] The more a subordinate feels that the supervisor is
someone to whom he can talk, the more open the lines of communication.

The effectiveness of the supervisor will be partly determined by
his integration into the management structure of the organization. Scott
sees five areas of discontent for today's supervisor:[161]

(1) Communication pertaining to policy matters
    seems to be weakest at the /supervisor/ level.

(2) /Supervisors/ feel they are given infrequent
    opportunity to voice their sentiments in labor
    negotiations.[162]

(3) One study shows that there exists a great
    deal of disagreement between the supervisor's
    and his boss's conception of the latter's job
    responsibility.

(4) Pay differentials are another problem area.
    Supervisors feel that there should be a
    greater differential between their pay and
    that of their subordinates.

(5) The old-line supervision finds the using of
    the supervisor's position as a training ground
    for upper-management positions extremely
    galling. By using it as a training position,
    the supervisor position is robbed of career
    status. It has now become an interim position.

From the preceding, it would appear that if management desires the
best in-line leadership, it will have to take many of these grievances into
consideration and prevent them from occurring.

---

[158] Ibid., p. 350.

[159] Ibid.

[160] William F. Whyte, op. cit.

[161] William G. Scott, op. cit., pp. 352-356.

[162] Ibid., cf. 18.

The Employee Counselor

The employee counselor is an outgrowth of the Hawthorne Studies
conducted by Elton Mayo.[163] An informal counselling organization was
established at the Hawthorne Western Electric Plant, and the counselors were
permitted to mingle with the employees and hold informal discussions on any
problem. This unstructured, nondirective approach to employee problems was
based on the belief that employees need the opportunity to talk out their
problems in addition to receiving advice.[164] The rationale behind this
approach is - since the problem was theirs, it was better that they arrive
at their own solutions rather than receive those of others. Many organizations have instituted such programs in their plants in the belief that
"(c)ounseling provides an effective means of clearing away troubles."[165]

The importance of collaborative planning in responding to employee
complaints was previously mentioned. This position is supported by the findings of an affiliate in the Bell System. The affiliate "...found that
participation-type meetings were most effective in /reaching/ employees."[166]
The company researchers concluded that "...belief and knowledge were best in
situations where employees said they had a whole lot of discussion."[167]

This employee commitment to change and the company has been
documented in several texts.[168] It follows that a commitment on the part of
management to participative management is desirable. By encouraging employee
participation in decision-making, it promotes "...a sense of partnership in
a responsibility for the affairs of the organization."[169] It allows, as
Peter Drucker sees it,[170] self-determination in place of conformity to the
whims of management.

There are several other reasons for encouraging employee participation. Cutlip lists four:

> Situations in which employees can fully participate
> can: (1) provide means of two-way communication,
> including feedback of employee questions, mistaken
> notions, and so forth; (2) provide individuals with
> means of self-expression and tap the creative ideas

---

[163]William F. Whyte, op. cit., p. 386, cf. 6.

[164]Ibid.

[165]Scott M. Cutlip, p. 235.

[166]Ibid.

[167]Ibid.

[168]See, e.g., Amitai Etzioni, Modern Organizations, (New York: Prentice-Hall,
1964).

[169]William G. Scott, op. cit., p. 265, cf. 12.

[170]Ibid., p. 58, cf. 25.

latent in any group; (3) uncover opposition and
obstacles to plans before they are put into
effect; (4) encourage a sense of responsibility
for the decisions made, and thus pave the way
for change.[171]

If such a program is carried out, management must be prepared to give these
views careful consideration and not just "lip service." A lack of positive
follow-up could result in greater employee resentment than that existing
before.

Physician-Patient and Nurse-Patient Relationships

Of equal importance with employee relations is the need for good
patient-doctor, and patient-nurse relationships. Traditionally, students
of the medical profession have been schooled in the use of therapeutic
techniques involving the administration of drugs and the application of
physical measures such as radiation therapy, and reni-dialysis.[172] Less
attention had been given to the therapeutic value of good patient-treator
communications.[173] Yet, any type of treatment necessitates communication
of some type.

Reliance on instruction in the social and psychological sciences
has not proven to be successful in developing needed communicative skills
in students.[174] As proof of this, two groups of students - one having little
schooling in the social and psychological sciences, and another having
extensive training in these two areas - were compared for their sensitivity
to patient needs. Bernstein reports, "/n/either had developed effective
skills in establishing meaningful relationships with patients, or in
recognizing and dealing with the emotional facets of illness."[175]

There has been a growing awareness of the emotional components of
illness. With this growing awareness has come a simultaneous increasing
emphasis on the social sciences in the medical and nursing school curricula.
"Particular attention has been given to interviewing skill as the basis for
establishing and maintaining both physician-patient relationships and nurse-
patient relationships."[176]

---

[171]Cutlip, loc. cit.

[172]Lewis Bernstein and Richard H. Dana, Interviewing and the Health
Professions, (New York: Appleton-Century-Crofts: Educational Division,
Meredith Corporation, 1970), p. vii.

[173]Ibid.

[174]Ibid.

[175]Ibid.

[176]Ibid.

One approach to the development of good patient-physician and patient-nurse relationships has been the following: Small tutor-student groups meet for four hours each day. During this time, students interview patients suffering from various types of ailments. Psychiatric patients are not included so as to establish the fact that emotional problems are not unique to psychiatric patients. After each student has interviewed a patient, he then decides which patient(s) presents a problem. At times, additional insight into the interviewing process is provided by watching the tutor interview the same patient(s) and making a comparison of the findings.[177]

The benefit of such an approach is that it also conditions the student to understand the patient-with-a-disease, rather than just understanding the disease.[178] Such conditioning enables the student to gain an overview of the disease's effect on the patient's entire life-style. This facilitates the development of a more positive relationship between physician and patient, nurse and patient, and as an added plus, physician and nurse.

Community Relationships

Community relationships are those relationships external to the organization. They are the interaction of the organization and the towns-people, or municipal government, local industry, civic groups, etc. They run the gamut of problems and opportunities for success. Unlike some, these relationships are inescapable and must be tended to with careful forethought and planning. Cutlip[179] discusses four tenets of responsible community relations.

The first tenet is that of an interdependency of H.M.O.'s on the teamwork and esteem of many people. Likewise, many people will be dependent upon the H.M.O. Without manpower, an H.M.O. would have to close its doors.

Where does it all begin? The way a community perceives any organization is through the eyes of the organization's employees. If they are satisfied with the organization, then this satisfaction will be reflected in their comments about the organization. If they are disgruntled, they will express this, also, and taint the organization's image, thereby hindering community acceptance. Therefore, public opinion will, in effect, begin at the top in the organization's policies towards its employees, its clients, its suppliers and competitors, filtering down and out into the community.

The old addage, "you can't expect something for nothing" applies to good H.M.O.-community relations too. The community provides the organization with manpower, housing, fire and police protection, transportation, health services, food, clothing, etc. In return, the community expects more than just "do-goodism." It expects a firm commitment by the firm to provide good jobs, adequate and fair wages, safe working conditions, pay their taxes, maintain the appearance of their buildings and grounds, participation in community affairs and contributions to worthwhile causes.

[177]Ibid.

[178]Ibid.

[179]Scott M. Cutlip, op. cit., pp. 251-252.

As part of its community relations efforts, Meadowbrook Hospital of East Meadow, N.Y., maintains suicide prevention and emergency services. The services provided include emotional first aid to lonely, frightened and confused individuals; brief emergency aid and emotional support for prior psychiatrically assisted persons; follow-up studies and short-term treatment; a ready referral source to physicians, lawyers, police, etc.

Lastly, it is the responsiblity of the organization to keep the community posted on events and developments occurring within. It is important that the good, as well as the bad news be made known so as to prevent exaggeration and misunderstanding. There are several ways of getting this news to the community, each of which will be covered at some later point in this chapter.

The local community can be viewed as the general public at large. It is stated that public opinion is born at the grass roots level and then permeates its way up through society.[180] In terms of its motivation, Dwight Sanderson, states, "The community includes not only individual persons but the organizations and institutions in which they associate. The real community is the devotion to common interest and purposes, the ability to act together in the chief concerns of life."[181]

According to Cutlip[182] and McCarthy,[183] this motivational force has caused community life to organize around interest groupings. Such groupings may be of people, organizations, businesses, etc. As George Simmel[184] describes it, when common threats or causes for concern arise, there occurs a natural and automatic alliance among those affected. When the problem has been attended to, then these affiliations dissolve. Consequently, there is a constant need to survey for the community influentials, so as to anticipate or discern those areas of community concern which the corporation can aid.

In identifying opinion leaders, Cutlip[185] warns us that decision-makers exist on different levels and that they may not be the nominal leaders. Floyd Hunter,[186] in his book Community Power Structure, developed a hierarchy of community decision-makers in civic affairs. He ranked them accordingly:

---

[180] Political science notes taken while student of Modern American Government given by Murry Levin, Professor of Political Science, Boston University, Boston, Mass., 1967. (Spring)

[181] Scott M. Cutlip, op. cit., p. 253.

[182] Ibid.

[183] See, e.g., E. Jerome McCarthy, Basic Marketing, (Homewood, Ill.: Richard D. Irwin, Inc., 1968).

[184] George Simmel, Conflict and the Web of Group Affiliations, (New York: Free Press, 1955).

[185] Cutlip, loc. cit.

[186] Floyd Hunter, Community Power Structure, (Chapel Hill, N..C.: University of North Carolina Press, 1953).

426

First Rank: Industrial, Commercial, financial owners
and top executives of large enterprises.

Second Rank: Operations officials, bank vice-presidents,
public relations men, small businessmen, top-ranking
public officials, corporation attorneys, contractors.

Third Rank: Civic organization personnel, civic agency
board personnel, newspaper columnists, radio commen-
tators, petty public officials, selected organization
executives.

Fourth Rank: Professionals such as ministers, teachers,
social workers, personnel directors, small business
managers, higher-paid accountants, and the like.

Identification of community decision-makers is the first step in
dealing with public-opinion leaders. The second step requires identification
of community prime movers. Millard Fraught[187] defines prime movers as being
those people who motivate the community to action. Fraught proceeds to
identify these prime movers as:

1. Employees' or members' families

2. The press, radio and TV, their editors and reporters.

3. Thought leaders, including clergy, teachers, city
   officials, prominent retailers, and professional
   men, union officials, bankers, civil workers and
   industrialists.

4. Organizations, including city planning commission,
   welfare agencies, youth groups, veterans, fraternal
   and service groups, cultural and political action
   bodies.

5. Crusaders, such as protest groups, petitioners,
   voice-of-the-people, special events, and the rumor
   factories.

Cataloging of decision-makers and prime movers leaves the identification of areas of community concern. These are the areas in which the
company can lend its support, employ its expertise, or make available its
resources. Cutlip[188] identifies ten elements usually seen as having
community interest. These ten are:

1. Commercial prosperity.

2. Support of religion.

---

187 Scott M. Cutlip, op. cit., p. 254.

188 Ibid.

3. Work for everyone.

4. Adequate education facilities.

5. Law and order.

6. Population growth.

7. Proper housing and utilities.

8. Varied recreational and cultural pursuits.

9. Attention to public welfare.

10. Progressive measures for good health.

The H.M.O. must try to identify with these interest and demonstrate to the community how it serves these interests.

The way in which an H.M.O. identified with the above interests will be seen in its overall organizational policies, the degree of participation and who participates in community affairs, the enrichment it can bring to the cultural and moral fibre of the community, and the openness and continuous exchange of information between itself and the community. The organization must not operate in a cloistered manner, but must be willing to receive the members of the community at all times. The H.M.O.'s management must remember that it is responsible not only for its own operation, but represents the medical industry as a whole. Because people judge the whole by the parts, they are likely to judge the entire industry by the actions of one of its members; a poor impression created here is a bad reflection on the whole.

An example of the type of community relations program that has been developed follows. It is a reprint of the Ansul Chemical Company's community relations program for the town of Marinette, Wisconsin.[189]

1. COMMUNITY AT LARGE. An emergency rescue squad available 24 hours a day at no charge to anyone in the community; participation in activities of Marinette Chamber of Commerce; a daily radio program which carries free social and civic announcements for all local groups; large fire demonstration to highlight Fire Prevention Week each fall; plant tours and open houses; weekly advertising support of "Go to Church" campaigns; periodic community advertising.

2. COMMUNITY THOUGHT LEADERS. Regular mailing of company publication, special tours for specific influence groups; special mailings, such as company annual report or an outstanding national publicity "break."

---

[189] As reprinted in Cutlip, op. cit., pp. 257-258.

3. LOCAL PRESS. Immediate dissemination of company news, both favorable and unfavorable; equitable, although modest, advertising support of all local communications media; impartial timing of news breaks, invitations to press to attend company functions; 24-hour-a-day availability to press; elimination of pressure to run company stories "as is."

4. CIVIC ORGANIZATIONS. Regular and proportionate donations to local charities; use of daily radio program; speaker's bureau, both for regular addresses and to fill emergency needs; free movies, projection equipment, and operator for use by nonprofit groups; plant tours and fire demonstrations for civic clubs.

5. STUDENTS, FACULTY, SCHOOL OFFICIALS. Plant tours by business, chemistry, and other school classes; regular advertisements in school yearbooks and newspapers; use of daily radio program by faculty; cooperation and leadership on Business-Education Day.

6. MUNICIPAL EMPLOYEES, OFFICIALS. Free fire equipment and recharging supplies to fire and police departments; use of fire test field for training and demonstrations; first aid training of firemen and policemen by Ansul Rescue Squad; availability of Ansul fire equipment for emergency use; personal leadership in city council, police and fire commission, civil defense, other municipal agencies; absence of pressure on tax assessments, zoning, special ordinances, and so forth.

7. LOCAL MERCHANTS, INDUSTRIALISTS. Mailing of Ansul Fuse Plug; avoidance of "pirating" employees from local business and industry; brief congratulatory letter when businessman is honored or promoted; welcoming visits to new merchants or industry officials; salutes to other industries in the company's employee publication.

8. NONEMPLOYEE LOCAL STOCKHOLDERS. Mailing of Ansul Fuse Plug; special mailing of periodic information about the company's progress; invitations to visit plant.

Ansul believes that building a reservoir of goodwill in its local community in these ways has helped to bring about dollars-and-cents returns:

1. Equitable tax rates, assessments, and other municipal actions which tend to regulate a company's operations.

429

2. Availability of labor, silled and unskilled.
   People prefer to work for a company that's
   liked and respected.

3. Public support in case of trouble - labor
   difficulties, layoffs, accidents, plant
   disasters.

4. Increased employee productivity. Employees
   tend to reflect favorable community attitudes.

Press Relations

Press relations can have very beneficial or very detrimental effects
on an H.M.O.'s reputation. Because the medical profession deals with life
and death situations, this becomes a vital news area. Just how cooperative
the H.M.O. is with the news media determines whether press relations will be
cordial or hostile. "A hostile newspaper or radio station can blast an
/H.M.O.'s/ reputation by the factual reporting of an unfortunate mistake
which cost a life."[190]

It is imperative that the H.M.O. work out procedures for the
release of information on patients to the press. Included in drawing up
these procedures should be some members of the press. By having them there,
they will understand why there must, at times, be some gap between what the
press wants and what the H.M.O. can release. This gap is determined to a
large extent by the medical profession's code[191] of ethics regarding the
private relationship of doctor and patient.

Numerous press codes have been worked out between the press and
the medical profession. One hospital press-code worked out in the state of
Wisconsin[192] admits to the need for willing, prompt and accurate information
on hospital affairs and the designation of those responsible for press
releases. Steps were also taken to educate the hospital staff on the
dissemination of any news.

An examination of several press codes by the Chicago Hospital
Council revealed that any press code should be guided by three major considerations:[193]

1. To safeguard the private rights of the individual,
   so that no subscribers will be caused embarrassment
   or discomfort or be made the object of scorn or
   ridicule.

---

[190]Scott M. Cutlip, op. cit., p. 364.

[191]Harold P. Kurtz, op. cit., p. 22.

[192]Scott M. Cutlip, op. cit., cf. 11.

[193]Ibid., cf. 12.

2. To report the news accurately, authoritatively, promptly.

3. To cooperate sincerely in all relationships.

These considerations are but an example of what may be needed, and should be adopted according to variances existing within organizational structures and approaches to medical care, public's need for information and the increasing demand for accountability and increased efficiency of operation.

The following is an example of how the U. S. Army evaluates its program and may serve as a model for similar plans:

1. Command Policy

a. Are the commander and his senior staff officers and subordinate commanders sold on the necessity for a sincere and consistent attitude toward the community?

b. Has a definite community relations program been outlined?

c. Is the community relations program under the direction of a qualified officer?

d. Has the community relations program been explained in detail to the senior staff officers and all subordinate commanders?

e. Does the commander take into confidence the officer directing the community relations program?

f. Has the officer in charge of community relations been given the opportunity to study and overhaul command policies and activities so that the command will always be on the right and ethical side of any argument?

g. Is the command in its operations guilty of any of the more common community complaints against a military installation:

(1) Local tax dodging.
(2) High Accident rates.
(3) Misconduct of military personnel.
(4) Waste of taxpayers' money.
(5) Failure of military personnel to participate in community projects and activities.

h. Does the command know what the public in the local civilian community thinks of it, its policies and its personnel?

i. Is there available an analysis of the community itself, its problems, its weaknesses, and its civic ambitions?

j. Have all points of citizen contact been checked for good community relations practice - the gate guards, military police, the telephone switchboard, the employment section of the Civilian Personnel Office,etc.?

k. Have all members of the command, particularly the officers and senior noncommissioned officers, been urged to take active part in community projects and activities?

l. Have all military personnel received an orientation on the local community as well as on the command community relations program?

m. Is there a continuing program to make members of the command more community relations-minded?

2. Publicity

a. Have arrangements been made to assure local press, radio, and television of a 24-hours source for command information?

b. Are command news releases written in good news reporting style, without padding, and angled for community interest?

c. Do local press, radio, and television reporters have easy access to the command and its senior officers on reasonable notice?

d. Does the commander hold frequent press conferences for the purpose of announcing important changes in command policies or activities?

e. Are local reporters invited to visit the command frequently on both a group and individual basis?

f. Are local news media representatives invited occasionally to command social functions?

3. Requests for Speakers

a. Has a routine been established for prompt handling of local requests for speakers?

b. Are military personnel given adequate assistance in preparation of speeches and of charts and other visual aids when asked to address more important gatherings?

c. Have several officers been selected because of their speaking ability to represent the command at meetings and gatherings not of sufficient importance to require the time of the commander or other senior officers?

d. Are all speech manuscripts cleared through one office for protection in matters of policy?

4. Open House and Tours

a. Is an open house held by the command at least once a year?

b. Does the command have an established plan for proper handling of visitors who "just drop in"?

c. Does the command have a souvenir booklet to give visitors to remind them of their visit to the command?

d. Is everything possible being done to encourage local schools and community groups to visit the command?

e. Are business and professional clubs being encouraged to occasionally hold their weekly luncheons at a military installation?

5. Contributions to Local Charities

a. Has the command made a careful study of local charities and annual community drives to determine its proper share of responsibility?

b. Does the command cooperate with local charity campaigns in other ways than by monetary contributions?

c. Has the command made any attempt to spearhead any such community drives with the initial gift?

d. Do any officers of the command serve on the boards of local charitable organizations?

6. Community Relations Plan

a. Is the community relations plan a flexible one geared to the changing needs and interests of the local civilian community?

b. Are command policies and the programs predicated on them explained frankly and in detail both directly and indirectly through all channels of communications to the opinion leaders in the community?

d. Is the community relations program completely humanized and personalized? In other words, the command must be interpreted to the community in terms of the attitude and character of all the individuals who are a part of its organization.

REACHING H.M.O. PUBLICS

The tools of communication are many and varied. They range from the printed word and personal appearances to audio-visual presentations. They may be internal, external or a combination of internal-external. Their intended use is the same - a telling of the H.M.O.'s story in as many ways as possible.

The word communication is derived from the Latin communis, meaning common. There are three basic elements in communication: the source, the message, and the receiver. Common knowledge and experience results from ongoing communications and is represented as an interlinking process.

Speakers Bureau

Personal contact is one of the most effective ways of communicating.[194] It provides the opportunity for clarification of intent, tonal inflection, rebuttal, elaboration and involvement on the part of the speaker and the audience. In each H.M.O., there should be some who are capable of telling the organization's story. You might find this ability in the H.M.O.'s administrators, department directors, board members, etc. Each may be a little unwilling at first, but with a little coaching, they will probably come around.

Providing these individuals with the opportunity to speak is not too difficult. In most towns, there exist several groups, such as the following: service clubs, church groups, school groups, and fraternal and social groups. Most of these organizations seek out speakers for their meetings or programs.[195] It might be preferable to have the speaker report on the topic with which he is most familiar; e.g., the administrator speaks on hospital management, or expenditures; the Nursing Director might speak on the rewards and direction of nursing as a profession.

Open House

The open house can be another effective and inexpensive means of reaching the public. It does require hard work in its preparation, but the rewards could be significant. Some guidelines, as suggested by Harold Kurtz,[196] are:

---

[194] William G. Scott, op. cit., Chapter VII.

[195] Harold P. Kurtz, op. cit., p.30.

[196] Ibid., p. 32.

434

1. Hold it when traffic will cause the least
    amount of interference with the H.M.O.
    schedule and in good weather.

2. Establish your purpose before announcing
    the open house.

3. Point out areas of concern on the tour.

Literature Racks

Literature racks are another inexpensive way of telling the H.M.O.'s
story. Each day, numerous people pass in and out of the H.M.O.'s facilities
and traffic areas. By stocking literature racks in these areas with the
H.M.O.'s publications and other related material, the reader not only has
the opportunity to "kill time" more pleasantly, but he can simultaneously
learn of the H.M.O.

Some items for inclusion are "...folders on the /H.M.O./, visitors
folder, copies of the /H.M.O./ publication, employees' magazine, folders on
H.M.O. costs, brochures on /H.M.O./ educational programs and similar
material."[197] It is important that the racks don't become dumping grounds
for outdated publications, and some form of regular check is advisable.

Hospital Week

Each year, the American Hospital Association sponsors a hospital
week.[198] This special event should be considered as part of the entire
public relations program and entered into the calendar of events. For
hospital week, the AHA mails a packet of "...editorials, news stories and
features."[199] How these are used will be determined, in part, by how many
other hospitals are in the area. If too many exist, there is the danger of
duplication of program, and this danger may warrant a prior conference among
those institutions concerned. Hospital Week will provide an excellent
opportunity to demonstrate needs and accomplishments and is worthy of much
planning and preparation.

Bulletin Boards

Bulletin boards are a good method of keeping the internal public
informed. Notices may be posted at regular intervals, directing attention

---

[197]Ibid.

[198]Ibid., p. 33.

[199]Ibid., p. 34.

at specific problems or events that are occurring within the organization. Policing of bulletin boards is as important as the policing of literature racks.

Posters

Posters are useful in drawing one's attention to issues of "...safety, housekeeping, economics, preparedness or security."[200] These issues should be ones of constant concern and can be covered briefly.

Handbooks, Manuals, Books

Indoctrination booklets, Reference guides and Institutional Booklets are useful.[201] The first is designed to orient the new employee or subscriber. It appraises them of the rules and regulations of the plan and tries to instill a team spirit - "...the feeling that he has joined a winning combination."[202] The reference guide concerns itself with facts and figures relevant to the organization. It is useful "...to the seasoned member as well as to the neophyte."[203] Institutional booklets are directed at "...the H.I.P., for example, publishes a comprehensive booklet for physicians interested in a prepaid group partnership practice with H.I.P. affiliation- (See Table VII - 3 for an outline of the booklet's contents).

Letters and Bulletins

Letters and bulletins serve to bridge the communications gap between management and employee, and company and the community. "Letters are used on a regular or spot-news basis to reach employees, dealers, alumni or workers in a fund raising or legislative campaign."[205] Quite often, the letter may be used as a supplement to the"..slower,less-frequently published house magazine."[206] Letters enable a more personal and intimate contact between the chief executive and the employee. "Typical content of letters for a business house would be policy statements, welfare programs, financial reports, product news and economic education."[207]

---

[200]Scott M. Cutlip, op. cit., p. 188.

[201]Ibid., pp. 184-185.

[202]Ibid.

[203]Ibid.

[204]Ibid.

[205]Ibid., p. 186.

[206]Ibid.

[207]Ibid., p. 187.

436

TABLE VII - 3

HEALTH INSURANCE PLAN OF
GREATER NEW YORK

TABLE OF CONTENTS

The Health Insurance Plan of Greater New York

The Medical Groups

H.I.P. Membership

General Functions of Physicians in a Group

Medical Center Facilities

H.I.P. Facilities Program

Working Relationships Between H.I.P. and

Contracting Medical Groups

H.I.P. Prepayment System

Special Services Fund

Services Provided to the Medical Groups by H.I.P.

Multiphasic Screening

Mental Health Service Program

Appendix A

    Professional Requirements for Physicians in an H.I.P. Group

Appendix B

    Medical Group Partnerships

Source: **H.I.P. of N.Y., N.Y., N.Y., Publication # 123 7C 2/71.**

Nassau County Medical Center, East Meadow, N.Y., and Long Beach Memorial Hospital, Long Beach, N.Y. use mailings to inform the public of special events. Direct mailings are used when direct contact and assured public awareness is desired. Announcements of this type may be directed at the opening of a new facility or clinic , or informing the community of an up-coming event.

Inserts and Enclosures

Inserts and enclosures are generally directed at an explanation of changes that may have occurred in payroll, vacation policy, work schedules or other job-related events. They could be items of interest pertaining to civic events, educational opportunities or community problems. These are usually enclosed in the employee's paycheck or subscriber's bill, or in other mailings.

Institutional Advertising

Institutional advertising has become the major way in which organizations publicize information about themselves.[208] The organization cannot only tell others about itself, but it can do so in its own words,and also choose its audience. George Hammond, President of the Carl Byoir firm, cataloged 14 possible uses of institutional advertising, ranging from (1) community relations efforts to "(14) presentations of industry or professional activities and points of view."[209] (See Table VII - 4).

The purpose of most institutional advertising is that of "...using this means to talk directly to the media gate-keepers by placing ads in the trade journals or press, magazines and radio."[210] The effectiveness of this approach is questionable, but evidence indicates that "...specific campaigns aimed at specific objectives by reputable sponsors are the most effective. Ads with a 'news' approach and using strong, human-interest pictures draw the biggest readership."[211]

The Metropolitan Diagnostic Institute of metropolitan New York, approach is to mail prospective subscribers an informative pamphlet describing the Institute's services, facilities, operations, and its three locations.

Audio-Visual

The telephone, public-address system, the phonograph and the film strip are audio-visual aids used in reaching people. The telephone can be programmed to automatically deliver messages to any who call that number.

---

[208]From lecture given by Dr. Cohen, Professor of Marketing, Hofstra University, Hempstead, N.Y., Spring 1971.

[209]Scott M. Cutlip, op. cit., p. 190.

[210]Ibid., p. 192.

[211]Ibid.

TABLE VII - 4

FOURTEEN USES OF INSTITUTIONAL ADVERTISING

1) Community relations - H.M.O. openings, H.M.O. expansions, H.M.O. open houses, H.M.O. anniversaries, annual reports, promotion of H.M.O. community activities, e.g, clean-up weeks, safety, community chest campaigns, etc.

2) Labor relations, including the H.M.O.'s side in labor disputes.

3) Recruitment of employees.

4) Promotion of art contests, scholarship awards, etc.

5) Statements of policy.

6) Elections of board members.

7) Consolidation of competitive position.

8) Records of accomplishments.

9) Service difficulty or public misunderstanding which must be cleared up immediately.

10) Promotion or opposition to pending legislation.

11) Consolidation of editorial opinion.

12) Supplier relations.

13) Celebration of local institutions, e.g., the press during National Newspaper Week.

14) Presentation of industry or professional activities and points of view.

439

In one Midwest hospital, "...(a) daily news bulletin is recorded in the morning and is accessible to all hospital employees, day or night."[212] Other hospitals can "...(use) the same device for special patient bulletins on facts about the hospital...(or)...utilize these for community health services."[213]

Audio-visual aids that employ sound films are being used more often in the training of employees, speakers bureau presentations and fund raising.[214] The reasons for this are many,[215] but due to the expense involved, not all organizations can afford their use. Depending on resources, the organization can make its own 35mm films or contract with a professional studio for a more-sophisticated production.

The public-address system is ideal for the announcing of special events, for paging personnel or for piping in music to employees or patients. It is mobile, useful for reaching large crowds and serves to link the boss in the front office to the man at the bench.

External Publications

External publications are those directed at the community, the general public or other businesses and affiliates. Its purpose should be to provide "...something over and above a rehash of H.M.O. news releases. It should emphasize interpretive comment, behind-the-scenes stories, first-person reports by H.M.O. officials and similar items. The external publication should not only answer the question of - What's happening at the H.M.O.?, but also the questions of Why? and How?

The Kaiser Foundation Health Plan, Inc., of California, publishes an annual report on the Medical Care Program Concept, the facilities, personnel, utilization, training programs, medical and technical developments in the treatment and approaches to medical care, growth projections, and historical highlights. Exhibit VII - 1 presents a graphic representation of the elements comprising the Kaiser Foundation Health Plan. This representation could serve as a graphic model for H.M.O.'s (having the same form) publishing similar reports.

Employee Publication

The employee publication is of utmost importance in developing good employee relations. Need for effective communication has been discussed in general. In an organization that operates 24 hours a day, seven days a week, there is less unity because of the shifts that exist and the number of personnel in transit.

---

[212] Harold P. Kurtz, op. cit., p. 35.

[213] Ibid.

[214] Ibid., p. 36.

[215] Association of National Advertisers, Inc., "The Dollar Sense of Business Films," (New York: ANA, 1954).

EXHIBIT VII - 1

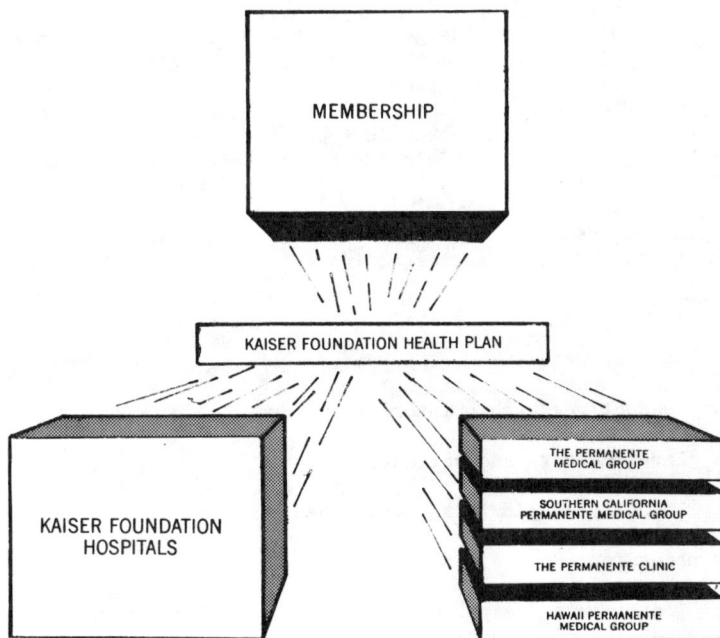

This chart illustrates the principal relationships involved in conducting the Program in its four Regions—

- Northern California: San Francisco Bay Area and Sacramento
- Southern California: Greater Los Angeles Area
- Oregon: Portland, Oregon—Vancouver, Washington and vicinity
- Hawaii: Island of Oahu.

Kaiser Foundation Health Plan, Inc., a California nonprofit corporation, undertakes to arrange for necessary hospital and professional care for subscribers and their dependents —the Health Plan members. In the Oregon Region this function is performed by a subsidiary, Kaiser Foundation Health Plan of Oregon, a Washington nonprofit corporation.

The Health Plan meets its commitment to arrange for health care services principally through two types of contracts—

■ A MEDICAL SERVICE AGREEMENT
In each Region one of four independent Permanente Medical Groups accepts responsi-

bility for professional care of Health Plan members in the Region. Three of the Medical Groups are organized as partnerships. The fourth, in Hawaii, is an unincorporated association.

■ A HOSPITAL SERVICE AGREEMENT
By a complementary agreement Kaiser Foundation Hospitals, a California nonprofit and charitable corporation, accepts Regional responsibility for necessary hospital services and facilities.

Because of their nonprofit and public service character, Kaiser Foundation Hospitals, Kaiser Foundation Health Plan, Inc., and Kaiser Foundation Health Plan of Oregon all are exempt from federal income tax.

In each Region one of four Permanente Services corporations performs centralized business and administrative services for the organizations cooperating in the Medical Care Program, and also operates prescription pharmacies at non-hospital locations. All Permanente Services capital stock is owned in equal shares by Kaiser Foundation Hospitals and Kaiser Foundation Health Plan.

To keep its medical staff informed of hospital events, and medical progress in the treatment of various diseases, as achieved by its physicians, South Nassau Communities Hospital, Oceanside, N.Y. publishes a medical staff journal. Also included are case studies on patients, and staff activities in the areas of publications, lectures, meeting presentations, and lastly, promotions.

Kurtz states that the "...employee publication should be issued regularly. It should outline the goals of the /H.M.O./ and show how the /H.M.O./ is attempting to achieve these goals. The periodical should attempt to show the roles of the various people and departments in the /H.M.O./. It should help employees recognize that while their jobs may be different, their goals are the same. An employee publication is the cornerstone of an employee communication program, but it should not be the total effort in employee communications."[216]

Kurtz also suggests some helpful hints in design and sources for ideas. Concerning hints, he suggests:[217]

1. Involve Administration.

2. Vary format.

3. Conduct readership interest surveys.

4. Experiment to add variety.

5. Identify people in the articles.

Suggested sources for ideas are:[218]

1. Departmental features with a different department spotlighted each month.

2. Monthly welcome to new employees.

3. A roving reporter with half-column photos of those being questioned.

4. Recipe box - a good place to get a person in the news who may not make news otherwise.

5. Monthly summary of what patients said about the hospital - both good and bad comments should be included.

6. Explanation of new equipment as it is purchased.

---

[216] Ibid., p. 42.

[217] Ibid.

[218] Ibid., p. 43.

Meetings and Conferences

Meetings and conferences provide the opportunity for a one-to-one, one-to-many or many-to-many information exchange.[219] It is an opportunity for individuals to gain and provide immediate feedback on issues of concern. Meetings can be informal or formal; they can be discussion groups or panels. They may consist of only staff, hospital personnel, outsiders or all of these. Attendance may be voluntary or compulsory (the former is preferred).

For example, Meadowbrook Hospital, East Meadow, Long Island, has scheduled regular, interdepartmental meetings into its employee relations program. These interdepartmental meetings are of vital importance in creating a team effort. In addition to the regular meeting of representatives from every department, individualized meetings of medical staff and administrative staff are held. What is sought out in these meetings is feedback and interaction of its members.[220] These people become key contacts for news stories, employee communications and many of the other hospital communications programs.

THE ECONOMICS OF A PUBLIC RELATIONS PLAN

Determining the cost of a Public Relations program is not an easy matter. It requires the same amount of planning and needs assessment, as does the budget for any other department in an organization. In determining the cost, Sallie Bright feels that the "...amount of time and money necessary for your public relations program will depend entirely on what the program is and what needs to be done about it. No generalization can be made as to what proportion of total budgets should be spent for public relations purposes."[221]

On the other hand, Alden B. Mills states that "... /a/ hospital might well spend for its public relations program between one and two per cent of its total budget."[222] It would seem that this point of view would be better received by planners. If an organization became incapable of assessing the cost of meeting its needs, then any kind of rationale operation could not exist. The entire operation would have to operate on uncertainty. Monies would have to be allocated on a "solve-the-problem-as-it-comes" basis. The success of this last-minute approach to budgeting seems quite questionable.

---

[219]Scott, op. cit., p. 159. (See, e.g., Jurgem Ruesch and Gregory Bateson, Communication: The Social Matrix of Psychiatry, (New York: W. W. Norton & Co., 1951), Chapter II.

[220]Interview with Robert K. Kushner, (See Supra, n. 158, p. 39).

[221]Sallie Bright, op. cit., p. 41.

[222]Alden B. Mills, op. cit., p. 305.

In terms of how to finance the public relations program, Mills cautions us not to treat it as a frill._ Rather, "...the public relations program is a legitimate part of /H.M.O./ operating expense...(as)...such it ought to appear in the /H.M.O./ budget."[223] If it comes to be considered a frill, it will receive only secondary or less consideration by upper management, and have, as was stated earlier, a secondary or less impact.

To assure it of its rightful place, Bright stresses the need for sound planning of a program. "Often, the lack of a careful plan is behind the indifference or hostility of a board, a budget committee, and even of a staff, to the idea of spending money for public relations."[224] A haphazard plan by any other department would be received the same way, and rightfully so.

The justification of the plan cannot easily be measured in terms of output. Unlike a factory producing Widgets, the output of which can be measured as well as the resulting sales, the product of a public relations is intangible. It is more of an effect on those to whom it is directed. Measuring the impact of this effect on the public is a behavioral measure in that the program is aimed at attitudinal problems and the behavior resulting from these attitudes. Consequently, many executives consider it an unproductive extra[225] because attitudinal changes are difficult to measure or detect.

Mills believes that any public relations plan can be justified by its effect on the publics under consideration. In the case of health care institutions, Mills[226] states several advantages accruing to subscribers, the medical staff, the employees and most importantly, the general public. His contention is that favorable attitudes resulting from the efforts of the public relations department's activities will have a beneficial effect on the success of the organization, and that the measure of this success is equal to the return on the monetary investment in the public relations program.

Concerning subscribers "...(p)robably 60 per cent of the effort put forth by the public relations staff will be directed toward improving the quality of care either physically, scientifically,psychologically or spiritually."[227] A first step in accomplishing this occurs because there is an individual (the P.R. Director) who is free to devote all his time to improving subscriber care. Generally, the H.M.O. administrator[228] is charged with this responsibility, and rightfully so. He is also responsible for many of the other operations and must spread himself around. This thinning of his

[223] Ibid., p. 306.

[224] Bright, loc. cit.

[225] Ibid.

[226] Alden B. Mills, op. cit., pp. 307-310.

[227] Ibid.

[228] See Supra, n. 150, p. 36.

attention prevents him from accomplishing as much as he would like to, and results in some problems not receiving the attention and correction needed.

Secondly, improved relations with the medical staff is another dividend. Physicians are interested in doing the most for their patients. Part of being able to do so means the H.M.O. must be progressive and alert to changes in medicine. "A progressive, alert /H.M.O./ is of much more aid to them in this endeavor than an institution that pays little or no attention to changing needs and advancing standards of medical and /H.M.O./ service."229 A progressive H.M.O. can mean better utilization of physician's services.

The effect of a good public relations program on H.M.O. employees can have profound results. First, the program should be able to educate the employee to the institution's purposes and functions. Secondly, the program should develop a sense of belonging or partnership in a vital community service. "As a result, they should serve the /H.M.O./ more loyally and more intelligently, and the /H.M.O./ should, therefore, be able to pay better wages and to provide better working conditions while still obtaining the same or a larger service for each payroll dollar."230

Public relations and community support can have a three-fold effect. First, there is the chance for increased patronage. This could arise from the creation of a favorable image in the eyes of the public. Also, as the public becomes more aware of the H.M.O.'s services and facilities, it will better be able to use them.

As Sallie Bright said, "...(a)ny organization, profit-making or nonprofit, exists only by the consent of the public."231 Therefore, it's important that public support exist. According to Mills, the second effect of a public relations program is that "...the public will more readily rally to the support of hospitals in their legitimate legislative ambitions and in the entire scope of their relations with governmental bodies."232 This means support for licensing, exemption from taxation, financial support, etc.

RESPONDING TO NEW CHALLENGES AND CHANGING PRIORITIES

A viable organization is one that is capable of effecting a harmonious adjustment between itself and its publics. This adjustment requires an

---

229 Alden B. Mills, op. cit.

230 Ibid.

231 Sallie Bright, "Management's Responsibility for Public Relations," Public Relations in Health and Welfare, Francis Schmidt & Harold N. Weiner, Editors, (New York: Columbia University Press, 1966), p. 1.

232 Mills, loc. cit.

awareness of each others needs and the ability to satisfy these needs. Not being able to adequately respond to or to measure correctly what the public wants can lend itself to the eventual demise of an organization. The technique of assessing public needs is that of opinion research and was pioneered by N. W. Ayer.[233]

Opinion Research

The process of opinion research has several implications for the organization. Cutlip lists six. First, "...Research provides much-needed emphasis on the listening phase of public relations and gives substance to the two-way street concept."[234] Research is both a listening and telling process. Historically, organizations have been only telling[235] and not listening for the values, viewpoints and language of its audience. "These values and viewpoints can only be learned through systematic and sympathetic listening."[236]

Secondly, "Research provides the objective look required to know thyself."[237] By determining what public opinions exist, a company simultaneously discovers itself. Public opinion is a mirror image of the company concerned.[238] It reflects just what exists and how favorably it is perceived. The practitioner must capture this public image and present it to the organization's policy-makers, just as the public sees it.

Thirdly, "Research earns support for counseling and programming around the policy-making table."[239] By carefully assessing public opinion, the practitioner can advise management on course of public action needed. Management is fact-minded and will respond to documented evidence, either in support of or against proposed action.

Fourth, "Research reveals festering trouble spots before they infect a large body of public opinion."[240] A basic tenet of prepaid group practice is that of preventive medicine. The same is true here. It is better to prevent trouble before it develops into crisis proportions. "Continuous fact-finding will uncover many problems while they are still small enough

---

[233]Edwin Emery, History of American Newspaper Publishers Association, (Minneapolis: University of Minnesota Press, 1950), pp. 125-130.

[234]Scott M. Cutlip, op. cit., p. 111.

[235]Ibid.

[236]See, e.g., "The Dewy and Almy Chemical Co. and the Chemical Workers," edited by Clinton Golden and Virginia Parker, (New York: Harper & Row, Publishers, 1955), pp. 100-120.

[237]Scott M. Cutlip, op. cit., p. 112.

[238]Ibid.

[239]Ibid.

[240]Ibid., p. 113.

to permit quiet handling...(and)...will permit the catching of rumors before they become widespread."[241]

Fifth, "Research increases the effectiveness of outbound communication."[242] Bombardment of the general public with organizational messages is not totally effective. The public is not a homogeneous, but rather, a heterogeneous grouping. Its needs, receptivity and responses will differ. Research will enable the practitioner to pinpoint his publics and narrow his target market. The effectiveness of his public relations effort will "...increase in...proportion to the specificity with which it is directed to a group."[243]

Lastly, "Research provides useful intelligence - an idea service for executives."[244] New ideas stem from the examination of what exists and then comparing this to what is needed. The difference is the opportunity for innovation. "Increasingly, administrators rely on the public relations department as a central source of information on the organization, the public's image, the industry or field, and the social, economic and political trends."[245] While this is a useful service in itself,executives often do not have the time to properly interpret these facts. The public relations department can assist here by analyzing these facts and presenting them in a lucid and cogent form for executive review.

An example of how the Sun Oil Company employs the research approach follows: (1) The company's research department maintains a library directed by a trained librarian and contains standard reference books on the oil industry and general business, public relations, legislative enactments and general news material. (2) A recording of daily and periodical press, radio and TV reports on the company, the industry, and business in general. (3) Special reports and surveys on topics vital to the company, the industry and general business, and the effectiveness of their public relations efforts.[246]

Fact Finding

The first step in measuring public opinion is the development of a fact file. A fact file is a collection of data on the organization, the industry, the organization's publics, and the general public. This information is of importance to a client or the organization. "From fact files come ideas and information for speeches, pamphlets, special reports,

---

[241]Ibid.

[242]Ibid.

[243]Ibid.

[244]Ibid.

[245]Ibid.

[246]Ibid., p. 114. (Reprinted without citation).

institutional advertising, exhibits, special events, and background information for special projects."[247]

Fact-finding may be done either formally or informally; the determining factors are generally time and money. A formal search for facts requires the employment of more sophisticated techniques, more time and additional personnel - all of which add up to a greater expenditure of money. Consequently, smaller organizations, or those just starting up, are forced, because of lack of funds, to use informal methods.

Informal Methods

Informal methods can be quite effective and consist of the following techniques: "(1) personal contacts by telephone or mail with persons you know; (2) advisory committees or panels; (3) analysis of an organization's incoming mail; (4) reports of field agents or salesmen on their evaluations of opinions about the organization; (5) press clippings and radio and TV monitorings on what has been said on a particular subject; (6) conferences of those involved in a particular problem or situation; (7) study of national public opinion polls... (8) study of election and legislative voting... on certain issues; (9) speeches and writings of recognized opinion leaders; (10) (use) records."[248]

There are two weaknesses inherent in informal methods. One is the lack of representativeness, and the other is a lack of objectivity.[249] These weaknesses do not preclude obtaining benefits from the use of informal methods but do require the need for careful interpretation of the results.

Formal Techniques

Formal techniques are based upon sampling methods. A sample is a representative group of people in each public.[250] It is hypothesized that this accurate miniature of the larger public will provide opinions representative of the general population in question. Several sampling methods exist for eleciting public bpinion.[251]

1. Cross-Section surveys. Three types of cross-section surveys exist - the probability sample, the area sample and the quota sample. Each sample is considered to be a cross-section of the given public. The questions asked this group are subject to some sampling error, but most important they

---

[247]Ibid., p. 116.

[248]Ibid., p. 119.

[249]Ibid.

[250]Webster's New World Dictionary, (New York: The World Publishing Co., 1966), p. 1289.

[251]Mildred Parten, Surveys, Polls and Samples, (New York: Cooper Square Publishers, Inc., 1950).

"...fail to reflect the depth and intensity of opinions expressed by respondents."[252]

        2. Survey panels. A cross-section of the given public is selected to participate in a survey panel. This panel is actually a controlled group and can be used as respondents to exposure to different projects in community relations, buying habits, brand preference, etc. Difficulties in administration and maintaining interest are common with this technique.[253]

        3. Depth interview. This is an informal, often unstructured, approach to opinion research. The respondent is interviewed individually and by a skilled interviewer. The primary benefit of this type of technique is that of being able to "...probe the attitudes underlying expressed opinions."[254]

        4. Content analysis. This method attempts to analyze and code the content of one or all of the mass media.[255] Looked for is qualitative and quantitative information on what is being said about the organization or any other area of concern. It can be a measure of effectiveness or record.

        5. Mail questionnaires. This is a less expense and less sophisticated method of measurement. Inherent in this technique is no guarantee that everyone will reply; the chance for misunderstanding as to what is desired; little flexibility in interpretation and the need for a homogeneous given public. "It is most effective in soliciting opinions...where the cleavage of opinion is decisive."[256]

        6. Semantic differential. This is a relatively new technique using bi-polar adjectives. An example might be a question on the wearing of hats. The respondent is asked whether he wears hats and is given a choice, consisting of Never - Always, with a scale of seven in between. A choice of four would be mid-way between never and always, and indicates that he wears hats 50 per cent of the time. Semantic differentials are "...designed to assess variations in the connotative meanings of objects and words, and is based on the premise that such meaning constitutes one of the most significant variables mediating human behavior."[257] A semantic differential scale representing the wearing of hats example is illustrated here.

        always _____ : _____ : _____ : _____ : _____ : _____ : _____ : never

---

[252]Scott M. Cutlip, op. cit., p. 122.

[253]Ibid.

[254]Ibid.

[255]Ibid.

[256]Ibid.

[257]Ibid.

Newer developments in the field of Multi-Variate Analysis[258] permits
a nonmetric comparison of responses to semantic differential questionnaire.
Through the use of Non-Metric Multi-Dimensional Scaling techniques, the
researcher is able to rank peoples' preferences relative to predetermined
ideal point. Those falling closest to the ideal point are closest in opinion
on the point in question.

The use of opinion research has been on the increase[259] since
World War II. It has come into its own recently in measuring political
opinion. The Gallop and the Harris Polls are two commonly-accepted measures
of public opinion. Concurrent with the acceptance of the predictability of
Gallop and Harris Polls is the acceptance of Marketing Research as a measure
of consumer opinion, and Opinion Research as a measure of public opinion.
The consequences for industry lie in employing these techniques to spot trouble
before it starts, to measure the pulse of their public, to serve as a means
of program evaluation and as a guide in long-range planning.

COORDINATING DEPARTMENTAL PUBLIC RELATIONS EFFORTS

The Marketing public and the Financial Lending public are two
groups whose support is vital to the success of the organization. The
Marketing public is the potential and actual subscriber population. Without
subscribers,there is no organization. The same is true of the Lending public.
Without the financial support of Financiers and Lending institutions, the
organization will not be able to meet its start-up costs. Start-up costs
are excessive and have historically been one of the major obstacles to H.M.O.
development and failure.[260]

One aspect of obtaining Lender support and subscriber enrollment is
the development of a public relations program directed at these special
publics. The program must convincingly communicate the organization's needs
to these groups, and inculcate in them a desire to satisfy these needs. The
program must also show how the organization will, in turn, satisfy its
publics' needs. It must insure that a sense of mutual exchange be felt by
both sides and strive to make this feeling a reality.

The design of this program must, in part, fall under the aegis of
the Public Relations Department. The added expertise of the public relations
department will provide direction, refinement and a professional touch to the
program. The P. R. Department will be the nexus for Marketing and Finance
public relations efforts. As such, it may facilitate interdepartmental
cooperation, coordination of the release of publications, interdepartmental
communication and understanding.

---

[258] See, e.g., Green and Tull, Research for Marketing Decisions,
(Englewood Cliffs, N.J.: Prentice-Hall, Inc., 1970), Chapter VII.

[259] Scott M. Cutlip, op. cit., p. 126.

[260] Interview with Leo Petit (See Supra, n. 88, p. 25.).

The assistance provided Marketing and Finance by Public Relations
may bear some similarities. This is because both departments must contend
with similar problems. Both departments will need to educate their respective
publics to the H.M.O. concept. Both will have media and publishing problems
in addition to other areas of mutual concern. Specifically, the Public
Relations department will assist each as follows. Cutlip lists six ways in
which P. R. can assist Marketing.[261]

1. By creating the belief that H.M.O. is a provider
   of quality medical care, this will increase brand
   preference.[262] The assumption here is that consumers are more apt to utilize a service provided
   by an organization with which they are impressed.
   This familiarity-at-a-distance breeds a sense of
   confidence and greater risk-taking.

2. Convert P. R. audiences into customers...[263]
   This means convincing employees and the families,
   friends and relatives of the employees, members
   of various trade associations, etc., to join the
   organization. These people are easily reached
   through the organization's publications or
   through direct on-the-job contact.

3. Establish a favorable identity in a new market
   to pave the way for acceptance of a new line
   of (services) or (benefits coverage).[264] New
   developments in medicine or the need for
   additional coverage as one's family grows in
   number and age often necessitates changes in
   plans. How favorably and how readily the public
   receives these changes depends on the preparation
   they've had. If they have been appraised in
   advance of the benefits they can derive from
   these innovations, they will probably be more
   receptive.

4. Build understanding of the (organization's) role
   and service to society by using its...services
   as examples in literature, speeches and so
   forth.[265] By showing how the organization serves

[261]Scott M. Cutlip, op. cit., p. 331.

[262]Ibid.

[263]Ibid.

[264]Ibid.

[265]Ibid.

society, you are more apt to enlist public
support for legislative enactments, manpower
needs, local zoning variances, etc. Most of
the benefits deriving from community support
were covered in a previous section on
Community Relations.

5. Build public demand for your (services).[266]
    The demand for medical services is normally
    a necessity and is not a derived demand. In
    the case of an H.M.O., the element of derived
    demand pertains to differentiating the H.M.O.
    as a provider of comprehensive, preventive
    health care from acute episodic and compulsory
    health insurance. National Health Week can
    provide the H.M.O. the opportunity to provide
    this differentiation by creating the excuse
    to include in its Community Publications
    articles on the advantages of H.M.O.'s over
    existing health care programs and to speak
    of developments within its own organization.
    This may bring added attention and may result
    in increased demand.

6. To overcome public opposition to (the H.M.O.).[267]
    Utilities have been faced with public opposition
    to the use of atomic power. To counter this
    opposition, the utilities waged on educational
    campaign on the benefits and safety of atomic
    energy.[268] A similar campaign could be waged
    showing the benefits (both economic and medical)
    of H.M.O.'s over the existing medical system.
    A recent wealth of publications have materialized
    and can provide much supportive data.

One way the Public Relations Department may help the Finance
Department is to increase Lender support by building an understanding of
the organization as a provider of quality health care. The inference here
is that by demonstrating that the H.M.O. can provide better health care than
other existing plans and that it will serve the "public good," the organization can appeal to the Lending public's sense of "Social Responsibility."
The Social Responsibility of Business is defined as an organization's commitment to serve the general public, in addition to its stockholders. This pre-
disposition to serve should assist the H.M.O. in obtaining a moral commitment
to help first, and a financial commitment second.

---

[266]Ibid.

[267]Ibid.

[268]Interview with G. Robert Odette, Associate Professor of Nuclear
    Engineering, University of California at Santa Barbara, Santa Barbara,
    Calif., January 1972.

Concurrent with gaining lender support should be the securing of lender enrollment. Lender enrollment will add an element of prestige to the plan that could make it more attractive to prospective subscribers or supporters. This follows,as it was stated earlier, that people view[269] members of the financial community as opinion leaders and trend setters and tend to follow suit. Lenders, as subscribers, will also provide an inside channel of communication to the professional market and might enable the H.M.O. to attract additional members of this group.

Imperative in gaining Lender support is creating the belief that the organization will be able to meet its financial obligations. The success of the H.M.O. must be seen as a virtual certainty. It must be shown that because of certain advantages and cost-saving features inherent in the system, the H.M.O. will be able to compete successfully for subscriber enrollment; recruit competent physicians and ancillary help; gain the cooperation of suppliers; enroll community support; and through the use of pooled resources, a multi-phasic screening process; and a preventive medicine approach to reduce costs and increase operational efficiency.

Public Relations can assist both the Marketing and the Finance Departments[270] in the preparation of publishable material. Public Relations is charged with identifying the various tools of communication, the selection of media, the choice of materials, layout and design, choice of color and type of print used, and the writing and editing of most internal, external, and internal-external publications. This familiarity with and acquired expertise in communications automatically lends itself to the communications needs of Marketing and Finance.

Public Relations can assist Marketing in the designing and wording of opinion surveys and questionnaires; the layout and content of a Monthly Newsletter to subscribers; the publication of information pamphlets for general inquiries from the public, or for recruiting special publics such as unions; the wording and design of application material; and lastly, the selection of mass media advertisers.

The need for publishable material by Finance is not as great as that of Marketing. Needed is assistance on the "...annual report and sub-scriber messages; arranging appearances before security analysts; helping with the speeches and preparing background materials for the financial press..."[271]

Public exposure in any large measure requires use of the mass media in one form or another. The cost of this type of exposure can be prohibitive. One way of avoiding this cost is to have the public relations department

---

[269] See *Supra*, n. 33, p. 13.

[270] See, e.g., O. M. Beveridge, *Financial Public Relations*, (New York: McGraw-Hill Book Co. Inc., 1963).

[271] R. W. Darrow, et. al., *Dartnell Public Relations Handbook*, (Chicago: Dartnell Press, Inc., 1967), p. 145.

obtain some free publicity for the organization. Quite often, this can be
accomplished by writing feature articles for reprint in the area newspapers.

To get publicity into newspapers, it is necessary to convince
editors that these feature articles will be of interest to their readers.
To do so, "(s)uch stories must be about people, places, events, organizations,
and other things in which readers are interested."[272] Executives of the
organization are the "...prime source of worthy information which can be
turned into publicity stories."[273]

[272]H. Stephenson, Editor, Handbook of Public Relations, (New York: McGraw-
Hill Book Co. Inc., 1971), p. 681.

[273]
Ibid.

BIBLIOGRAPHY

Books

_____, Webster's New World Dictionary, New York: The World Publishing
      Co., 1966.

Bernstein, Lewis, and Dana, Richard H. Interviewing and the Health
      Professions. New York: Appleton-Century-Crofts: Educational
      Division, Meredith Corporation, 1970.

Beveridge, O.M. Financial Public Relations. New York: McGraw-Hill Book Co.
      Inc., 1963.

Bright, Sallie, Public Relations Programs. New York: National Public
      Relations Council, Inc., 1970.

Cutlip, Scott M. and Center, Allen H. Effective Public Relations.
      Englewood Cliffs, N.J.: Prentice-Hall, Inc., 1964

Darrow, R. W. et. al., Dartnell Public Relations Handbook. Chicago:
      Dartnell Press, Inc., 1967.

deKruif, Paul. Kaiser Wakes the Doctors. New York: Harcourt Brace, 1943.

Emery, Edwin. History of American Newspaper Publishers Association.
      Minneapolis: University of Minnesota Press, 1950.

Etzioni, Amitai, Modern Organizations. New York: Prentice-Hall, 1964.

Festinger, Leon. A Theory of Cognitive Dissonance. Evanston, Ill.: Row,
      Peterson, 1957.

Galbraith, John Kenneth, American Capitalism. Boston: Sentry Editions,
      Imprint of Houghton Mifflin Co. 1956.

Green and Tull, Research for Marketing Decisions. Englewood Cliffs, N.J.:
      Prentice-Hall, Inc., 1970.

Harrington, Michael. The Other America. New York: MacMillan Co., 1970.

Hoffer, Eric. The Ordeal of Change. New York: Harper and Row Publishers,
      Inc., 1963.

Hunter, Floyd. Community Power Structure. Chapel Hill, N.C.: University
      of North Carolina Press, 1953.

Kassarjian, Harold H. Perspectives in Consumer Behavior. Atlanta, Georgia:
      Scott, Foresman and Company, 1963.

Katz and Lazarfield, Personal Influence: The Part Played by People in the
      Flow of Mass Communications. New York: The Free Press of Glencoe,
      Inc., 1955.

Kurtz, Harold P. _Public Relations for Hospitals._ Springfield, Ill.: Charles C. Thomas, 1969.

Larson, John A. _The Responsible Businessman._ New York: Holt, Rinehart & Winston, Inc., 1966.

McCarthy, E. Jerome. _Basic Marketing._ Homewood, Ill.: Richard D. Irwin, Inc., 1968.

Mills, Alden B. _Hospital Public Relations._ Chicago: Physicians' Record Company, 1939.

Olmsted, Michael S. _The Small Group._ New York: Random House, 1959.

Parten, Mildred B. _Surveys, Polls and Samples._ New York: Cooper Square Publishers, Inc., 1950.

Riesman, David. _The Lonely Crowd._ Garden City, N.Y.: Doubleday & Company, Inc., 1950.

Ruesch, Jurgem and Bateson, Gregory. _Communication: The Social Matrix of Psychiatry._ New York: W. W. Norton & Co., 1951.

Scott, William G. _Organizational Theory._ Homewood, Ill.: Richard D. Irwin, Inc., 1967.

Simmel, George. _Conflict and the Web of Group Affiliations._ New York: Free Press, 1955.

Stephenson, H., Editor, _Handbook of Public Relations._ New York: McGraw-Hill Book Co., Inc. 1971.

Whyte, William F. _Organizational Behavior: Theory and Application._ Homewood, Ill.: Richard D. Irwin.

Articles

_____, "American Medical Association: Power, Purpose and Politics in Organized Medicine," _Yale Law Journal_, #63, (1954).

_____, "AOA House of Delegates OK's National Health Insurance," _AOA News Review_, 13:1, (September 1970).

_____, "The Columbia Medical Plan and the East Baltimore Medical Plan," _Hospitals_, (Journal of the American Hospital Association, March 16, 1971).

_____, "Expulsion and Exclusion from Hospital Practice and Organized Medical Societies," _Rutgers Law Review_, #15, (1961).

_____, "Further Testing of H.M.O.'s Urged," _American Medical News_, 14:7, (July 5, 1971).

_____, "Group Health Plans: Some Legal and Economic Aspects," _Yale Law Journal_, No. 53, (1943).

456

_____, "H.M.O.'s - Past and Present," <u>California Medical Association News</u>, Vol. 16, (May 7, 1971).

_____, "NIN Convention Resolutions," <u>Nursing Outlook</u>, 19:393, (June 1971).

_____, "The Non-Profit Medical Corporations Act," <u>Newsletter, Medical Societies' Reference Committee</u>, (1971).

Abeshouse, Jack. "Manpower Development," Chapter VII.

Association of National Advertisers, Inc., "The Dollar Sense of Business Films," New York: ANA, 1954.

Bright, Sallie. "Management's Responsibility for Public Relations," <u>Public Relations in Health and Welfare</u>, Francis Schmidt & Harold N. Weiner, Editors, New York: Columbia University Press, 1966.

California Medical Association, Bureau of Research and Planning, Division of Socio-Economics and Research, "Survey on Medical Student Attitudes," <u>Socio-Economic Report</u>, Vol. 9, (September 1969).

Chase, "The Politics of Medicine," <u>Harper's</u>, (October 1960).

Dearing, W. "Developments and Accomplishments of Comprehensive Group Practice Payment Programs," <u>Group Health Association of America, Inc.</u>,Booklet #16, (1970).

Dodds, Richard W. "A Framework for Political Mapping of Conflict in Organized Medicine - Especially Pediatrics," Washington, D.C.: U. S. Government Printing Office.

Ellwood, Paul M. Jr., "Concept and Strategy," <u>Hospitals</u>, (Journal of the American Hospital Association, March 16, 1971).

Faltermayer, Edmund K. "Better Care at Less Cost Without Miracles," <u>Fortune</u>, (January 1970).

Fleming, Scott. "Kaiser Foundation-Permanente Program," <u>Hospitals</u>, Journal of the American Hospital Association, (March 16,1971, Vol. 45).

Forgotson, Roemer & Newman. "Innovations in the Organization of Health Services: Inhibiting vs. Permissive Regulation," <u>Washington University Law Quarterly</u>, (1967).

Garfield, Sydney. "The Delivery of Medical Care," <u>Scientific American</u>, (April 1970).

Golden, Clinton and Parker, Virginia, Editors, "The Dewy and Almy Chemical Co., and the Chemical Workers," New York: Harper & Row Publishers, 1955.

457

Greenberg, Ira G. and Rodburg, Michael L. "The Role of Prepaid Group Practice in Relieving the Medical Care Crisis," Harvard Law Review, (February 1971).

Greenberg, Ira G. "The Decline of the Healing Act," Harper's, (October 1960).

MacColl, William. "Group Practice and Prepayment of Medical Care," Washington, D.C.: Public Affairs Press, 1966.

Neely, James R. "Guidelines for Implementation," Hospitals, (Journal of the American Hospital Association, March 16, 1971).

Perry, Glen. "Which Public Do You Mean?" Public Relations Journal, Vol. 12, (March 1956).

Reed, Jim. "Basics in Medical Public Relations," Arizona Medicine, (October 1968).

Swan, Lionel F. "Group Approach to Medical Care," Nursing Outlook, Vol. 18, (January 1970).

Tannenbaum, Percy. "Communication of Science Information," Science, Vol. 14, (May 10, 1963).

Werner, William G. "Person to Person," Public Relations Journal, Vol. 12, (April 1956).

Wilcox, "Hospitals and the Corporate Practice of Medicine," 45 Cornell Law Quarterly, 432, (1960).

Williams, Greer. "Kaiser: What Is It?, How Does It Work?, Why Does It Work?" Modern Hospital, (February 1971).

Wilson, "Health Legislation in Ohio," American Journal of Public Health, Vol. 51, (1961).

Reports

AMA Judicial Council Opinions and Reports, 2:'69, (disciplinary action may depend on local attitudes).

Kaiser Foundation Medical Care Program, Annual Report, 1969, at II: Criteria for Expansion.

Report of the National Conference on Group Practice, Promoting the Group Practice of Medicine, Keynote Address by William H. Stewart, M.D., Surgeon General, U. S. Public Health Service (1967 PHS publication).

United States Employment Service: Job Descriptions and Organizational Analysis for Hospitals and Related Health Service, Washington, D.C.: U. S. Government Printing Office, 1952.

Yedidia, A. "Planning and Implementation of the Community Health Foundation of Cleveland, Ohio," Washington, D.C.: U. S. Government Printing Office, 1968.

Interviews

Benton, Louis. Professor of Management, Hofstra University, Hempstead, N.Y.,
February 1972.

Kushner, Robert K. Public Relations Director, Meadowbrook Hospital,
East Meadow, N.Y., December 1971.

Odette, Robert G., Associate Professor of Nuclear Engineering, University
of California at Santa Barbara, Santa Barbara, Calif.,
January 1972.

Petit, Leo. Director of Operations, Providence, R.I.: Rhode Island Group
Health Association, December 1971.

Sands, Saul. Professor of Marketing, Hofstra University, Hempstead, N.Y.,
November 1971.

Saposnick, Shelly, Reporter, Fairchild Publications, New York, N.Y.,
January 1972.

Zeeman, Barry. H.M.O. Planning Director, L. I. Jewish Medical Center,
Lake Success, N.Y., November 1971.

Miscellaneous

_____, Article 44, Public Health Law, "New York's Approach to Prepaid
Comprehensive Group Practice - Considerations for Applicants,"
New York State Department of Health, (July 1971).

_____, "Resolutions Adopted by House of Delegates, April 17, 1971,
Associationof American Physicians and Surgeons: Chicago, Ill.,"
Association of American Physicians and Surgeons, Inc. (April 17,
1971).

AMA News, (April 5, 1971).

AMA News, (June 28, 1971).

AMA vs. United States, 317 U.S. 519, 1943: Group Health Cooperative v.
King Medical Society, 39, Washington, 2nd 586, 237 p. 2d. 737,
(1951).

Auerbach, Stuart. "AMA President Pushes Aid for Group Practice,"
Washington Post and Times Herald, 93:24a, (September 10, 1970).

Kornfield, A. Memorandum on the Critical Need for New Legislation to
Encourage the Organization, Promotion and Expansion of Prepaid
Group Health Care Plans 10 (1970), (Submitted to the New York
State Legislature).

Lecture given by Dr. Cohen, Professor of Marketing, Hofstra University,
Hempstead, N.Y., Spring, 1971.

Medical Group News, (July 1970).

CHAPTER VIII

THE QUALITY ASSURANCE PLAN

Jeffrey M. Caro

INTRODUCTION

Monitoring Health System Performance

A Health Maintenance Organization can and must maintain effective quality at all levels. It should have goals for preventing medical crises and for economically meeting patient needs for access to high quality care. Several means designed to help monitor goal achievement are discussed in this chapter, which contains the following sections:

1. Goals of the health care plan;
2. Description of the system;
3. System standards;
4. Techniques of monitoring standards;
5. Corrective measures for excessive deviations;
6. Cost versus system performance.

If the suggestions contained in this chapter are followed, it should be possible to achieve improved control over the quality of health care delivery in a Health Care Maintenance Organization.

H.M.O. GOALS

Overall Aims

It is desirable that an H.M.O. achieve the following goals:

1. To affect favorably the health, morbidity and mortality of the membership;
2. To decrease unnecessary treatment, malpractice suits and medico-legal problems;[1]

---

[1]U.S. Government, AMHT Advisory Committee to the National Center for Health Services Research and Development, Provisional Guidelines for Automated Multiphasic Health Testing and Services, Report (Washington, D.C.: U.S. Government Printing Office, 1970), Extract.

3. To aid in achieving significant economies in the
    delivery of quality health care;
4. To improve the quality, effectiveness and avail-
    ability of health services.[2]

Health Status Measures

A goal of the quality assurance (synonym: Quality Control, Q.C.)
system is to provide reliable data on the health status of H.M.O. members.
Considerable emphasis is placed on factors known to be related to health
status - for example, immunization status among children, family planning
practices, prenatal care, responsiveness to symptoms, smoking and poor
diet.[3]

Physician Goals

Systematic Methodology. By use of standardized formats and testing
procedures, a system can provide guidance for the physician in his work-ups
for patient diagnosis and treatment.[4]

Increased Productivity. Comprehensive preventive medicine requires
periodic health examinations, but the enrollment of 50,000 participants pre-
cludes individual periodic checkups by the staff physicians. Doctors presently spend much too much of their time in routine work that permits no
exercise of professional competence.

Automated methods for performing repetitive tests, recording
measurements, collating and processing findings permits physicians to increase both the number of patients examined and the amount of productive
time spent with each patient.[5]

More Comprehensive and Accurate Information. Taking a detailed
medical history is costly in physician and patient time. A digital computer,
programmed for medical histories and linked by telephone line or other
terminal to the regional medical centers and hospitals, can help cut this
cost. Information is not lost or misfiled. Data are retrievable at the
touch of a button, and updates to a medical history can be made instantly
with no file errors.[6]

---

[2]S. Shapiro, "Efficacy of the Concept," Hospitals, J.A.H.A., Vol. 45,
March 1, 1971, pp. 45-47.

[3]Ibid.

[4]U.S. Congress, Senate, Subcommittee on Health of the Elderly, Detection and
Prevention of Chronic Diseases Utilizing Multiphasic Health Screening
Techniques, Hearing, Sess. of 89th Congress, (Washington, D.C.: U.S.
Government Printing Office, 1966), Finding 7.

[5]Ibid., Finding 6.

[6]Ibid.

Patient Medical Profile. Information can be stored accurately by computer, and, therefore, the doctor has on call a total medical profile of each patient. This data is important for continuous monitoring of the patient's health. The physicians need up-to-date data for diagnosis and treatment, also. The system makes it much easier to compare actual medical action against accepted standards.[7]

Lower Costs of Service

Both the H.M.O. and its patients realize lower costs when early diagnosis and accurate treatment reduces the amount of time the patient spends undergoing treatment.[8] Pain and suffering, loss of pay from medical absenteeism and other patient costs can be reduced through the application of preventive medicine.[9]

DESCRIPTION OF THE SYSTEM

The quality assurance plan described in this chapter is a closed-loop system that monitors actual performance to established standards. Figure XI - 1 shows the overall flow of information in the system.

A workable quality control system depends heavily on quantitative data. Consequently, a part of the quality assurance plan assumes the existence of an AMHT (Automated Multiphasic Health Testing) center and associated data processing equipment. This technique[10] gives the H.M.O. reliable quantitative data for comparing medical action with standards and producing variances that are prerequisite for taking timely and appropriate corrective action.

Quality Assurance: Management Involvement

The promotion of excellence has always been a primary concern to the medical profession. Quality control in industry is usually a specific function assigned to a designated individual on a management team, but in H.M.O.'s it becomes everybody's business.[11]

But even in H.M.O.'s, excellence in medicine can best be achieved if the responsibility for the development and maintenance of the quality

---

[7]Ibid.

[8]Morris F. Collen, et al., "Provisional Guidelines for Automated Multiphasic Health Testing and Services," Operational Manual, (Washington, D.C.: U.S. Government Printing Office, 1960), Entire.

[9]Ibid.

[10]Author's opinion.

[11]J.E. Smits, "Strong Management and Quality Control," Hospital Progress, February 1969, p. 56.

FIGURE VIII - 1

FLOW DIAGRAM OF MONITORING SYSTEM[a]

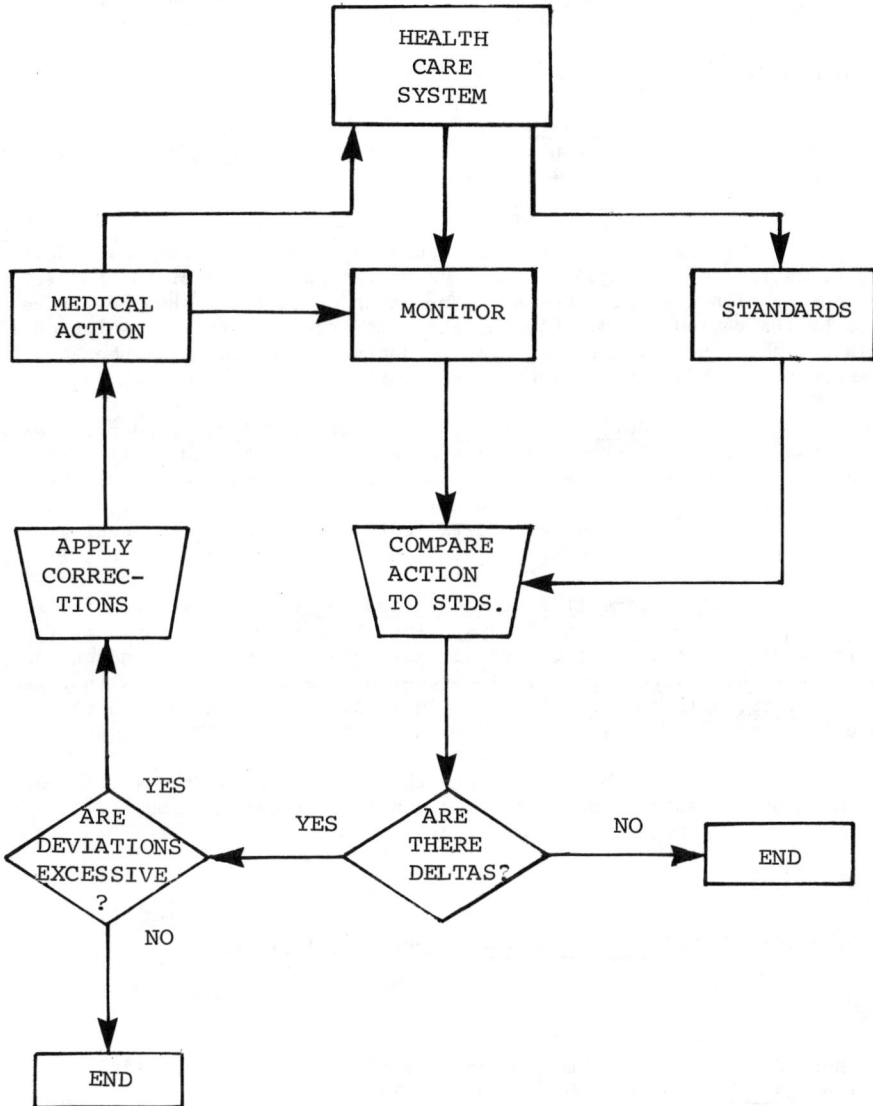

(a) Author's diagram

control program is the responsibility of one individual with complete accountability for results. Such a program would not only encompass the quality control measures now practiced in most hospitals and H.M.O.'s: chart review, medical audit, nursing audit, patient care committee activity, tissue committees, etc. - but would encourage the adoption of new techniques for measuring quality. The maintenance of high standards of health care would continue to be everybody's business, but control would be on a rationally organized basis. Then management could be at least as well informed on quality of care as it is on cost of care, and it could devote as much attention to quality as it traditionally does to cost control.[12]

Control Groups

Principle of Peer Review. An underlying principle of peer review is that the medical profession should keep its own house in order - and let the public know that it is doing so - rather than let others do it for them.[13]

The medical community establishes review boards which meet periodically to review and pass judgment on the medical practices of the physicians under the panel's control. Unethical practice could bring about punitive action by the review board. For instance, referral to ethics committees for possible discipline, or perhaps to State Boards of Medical Examinees for suspension or revocation of license is possible.[14]

Utilization Review. This is, in general, a part of peer review in which certain groups of physicians evaluate the need for and utilization of diagnostic, therapeutic and attendant services ordered by fellow practitioners. The primary purposes for utilization review are to provide quality control of patient care, reduce hospitalization time and corresponding medical costs, and eliminate unnecessary and inappropriate treatment.[15]

Utilization Committee Structure and Power. The typical utilization committee is composed of several physicians, the director of nursing, the hospital administrator and a recording secretary, who meet to conduct business no less than twice a month. The power of the committee lies in persuasive authority, with the aim of continuing staff education through construction criticism.

However, it is possible, with the concurrence of the staff, for the committee to restrict privileges of continually erring members.[16]

---

[12]Ibid.

[13]"Peer Review," Medical World News, August 20, 1971, p. 46.

[14]Ibid.

[15]Stephen Daiger, "Peer Review - Cost Control or Quality Control?" California Medicine, December 1970, p. 75.

[16]Ibid., p. 76.

The Standards Committee. This is one of the groups that work to achieve quality control in medicine. This particular group has two broad functions:

1. Establishment of standardized procedures to be employed in the hospital;
2. Analysis of the value of therapeutic products for purchasing and cost reduction purposes.[17]

A workable committee has five or six permanent members plus departmental specialists who can be called on when their disciplines are under consideration. In the core group would be: the assistant administrator, the controller, the purchasing director, the nursing service director, the central supply supervisor and medical staff members.[18]

Medical Testing Group

To ensure the ability to process an adequate volume of patients and for proper quality control of patient testing, it is best to have an AMHT laboratory with the medical center. Giving ambulatory hospital patients a preadmission AMHT checkup will shorten their hospital stay, decrease hospitalization costs, and ensure a level daily load for the AMHT laboratory.

An organization chart for an AMHT operation is shown in Figure VIII - 2.[19]

The AMHT Director. The AMHT director should be a man with a strong commitment to preventive medicine. He should have background in the physical sciences, to aid his understanding of the technological aspects of AMHT.[20]

He is responsible for all administrative and medical aspects of the testing center and only he can authorize changes and additions to standard operating procedures and personnel. He consults with the advisory committee on all policy matters. The director aids in maintenance of quality control and performance standards by making regular rounds of the facility for personal inspection of procedures and data handling.

The director also functions as liaison between the AMHT and the physicians in the group practice, keeping them informed of all problems and changes. He is responsible for incorporating new tests required by the physicians of the group, if such are warranted for maintenance of high quality medical care.[21]

---

[17] J. A. O'Connell, "Product Analysis Committee, Yes, Standards Committee, No," Hospital Progress, February 1969, p. 68.

[18] Ibid., p. 72.

[19] Morris F. Collen, "The Multitest Laboratory in Health Care of the Future," Hospitals, J.A.H.A., Vol. 41, May 1967, p. 119.

[20] Ibid.

[21] Ibid.

FIGURE VIII - 2

Suggested Organizational Chart for the AMHT[a]

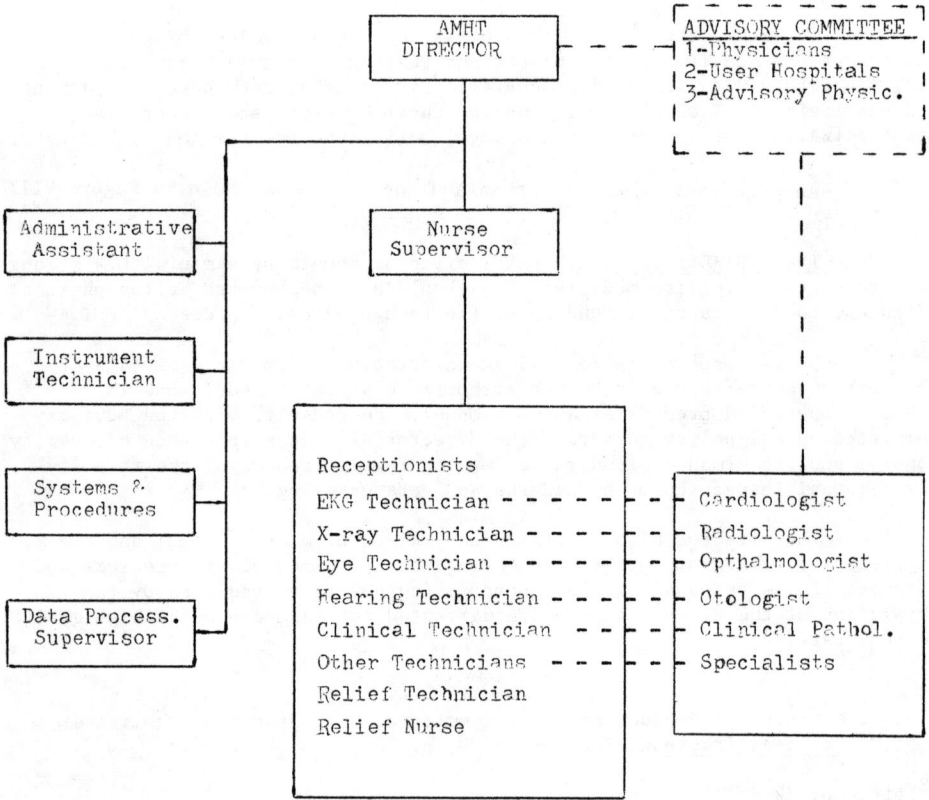

(a) Collen, M.F., "Implementation of a System - Automated
    Multiphasic Health Testing", Hospitals, J.A.H.A.,
    Vol. 45, March 1, 1971, p. 56.

The Advisory Committee. A special committee advises the AMHT director on policies, objectives, and operations. The Committee represents users of the AMHT facility, including the physicians of the medical care group and user hospitals. The committee also represents the physician-specialists who are suppliers of the professional and technical parts of the various AMHT stations (for example, the consulting cardiologist for the EKG test station, the radiologist for the X-ray phase, and the clinical pathologist for the laboratory phase).[22]

The advisory committee acts not only on policy matters, but also monitors the quality of services offered by the testing center by acting as a peer review group. They have the responsibility for judging the performance and capabilities of the personnel connected with the AMHT center.[23]

The Nurse Supervisor. One key individual for maintaining good day-to-day AMHT operation is the nurse supervisor (abbreviated N.S.) N.S. supervises and coordinates the AMHT under the aegis of the director. N.S. is responsible for supervision and coordination of all technicians and the training of personnel. Staff schedules appropriate for the patient load are prepared by the N.S. who also monitors the flow of patient traffic and makes adjustments in staffing of phases as necessary to ensure a smoothly operating unit.[24]

Technical NonMedical Personnel. Medical technicians, thoroughly trained in instrumentation, systems and procedures, and data processing are essential for a complex system such as AMHT. It is best for the project to have in-house expertise, full or part-time, in these fields to help carry out specific functions and to assist the director in making technical decisions.[25]

Instrument Technician. One or more instrument technicians are necessary to maintain AMHT laboratory equipment in proper working order. They establish an adequate preventive maintenance program and monitor the accuracy and reliability of equipment, advise appropriate personnel concerning equipment modification to improve reliability and accuracy, advise and assist in planning, designing and building (or selecting) new equipment and maintain an inventory of calibrated standby equipment.[26]

Systems and Procedures. A full or part-time expert is necessary for the establishment of an AMHT. He assists with the design of forms, is responsible for maintaining a standard operating procedures manual, advises on patient flow and scheduling, and conducts systems and procedures analyses.[27]

---

[22]Ibid.

[23]Ibid.

[24]Morris F. Collen, op. cit.

[25]Ibid.

[26]Ibid.

[27]Ibid.

Data Processing Personnel. A data processing computer programmer is usually necessary to create and maintain computer programs for AMHT. He also advises on interfacing requirements between test equipment and data processing equipment.

Computer operators are needed to operate the data processing equipment. They are responsible for proper utilization and throughput of the machines and data.

Control personnel who work to ensure validity of input, accuracy and totality of output, and distribution of reports may also be necessary for efficient operation of the computer and peripheral equipment. These and all other data processing personnel report to a data processing supervisor.[28]

Resources Required for Control
System Hardware

A complete system will have the equipment shown in Table XI - 1 or its equivalents.[29]

A typical AMHT system will be capable of accommodating 20 medical history devices (MHD) and data entry keyboards (DEK), two cathode ray tube (CRT) displays and one mark sense document reader (MDR). The system permits the addition of a data communications set to communicate, via synchronous modems, through telephone lines to remote stations or to other center or centers. Keyboard entry permits instant visual retrieval of medical records, which are backed up by duplicate micro-film files.[30]

Data Entry Terminals

Five types of data entry terminals are included in the system: CRT displays, data entry keyboards, medical history devices, a mark sense document reader, and a keypunch.[31]

CRT Displays. A CRT serves each reception station to collect demographic data. The system generates displays identifying each item of data. A cursor is automatically positioned on the display so that an operator, using the display keyboard, can type the described data and command its transmittal.

The display is also able to correct or modify demographic data in a "real time" mode. Also included are means to advise an operator that a computer message is waiting. This feature is necessary so that when the operator responds, the CRT will display the identity of a faulty equipment or a software failure.[32]

---

[28]Ibid.

[29]Marketing Paper on "Specification for the MS5110 AMHT System,"(New York: Sperry-Rand Corp.) March1971, p. 1.

[30]Ibid., pp. 3-5.

[31]Ibid.
[32]Ibid.

TABLE VIII - 1

Data System Equipment ^(b)

Unless otherwise noted, one each of the following items shall be provided:

Item	Source	Identification
9200- 11 Processor and 250 line per		
minute printer	Univac	3030-94
Multiply, divide and edit feature	Univac	F0882-00
Storage - Plated Wire		
16,384 bytes	Univac	7007-91
8,192 byte expansion	Univac	F0890-95
Card Punch	Univac	0603-04
Card Reader	Univac	0711-00
Data Communications Set		
Line Terminal Control - 1	Univac	F1000-00
Line Terminal, Synchronous,Checking	Univac	F1005-98
Longitudinal Redundancy Check	Univac	F1008-99
Communications Interface, Private		
Line	Univac	F1002-03
8410-Disc		
Dual Disc Drive	Univac	8410-00
Disc Control	Univac	F1023-00
Fastband Buffer	Univac	F1015-00
Modem Eliminator	Univac	TBA
Terminal Multiplexer	Univac	8538-00
RS232C Synchronous Interface	Univac	F1266-00
Special Multiplexer	SSMD	MS5203
Interface	Univac	F1245-01
Uniscope 100		
Display Terminal	Univac	3536-99
Interface	Univac	F1245-01
Keyboard, Alphanumeric	Univac	F1242-01
Mark-Sense Document Reader	Motorola MDR	8340S
Data Entry Keyboard*	SSMD	MS 5202
Medical History Device*	SSMD	MS 5204
Interpreting Keypunch	Univac	VIP1710-04
Computer Cables	SSMD	
Mating Connectors	SSMD	
Disk Packs*	Univac	F1102-00
Program Card Decks	SSMD	
Mark Sense Card Forms*	SSMD	
Medical History Film Strips*	SSMD	
Patient Identity Cards*	SSMD	
Medical History Backup Forms*	SSMD	
Punch for Medical History Backup Forms	SSMD	

*Quantities per contract

(b) "Specification for the MS5110 AMHT System," Sperry-Rand Corp., March
1971, p. 4.

Data Entry Keyboards. The DEK's serve to enter all clinical data to the computer, together with positive patient identification. The system requires operator re-confirmation of all abnormal data and permits entry of corrected data.[33]

Medical History Devices. Medical history questions and branching sequences are alterable by modification of medical history film-strips. The AMHT accomodates at least 500 different frame numbers that result in print-outs, and provides for at least 1,500 total frames. Thus, for example, 500 questions may be asked in each of three languages. The patient can be given a choice between an initial full history or an abbreviated interval history, when the total number of questions does not exceed 500.

Modification to the programming provides an increase in the number of questions to 1,000 different frame numbers with printouts.[34]

Mark Sense Document Reader. A mark sense document reader (MDR) is employed to transfer data from cards or forms that are manually marked, keypunched, printed (or a mixture of all three), during a "transitional time" period after other terminals are no longer in use.[35]

Keypunch. A verifying and interpreting punch is included to: permit duplication or generation of computer control cards; serve as a back-up point-of-entry for demographic data; enter physician's and technicians' english language comments.[36]

Data Storage. Patient examination, history and treatment records are stored on disk cartridges, with at least 1,000 records on each of the two surfaces of a disk. The storage permits regeneration of reports and access for statistical analyses of selected entries. On-line microfilm (or micro-fiche) interface equipment provides a duplicate set of records that are maintained in the group's central files.[37]

Figure VIII - 3 shows a simplified flow diagram of the H.M.O. system hardware linkage.

SYSTEM STANDARDS

Lack of Quality Standards

H.M.O. management decisions must always include consideration of quality for which no precise measurements may exist. Speaker after speaker at the National Health Forum in Los Angeles, March 15-17, 1968, mentioned the absence of quality standards for health care:

---

[33]Ibid.

[34]Ibid.

[35]Ibid.

[36]Ibid.

[37]Ibid.

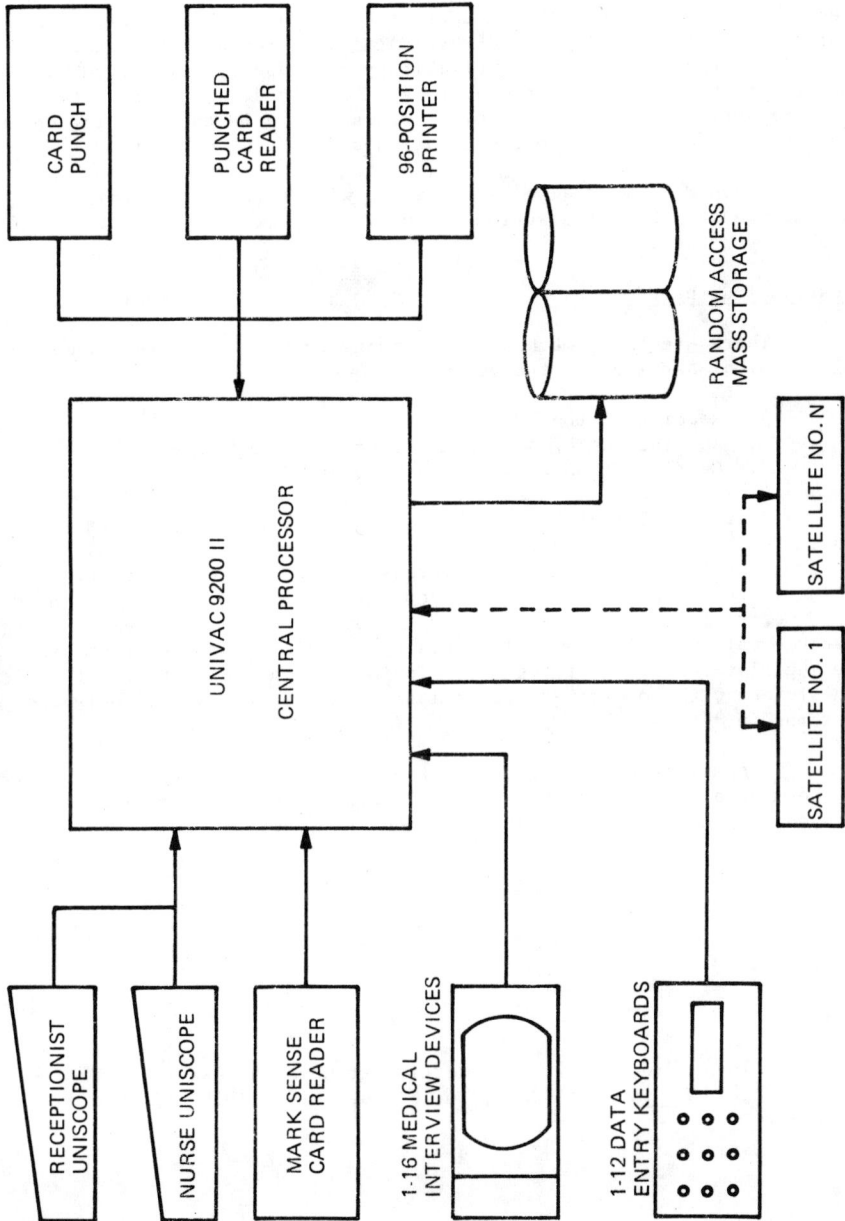

FIGURE VIII - 3

H.M.O. SYSTEM HARDWARE LINKAGE (c)

(c) Sperry-Rand, "Multiphasic Testing Center," Unpublished Report, 1971, p. 26.

471

"It is much more difficult, perhaps impossible, to specify what is goodness. This is because the judgment of what is good or bad derives, in the main, from the standards of management acceptable to the leaders of the profession at any given time."[38] In spite of the obvious difficulties it is incumbent on management to insure that the staff is diligent in the pursuit of excellence.[39]

Aside from the excellence of the individual practitioners and those who assist them in direct patient care, there is a myriad of detail that contributes to quality or its lack. Physical facilities and maintenance can be a major influence on quality. Availability of properly calibrated equipment, prompt lab service, even the temperature of the food, are factors to be weighed in evaluating quality. And of course there is the need for unflagging attention to infection control, sanitation and patient comfort.[40]

The H.M.O. must also be concerned with a larger dimension of quality which encompasses the satisfaction of the subscriber regarding scope and availability of services.

Professional Competence

There are three methods of defining professional competence to provide medical services to the public:

    A. Receipt of the MD degree;
    B. Acquisition of a license to practice medicine;
    C. Certification by a specialty board.[41]

Board certification, unlike the MD or state licenses, have no legal status. Yet, such certification is widely accepted by the medical profession as a recognizable index of minimal professional competence to practice medicine in the specialty areas. Leaders of the medical profession hold that several years of graduate education in approved teaching programs are required to produce safe practitioners of specialty medicine. On the other hand, State legislatures in 11 States are allowing issuance of unrestricted licenses to physicians with no graduate education and in 39 States with only one year of internship.[42]

Because of the limited education and experience required for licensing, the medical profession has created boards of experts to thoroughly test the physician who wishes to practice a medical specialty, and certify his

---

[38]J. E. Smits, op. cit.

[39]Ibid.

[40]Ibid.

[41]William Holden, "Specialty Board Certification as a Measure of Professional Competence," J.A.M.A., Vol. 213, No. 6, August 10, 1970, p. 1016.

[42]Ibid., p. 1018

competency in that area. The practice is so widespread that positions on the active staff of many hospitals are available only to board certified physicians. In some University Medical Centers and federal institutions, promotions and increments in salaries are tied to certification.[43]

Board certification designates, in a variety of ways, a degree of professional competence in a specialty. It has always been intended by the boards to denote minimal qualifications and competence for practice. In order to qualify for the examinations conducted by a specialty board, a physician must have satisfactorily completed a prescribed educational program that has been surveyed and accredited by a residency review committee. The educational requirement has been of considerable importance in enhancing the status of certification itself and, when obtained in some teaching hospitals, is the equivalent of successfully completing the examinations. Not only must the physician have completed the residency but the director, at the time of application, must certify to the board in writing the adequacy of the individual's experience and his competence in relationship to his peers.[44]

A time will come when physicians must be licensed to practice what they are educated and trained to do. It is in this area that the overlapping interests and privileges of state licensing agencies, the National Board of Medical Examiners, and the specialty boards will be amalgamated to provide:

1. Examinations which assess the professional competence
    of physicians in the areas in which they have been
    educated;
2. Examinations that are standard and applicable to all
    states;
3. Licenses to practice medicine that reflect the fact
    that the individual physician has met all of the
    criteria established by the medical profession for
    a general education in medicine and for the develop-
    ment of special competence in a particular field of
    medicine.[45]

Peer Review

Definition. The AMA urges all of its component societies to under-take peer review, and officially defines peer review as, "Evaluation by practicing physicians of the quality and efficiency of services ordered or performed by other practicing physicians. Peer review is the all-inclusive term for medical review effort."[46] Thus, it includes such functions as utilization review, claims review and medical audit.

---

[43]Ibid., p. 1017.

[44]Ibid.

[45]Ibid., p. 1018.

[46]"Peer Review," Medical World News, August 20, 1971, p. 45.

The process of peer review is educational, both for the reviewed and the reviewer. It helps to improve the quality of care, even when its primary purpose is economic, as in utilization and claims review, which constitute most of present-day reviewing.[47]

Background. Peer review began with the Screening and Discharge Committee at the Jewish Hospital of Cincinnati in 1951. It became necessary when some California Medical Societies contracted with insurers to deliver health care and began to find disparities in claims. It grew in importance when Blue Cross and Blue Shield began referring problem cases to review committees.[48]

Historical Problems. There have been several problems connected with the process of peer review. Among them are:

1. Physician fear that the punitive aspects of peer review overshadow the educational value;
2. Personal relationships among the physicians make effective review difficult;
3. Peer review is often practiced best where it is least needed;
4. There are conflicts between professional standards and self-enrichment in doctor-owned profit-making health facilities.[49]

The Medical Audit

From 1918 to 1952, the American College of Surgeons based its hospital standards on a publication called the Minimum Standard for Hospitals. The activities covered in this document include: medical staff organization, qualifications for medical staff organization, qualifications for medical staff membership, rules and policies governing the professional work of the hospital, medical records, and diagnostic and therapeutic facilities.[50]

Faithfully construed, the principles required a staff of thoroughly trained physicians, supplied with adequate facilities, working within the limits of their professional competence, following generally accepted procedures, being advised by their colleagues in serious or doubtful cases, and undergoing professional scrutiny of their performance through regular review of the medical records of their cases. However, this does not necessarily guarantee medical care of good quality, because:

A. Compliance is widely variable;

---

[47] Ibid.

[48] Ibid., p. 47.

[49] Ibid., p. 52.

[50] "Manual of Hospital Standardization," Chicago: American College of Surgeons, 1946, p. 8.

B. Such standards as those concerning staff organization
    or completeness of medical records are not related
    directly to patient care as the clinican sees it;
C. The criteria for performance are not explicit.[51]

The medical audit deals with these points in a scientific manner.
Objective criteria are employed related closely to end results, and standards
are established for degrees of compliance based on empirical observations in
the leading hospitals.[52] The Joint Commission on Accreditation of Hospitals
has stimulated interest in the medical audit through the criticism they level
at individual hospitals found to be out of line in the check on quality of
care made in the course of inspecting hospitals for compliance with the
Commission's standards for organization, facilities and procedures.[53]

Analysis of Professional Activities

Various indices developed by the Commonwealth Fund staff[54] were
employed to determine whether and to what extent their educational and
advisory programs were contributing to the improvement of hospital and
medical care.

The "Reports of Professional Activities," as these analyses were
called in the Rochester, New York Region, contained such indices as:

1. Total death rates;
2. Institutional death rates, based on deaths occurring
    48 hours or more following admission to the hospital;
3. Death rates among such specific groups as: medical
    cases, surgical cases, etc.[55]

Such indices do not account for variation in types of disease and
kinds of patients cared for. Further, there was no discernible relationship
between death rates and the proportion of cases having reasonably complete
history, physical examination, laboratory diagnosis and consultation. The
indices that seemed meaningful in the Rochester region experience were those
showing frequency rates of X-ray, electrocardiographic, clinical laboratory
examinations, and blood transfusions. High rates were directly correlated
with subjective impressions of a good quality of hospital care.[56]

Rates of Surgical Operations as Index of Quality

There was marked variation among the hospitals of the Rochester
region in the terminology employed in pathology reports. In many instances
there was a tendency to use euphemistic terms or anatomical descriptions,

---

[51]Paul A. Lembcke, "Evolution of the Medical Audit," J.A.M.A., Vol. 199,
   No. 8, February 20, 1967, p. 114.

[52]Ibid.

[53]Ibid.

[54]H.J. Southmayd, et al., "Small Community Hospitals," New York: Commonwealth
   Fund, Div. of Publications, 1944, pp. 159-164.

[55]Paul A. Lembcke, op. cit.

[56]Ibid., p. 115.   475

presumably to avoid giving offense to the surgeon by reporting surgical tissues as essentially normal. High correlations between post-operative, preoperative and tissue diagnosis were obviously artificial in many instances. Thus, in making a comparative study of surgery for appendicitis, it was felt necessary to employ primary appendectomy rates in the general population of hospital service areas as an index, rather than to evaluate individual cases on the basis of hospital records.[57] They did not adequately distinguish between the quality of care in individual hospitals where there was more than one hospital in the community.[58]

Development of Criteria and Standards

The need for objective criteria and for standards by which to measure compliance with the criteria is obvious. There are scientific methods of medical auditing that can be used with common understanding by hospitals and doctors whose work is to be audited and by persons or agencies conducting audits.

Criteria. The first step in developing criteria is the preparation of written definitions and rules from the information available in current medical literature. Considerable emphasis is placed on textbooks as expressing conservative medical opinion, generally representative of the theory and practice accepted by a majority of competent physicians.[59]

Cardinal points applicable to all criteria are the following:

1. Objectivity - stated in writing with sufficient precision and detail to make them relatively immune to varying interpretations;
2. Verifiability - so framed that points on which they rest could be verified by laboratory examination, consultation, or documentation;
3. Uniformity - independent of such factors as size or location of hospital, qualifications of the physicians, or social and economic status of patients;
4. Specificity - specific for each kind of disease or operation to be evaluated, and all significant and closely related diseases or operation in the same patient considered as a unit;
5. Pertinence - pertinent to the ultimate aim of the medical care being evaluated, and based on results rather than intentions;

---

[57] Paul A. Lembcke, "Measuring the Quality of Medical Care Through Vital Statistics Based on Hospital Service Areas: 1. Comparative Study of Appendectomy Rates," American Journal of Public Health, Vol. 42, March 1952, pp. 276-286.

[58] Paul A. Lembcke, op. cit., p. 115.

[59] Ibid., p. 117.

6. Acceptability - conform with generally accepted levels of
    good quality as set forth in textbooks and articles based
    on scientific study.[60]

Testing the Criteria. Next, the criteria derived from the literature
should be tested on several hundred cases in teaching hospitals and others, to
make sure that the data to which they apply are available in most instances.

Observations should also be made as to feasibility of compliance -
whether medical staffs can or will comply without resorting to such subter-
fuges as taking doubtful or borderline cases to other hospitals while one
particular hospital is undergoing rigid scrutiny.[61]

An interesting validation of certain criteria consists of observing
the changes made independently by physicians when a medical audit is begun.
For example, in one hospital where the staff knew only that an audit was to
be made, there was a sharp reduction in unnecessary surgery corresponding
closely with what would be expected by application of the as yet unannounced
criteria. This indicated a generally similar interpretation of good medical
practice by both the medical staff and the person establishing the criteria.[62]

Whenever possible, the effect of the new criteria on such important
matters as mortality, discovery of cancer, etc. should be measured. It is
here that community incidence rates are of great importance.[63]

Standards. The degree or percentage of compliance with criteria,
and the appropriate rates for mortality, etc. are used as standards. This
represents the usual performance at a center for medical teaching and research
as well as medical practice. It is a genuine standard, representing the best
that can be done, without any special incentive. Compliance with these
criteria are calculated for each hospital and each physician.[64] Standards
are seldom 100 per cent; allowance must be made to accommodate the inexactness
of criteria and the exercise of clinical judgment.

Value Analysis

Value analysis is new to hospitals, and is an important factor in
control of quality.[65]

Product analysis and review is a necessity. There are scores of
suppliers, offering a wide variety of disposables in sterile, convenient
packages. It is no longer sufficient to buy merely a quality product. The
product must be perfectly suited to its intended usage. It must be conveniently packaged for storage, distribution, or use. It must be readily disposable

---

[60]Ibid.

[61]Ibid.

[62]Ibid.

[63]Paul A. Lembcke, "A Scientific Method for Medical Auditing," Modern Hospitals,
    Vol. 33, June 16, 1959 & July 1, 1959, pp. 65-71.

[64]Paul A. Lembcke, op. cit., p. 117.

[65]J. A. O'Connell, op. cit.

by crushing, incineration, or by other disposable methods. The product that cannot be conveniently opened by the nurse, or cannot be easily stored or easily disposed of is not acceptable.[66]

The purchasing director alone cannot decide what is of most value to the hospital. He needs an analysis by the nurse who unpacks and uses the product, or by the physician who uses it, or by the housekeeper who must pour it from one container to another or carry it in a large bottle. The director needs the housekeeper or the engineer to advise him on disposition of the goods after their use, and the expertise of the controller who can evaluate dollar savings against manpower costs. Furthermore, the director must heed the evaluation of a product by the infection or safety committee. Other valid inputs should come from the patient who uses the product and by the public relations people. All of these parties have something to contribute to a better understanding of the real value of a product. Yet, it is impractical to discuss with each party the pros and cons of every new product offered. This is where the standards committee can be of assistance to the purchasing department.[67]

The purchasing director or his staff should research the products under analysis in advance. In many situations evaluation can be made in a brief discussion when only a few departments are involved.[68]

The committee approach serves also as an educational tool for all departments concerned. Each has a better understanding of the cost and value of supplies throughout the hospital, and of the advantages that come from doing a thorough research job on the product.[69]

Pharmacy Control

The objectives of this control program are:

1. To provide an automated inventory system to eliminate the manual counting of stock;
2. To provide the pharmacy with a larger volume of more accurate information for tighter control;
3. To avoid or minimize cost increases.[70]

Drug Control Procedure

Only one form is used in this system: the purchase order. Drugs are ordered in predetermined base units, such as ampules, vials, tubes, tablets

---

[66]Ibid., p. 70.

[67]Ibid.

[68]Ibid.

[69]Ibid.

[70]J. E. Moon, "Computerized Pharmacy System Solves Hospital Drug Inventory Problem," Modern Hospital, November 1969, p. 118.

and bottles. The base unit of each medication conforms to the units dispensed for patient treatment. Current unit prices are supplied by the vendor.[71]

Drugs are requisitioned from the pharmacy by three methods: a patient charge, a prescription, or a requisition from another department, such as the operating room or the delivery room. A charge ticket is sent to accounting for the drugs administered. About 70 per cent of all drugs dispensed to patients on the nursing units go through a machine which automatically imprints the charge ticket with all the information necessary for proper accounting of charges and for crediting the inventory. One copy of this two-part form is sent to data processing, where the appropriate account is charged and the inventory credited by computer.[72]

If a drug is not contained in the machine, all information except the drug name is written by the machine. The drug name is written on the charge ticket by the nurse, who sends the requisition to the pharmacy to be filled. The pharmacist, when he fills the prescription, writes in the drug code and units. This procedure, when put through the computer, automatically prices the drug, charges the proper account, and removes the drug from the inventory.

The second method of removing a drug from inventory is by prescription issued to an employee, intern, resident, nurse, or a patient who has been discharged and wishes to obtain drugs from the H.M.O. pharmacy. When a prescription from one of these sources is presented to the pharmacy, the prescription issue form, including date, drug code, base units and price, is completed.[73]

The last method of removing a drug is a charge to another department, which requires the use of a departmental pharmacy requisition form. Departments which routinely requisition drugs have preprinted forms for common items. When drugs are requisitioned, the department requesting them is charged with the cost (purchase cost). The departments then charge for the drugs when they are administered to the patients, with the exception of floor stock. When the department pharmacy requisition form is processed through the computer, the drugs are removed from inventory.[74]

Medication Distribution

The provision of pharmaceutical services in the hospital environment is influenced by several factors, among which are:

1. Available nursing staff;
2. Results of medication error studies;

---

[71] Ibid.

[72] Ibid.

[73] Ibid.

[74] Ibid.

3. Improved medication service;
4. Third party payment plans;
5. Role of the pharmacist.[75]

Available Nursing Staff. Usually, nurses spend a considerable amount
of time with medications, doing such things as adding medications to intravenous fluids, diluting lyphoized powders and supplying drug information to
physicians and patients. In addition, they perform many mechanical tasks,
such as charging medications to accounts and controlling narcotics. If
responsibility is assumed by another agency, such as the Department of
Pharmacy, the available nursing staff is more effectively employed in patient
monitoring tasks.[76]

Results of Error Studies. In-house studies, such as the Barker-
Macconnell Medication Error Study, may indicate a need for a full review of
the medication distribution quality control system.[77]

Improved Service. Traditional problems, such as limited floor
stocks, with individual patient orders, indicate a system that exists for
convenience of posting charges to patients' accounts, rather than for patient
safety or quality control.[78]

Third Party Payment. The implementation of Medicare made it clear
that the Federal Insurance Program would scrutinize the contribution that
each of the health team members made in relation to the cost of their
services.[79]

Role of the Chief Pharmacist. Elaboration of a few of the chief
pharmacist's responsibilities illustrates the impact of the medication distribution system. These include:

1. Viewing the original order as written by the physician;
2. Reviewing the entire patient medication therapy on a
   continuing basis. Specific areas to be reviewed include
   drug sensitivities, therapeutic incompatibilities, adverse
   drug reactions, etc. This kind of information enables the
   chief pharmacist to assist in selecting the most efficacious
   therapeutic agent;
3. Preparing and identifying the ultimate dosage form for
   administration;
4. Ensuring that medication is administered properly in
   terms of patient, drug, dose, route and time;

---

[75]Winston Durant, "A New Medication Distribution System," Hospital Progress,
(May 1969), p. 104.

[76]Ibid.

[77]Ibid.

[78]Ibid.

[79]Ibid., p. 105.

5. Serving as a source of drug information, including
    statistical data on drugs, for physicians, nurses,
    patients, etc.;
6. Supervising the selection, procurement and storage
    of pharmaceuticals.[80]

For quality control, the key factor in this system is the pharmacist's responsibility for medications from the time of selection up to the time of administration.[81]

Quality Control in the Laboratory

In the hospital laboratory, many specimens from all areas of medicine are sent for examination and analysis. A partial list of departments involved with laboratory testing include: microbiology (including bacteriology, mycology and parasitology), serology, clinical chemistry, immunohematology (blood banking), hematology, anatonic pathology, cytology and radio bio-assay.[82]

A laboratory inspection program begins with provision for monthly checking of unknown specimens from the State Board of Health and State Board of Hygiene. These agencies check every phase of laboratory work.[83] To enable the laboratory to accept specimens arriving across state lines, it is necessary to have licensure from the Department of Health, Education and Welfare under the Federal Clinical Laboratories Improvement Act of 1967. Exceptions to this necessity are those laboratories accredited by the College of American Pathologists (CAP) or by any other national accreditation body approved by the HEW Secretary and any laboratory whose interstate operations are so small or infrequent as to pose no significant threat to the public health.[84]

As part of external quality control, the laboratory checks the reliability of its performance weekly on test specimens received from the State Society of Pathologists, the CAP, the State Board of Health, and HEW. Such specimens, or "unknowns," are regularly introduced into every department of the laboratory in order to determine whether or not all procedures are being performed with accuracy and precision.[85]

An internal quality control program requires the technologist to include one or more specimens whose value is already known with every batch

---

[80]Ibid.

[81]Ibid.

[82]Marty Juel, "Maintaining High Lab Standards Through a Quality Assurance Program," Hospital Progress, (July 1970), p. 14.

[83]Ibid.

[84]Ibid.

[85]Ibid.

of specimens.[86] Two distinct kinds of control samples are tested, along with each patient's specimen. Samples with a known value are collected in the laboratory, along with the unknowns being tested. If results of tests on the unknowns do not compare with one of the known specimens, the test is repeated.[87]

The second kind of control sample is the manufactured specimen. These specimens are purchased from any of the several pharmaceutical houses in the country. They can be tested in the same way as the known specimens collected in the laboratory.[88]

With this emphasis on controls, it would appear that frequent errors are discovered. However, through application of such a rigid control program, the laboratory maintains a close check to monitor the tests and spot any variation the moment it occurs. For instance, if a certain reagent is weak, the quality assurance program will reveal this before serious error involving its use is made.[89]

Statistical Controls

The objectives of the statistical program are:

1. To utilize the resources of the H.M.O. for the development of improved methods and procedures, and to disseminate collective and individual accomplishments to all participating units;
2. To establish average standards of job performance for departmental operations reflecting proper utilization of personnel and adherence to high levels of care and service. Such standards are utilized to assist in establishing staffing and quality requirements for each department of the hospital;
3. To train administrative and supervisory personnel in the principles and use of scientific management and industrial engineering techniques, and to assist them in applying these techniques to the H.M.O. environment.[90]

Standards

Quality control check sheets are prepared for each department: dietary, business office, admitting, central supply, surgery, laboratory, pharmacy, maintenance, radiology, medical records, laundry, etc. Although

---

[86]Ibid.

[87]Ibid., p. 16.

[88]Ibid.

[89]Ibid.

[90]Carron Herring, "Ohio Hospitals' Quality Control and Staff Utilization Program," Hospital Progress, July 1970. p. 38.

too extensive to list in its entirety, examples of the types of criteria
applied are found in medical/surgical/gynecological:

A. Patient care:

   1. Have adequate measures been taken to make the
       patient as comfortable as possible with no
       need for immediate attention?

   A. The patient is comfortably situated in bed.
   B. Signs and symptoms requiring immediate attention
       are absent (pain, dyspnea, bleeding, incontinence,
       cyanosis, etc.).

   2. Appropriate infection control procedures and safety
       precautions by both staff and patient?

       A. Proper hand washing technique is utilized between
           patients, before and after treatments by staff.
       B. If indicated, patient has received instruction as
           to infection control procedures and safety pre-
           cautions, especially when being attended by
           physician and other staff.
       C. Used material is removed from the room unless
           contraindicated.
       D. Isolation procedures are being followed - the
           equipment and supplies are properly placed and
           adequate in numbers.[91]

AMHT Standards

Medical Protocol. Chart VIII - 1 shows the suggested medical protocol
for the AMHT to be applied to the H.M.O. The sequence is a result of experiences learned from other operating AMHT centers, particularly that of Kaiser-
Permanente.

The patient, after passing the receiving area, gives a complete
history, including:

   1. Demographic data;
   2. Genetic characteristics;
   3. Habits;
   4. Social background;
   5. Medical complaints.[92]

---

[91]Ibid., p. 41.

[92]B.D. Schapiro, "Multiphasic Testing in the Hospital Environment," AMHT
Workshop Joint Meeting of College of American Pathologists and the
American Society of Clinical Pathologists, September 17-18, 1970, p. 20.

CHART VIII - 1
Suggested Test Sequence for AMHT[d]

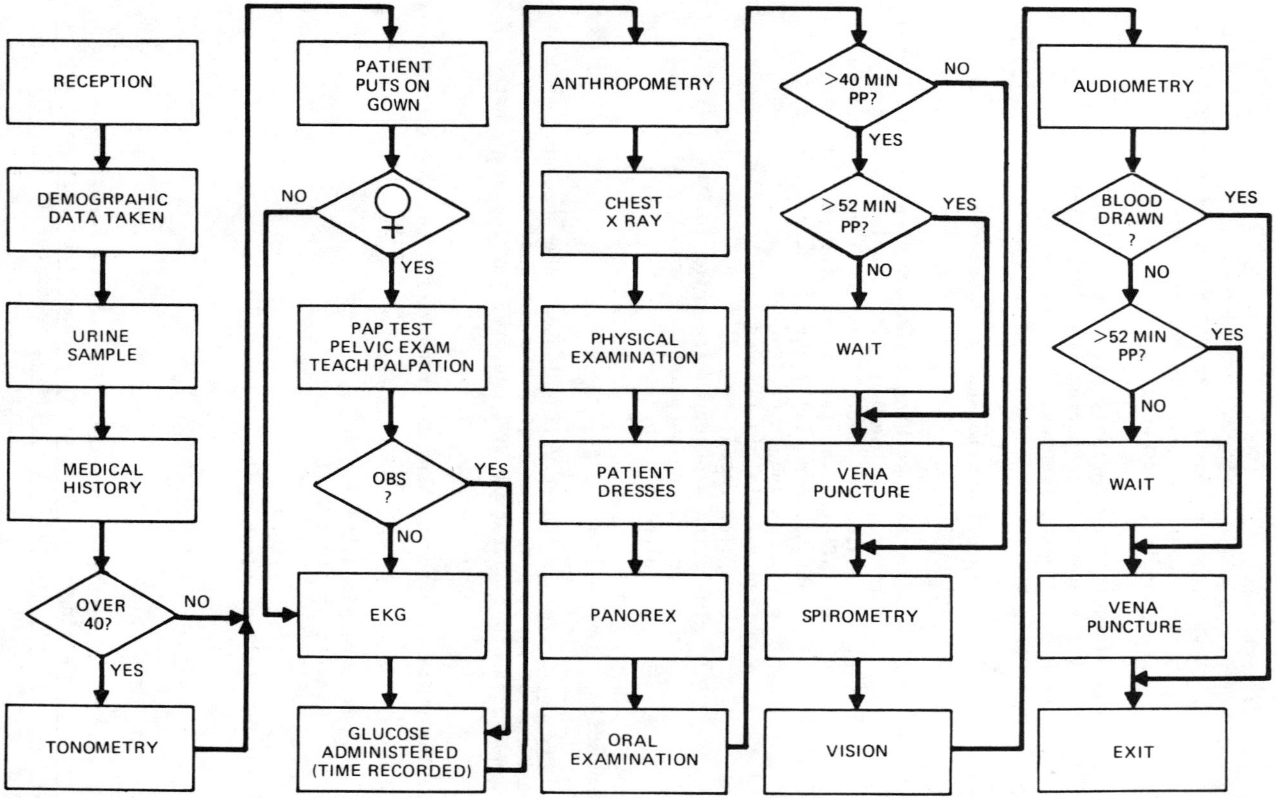

(d) Schapiro, B. D., "Multiphasic Testing in the Hospital Environment," AMHT Workshop Joint Meeting of College of American Pathologists and the American Society of Clinical Pathologists, September 17-18, 1970, p. 20.

484

Tonometry measurements are provided if the patient is over 40 years of age, followed by tests against known standards in a prescribed sequence:

1. Urine analysis;
2. PAP smear and pelvic examination for females;
   EKG for males;
3. EKG for females;
4. Glucose administration (time recorded);
5. Anthropometry;
6. Chest x-ray;
7. Complete physical examination by internist;
8. Panorex tests;
9. Oral examination by dentist;
10. Blood chemistry;
11. Blood and RH type determination for surgery and obstetrics;
12. Spirometry;
13. Vision;
14. Audiometry;
15. Vena puncture for further blood chemistry analysis.

As a patient progress through each testing phase, the mark sense cards are read into the computer for an analyses of the test values compared to normal values established by the physicians. The history data, completed early in the testing sequence, is made available at the physical examination station via computer printout. The physician uses the data as a guide when conducting the initial examination.

The AMHT system, based upon results obtained, makes additional recommendations for further tests, if needed. These are scheduled by the nurse supervisor at the completion of initial testing.[93]

TECHNIQUES OF MONITORING STANDARDS

Inputs/Outputs/In-process

Entry. When a patient subscribes to the medical group, a plastic charge card is created, containing his name, patient number, age, sex and physician assigned. This card is machine readable and provides the entry point for all demographic data.

All new patients are sent to the screening center for testing prior to any personal examinations by the assigned physician. This procedure allows the patient's initial medical history to be created.

At the screening center, the charge card information is transferred to mark sense cards used to initiate the testing process. These cards contain:

---

[93]
Ibid., pp. 17-19.

patient number, test station number, date andcard type (including spaces for results of tests at that station).[94]

A patient who is not a subscriber to the H.M.O. and is admitted on an emergency basis, will have the same basic data created. This allows the proper medical records and billing information to be generated.

Outputs

Output Reports. The combination of medical history, mark-sense cards, testing stations, technician and physician input provide the data base for medical reports that assist the physician in diagnosing and treating his patients. The computer-generated output from the testing and physician input include:

1. Results of initial tests (demographic, history, actual results versus standards, complaints);
2. Patient medical summary for cardiologist;
3. Patients with missing reports (for control of data);
4. Additional activity records requested.[95]

In-process

Doctor/Patient Interaction. The patient is given an appointment with his physician following completion of all testing. The physician does his own workup, using the results provided by the AMHT. Problems are diagnosed and treated. The patient is given followup appointments with the doctor as often as is necessary to ensure that corrective action is effective.

To enhance quality of diagnosis and treatment, the patient is scheduled to undergo the multiphasic tests once a year as a minimum, in order to provide base-line data and health trends. The physician may schedule partial AMHT workups at more frequent intervals, if such is deemed advisable for control of specific problems.[96]

Patient/Educator Interaction. Following diagnosis and treatment for a problem or problems, the patient is seen by the health educator member of the group. This individual enlightens the patient on the care regimen required and assists with health care information and guidance appropriate to the patient's condition.[97]

Auditing Procedures

Advisory Committee. Weekly, members of the committee and assisting nurses make unannounced observation visits to each unit on each shift, filling

---

[94]"Laboratory Information System," Systems Management Division, (New York: Sperry-Rand Corp. March 1971, pp. 9-12.

[95]B. D. Schapiro, op. cit., p. 20.

[96]Ibid.

[97]Ibid.

out the check sheet for that area. The examiner rates the condition of the unit as it appears at the time of inspection.

The results of weekly inspections are fed into the computer and tabulated into an over-all weekly quality control index report. A weekly quality index is computed and plotted on a weekly performance chart to provide a graphic display of relative trends. Identifiable deficiencies are brought to the attention of the area involved and corrective action taken.[98]

Analyzing each item on every check list weekly is highly desirable, but poses a problem in staff utilization and having the available time. Consequently, sampling different criteria within an area is more practical, given the staff and time limitations. Areas shown to be chronic quality control problems should be checked more frequently. Standards are not frozen, but change as the profession, equipment and knowledge change.[99]

The Medical Audit. This should make use of three methods that have been found desirable and feasible:

1. The individual case analysis, with evaluation based on objective, written criteria;
2. The assemblage of epidemiologic data, chiefly community-wide incidence rates, to provide an independent check on the results obtained by the case analysis method;
3. A comparative analysis to determine the accuracy of the tissue, x-ray, and clinical laboratory examinations that are employed for preoperative and postoperative diagnosis.[100]

These recommendations do not yet include the checking of results at intervals after the patient has left the hospital, however desirable that may be, because appropriate methodology and favorable public attitudes have yet to be developed on a broad scale.[101]

The individual H.M.O., like a bank, should maintain its own con- tinuous, internal audit according to uniform, generally accepted methods. An independent outside agency, like the Joint Commission, should do a periodic external audit. Due to the lack of personnel trained for this purpose, and the relatively limited resources of small H.M.O.'s, it may be desirable to utilize the services of a regional organization.[102]

---

[98]Carron Herring, op. cit., p. 41.

[99]Ibid., p. 44.

[100]Paul A. Lembcke, op. cit., p. 115.

[101]Ibid.

[102]V. N. Slee, "Statistics Influence Medical Practice," Modern Hospital, Vol. 83, July 1954, pp. 55-58.

The same uniform standards should be used for both internal and external audits. Persons doing routine external audits should, in most instances, represent an agency such as the Joint Commission. Where independent audits at frequent intervals are desired, however, an auditor accredited by the American Hospital Association or the American Association of Hospital Consultants should be employed, since this is somewhat akin to the standing of a Certified Public Accountant.[103]

Methodology. The ingredient for a common understanding by the H.M.O.'s and doctors whose work is to be inspected, and by the person or agency making the inspection, is an acceptable methodology. Such a methodology should include:

1. Practical methods for abstracting and classifying cases;
2. Criteria by which the cases could be judged;
3. Standards by which satisfactory performance could be measured.[104]

Abstracting and Tabulating. Abstracts of all medical records are created and sorted to present a statistical analysis indicating what kind of cases or phases of patient care should be selected by the medical staff audit committee for deliberation. The audit committee's analysis is, in turn, recorded on special sheets for computer processing.[105]

These case abstracts are sent to the Office of the Commission on Professional and Hospital Activities at monthly intervals. Reports such as diagnostic, operative, physicians' indexes and administrative service are prepared. Other tabulations are made from time to time comparing participating hospitals with each other in respect to such items as what proportion of the diagnoses of diabetes was supported by blood chemistry findings, what proportion of cases diagnosed as pneumonia had chest x-ray examination, etc.[106] In addition, more detailed abstracts are completed by some hospitals for additional tabulations that serve as ground for medical audit. The criteria and standards for analyses are worked up by each individual hospital for its own use.

Self-evaluation by other methods, with individual formulated criteria and standards are employed by the tissue committee in numerous hospitals.[107]

C. W. Eisele applied medical auditing based upon expert knowledge to an evaluation of individual cases.[108] In a 75-bed hospital that Eisele was

---

[103]Lembcke, loc. cit.

[104]Ibid.

[105]R.S. Myers, et al, "Medical Audit," Modern Hospital, Vol. 85, September 1955, pp.77-83.

[106]V.N. Slee, et al., "Can the Practice of Internal Medicine be Evaluated," Ann. Intern Med., Vol. 44, January 1956, pp. 144-161.

[107]Paul A. Lembcke, op. cit., p. 116.

[108]C.W. Eisele, "Methods of Evaluating Medical Care in Hospitals," Rocky Mountain Medical Journal, Vol. 53, December 1956, pp. 1117-1121.

associated with for over seven years, a combination of continuing medical audit and an educational program for the medical staff reduced the number of appendectomies and tonsillectomies by one-half, and he reported that improvement had taken place in the quality of other areas of medical care. In a number of cases, the findings are expressed in objective terms as incidence of operations.[109]

L. S. Rosenfeld rated or scored the quality of medical care in eight selected diseases and operations with partly objective but largely subjective judgments to arrive at an overall rating of superior, good, fair or poor.[110] Medical specialists served as medical auditors. The most important finding was that in spite of the large subjective element in the scoring, in the three areas studied - medicine, surgery and obstetrics-gynecology - each of a pair of specialists arrived at essentially similar findings on the same series of cases.[111]

H. B. Makover describes the methodology of a survey of medical groups associated with H.I.P. of Greater New York, in which he scored the quality of medical care as shown in 3,148 records from 26 medical groups.[112] Four diseases or conditions were studied: health examinations; the care of the infants; the diagnosis and treatment of cancer; and the diagnosis and treatment of gastro-intestinal diseases. Makover pointed out that the method employed was a comparative one not based upon absolute standards and that the subjective element in rating was relatively great.[113]

Peer Review Monitoring

Steps for Effective Review. Dr. Robert H. Barnes, Jr., internist and Director of Medical Education at Doctor's Hospital in Kings County has the aim of using peer review as the basis for second medical education.[114]

Phase 1 of his plan is to pin down exactly what part every member of the review team is to play. It is not enough to have a committee composed only of physicians. Review should be accomplished by people who do not know the physicians. These may be men who are semi-retired physicians and specialists and can give time to it. Other individuals who are good candidates for review committees are board members of hospitals or the prepaid medical group, as they are legally responsible for the quality of care at their respective facilities. At the same time, this gives the board member a greater understanding of doctor's problems, aids in evaluating them and in choosing priorities.[115]

[109]Lembcke, loc. cit.

[110]L.S. Rosenfeld, "Quality of Medical Care in Hospitals," American Journal of Public Health, Vol. 47, July 1957, pp. 856-865.

[111]Paul A. Lembcke, op. cit., p. 117.

[112]H.B. Makover, "The Quality of Medical Care, Methodology of Survey of the Medical Groups Associated with the Health Insurance Plan of New York," American Journal of Public Health, Vol. 41, July 1951, pp. 824-832.

[113]Lembcke, loc. cit.

[114]"Peer Review," op. cit. pp. 45-46.

[115]Ibid.

Phase 2 is to train each member of the review team in the use of the problem-oriented medical record system. The board then has a concise, standardized procedure for reviewing the history, problems, diagnoses, treatment and results. Given the total picture, evaluation by the board is easier, with greater equity in applying judgment.[116]

Phase 3 is to establish a medical audit system based on the records. This encompasses the use of Model treatment programs, such as those of the Santa Clara Foundation. These detail standard treatments and flag certain items, such as underutilization (for example - a patient has been visiting a doctor for persistent rectal bleeding and no barium enema has been ordered). By using available data of this type and tables of usage rates established by the Commission on Hospital Activities as a base, the medical audit by the committee, provides a wealth of quality control data.[117]

Phase 4 is a strategy of continued physician education based upon the deficiencies uncovered by the medical audits. Deficiencies and suggested corrections are documented and distributed to the members of the Health Care Delivery Team for review and educational purposes.[118]

Lastly, phase 5 is the review and evaluation by the board, on a monthly basis, of corrective actions taken on deficient items to close the loop on the entire system.[119]

Application. When a member of the H.M.O. enters the system for an elective procedure, his assigned physician completes a certification request identifying the patient and his medical needs. This document is part of the medical history data provided by the AMHT system. The request is forwarded to the committee for determination of "medical necessity."[120]

Utilizing averages based on a study by the Commission on Professional and Hospital Activities of Ann Arbor (known as PAS),[121] the committee approves hospital stay up to the 50th percentile for the stay of an average patient of the same age with the same diagnoses. Emergency cases are certified in a similar manner on the first working day following admission.[122]

Registered nurses assigned to the hospital review the correctness of the certification request on each admission, and review the need for

---

[116]Ibid.

[117]Ibid.

[118]Ibid.

[119]Ibid.

[120]Stephen Daiger, op. cit., p. 77.

[121]Commission on Professional and Hospital Activities: Length of Stay in PAS Hospitals, United States, Pre- and Post-Medicare, Ann Arbor, Michigan, 1969, extract.

[122]Daiger, loc. cit.

medical services daily. Inappropriate care rendered the patient results in referral to the review committee. Similarly, requests for extension of stay are evaluated by the reviewer. When a request is denied, the committee has the option to appoint a consultant to review the case.[123]

Review in the Extended Care Facility. In this environment, the methods of the utilization review board are modified to effect quality control.

Initial care evaluations and recommendations are made during on-site visits by an individual reviewer who is one of a large number of physicians forming a subcommittee of the review committee. The reviewer transmits his findings to the executive group which makes a final determination or seeks further information. The reviewer is empowered to disapprove patient stays on the spot when indicated, to help overcome the time-lag problem inherent in such proceedings. In addition, a full-time "utilization review coordinator" helps to establish uniform procedures and provides essential coordination.[124]

This type of program will lead to:

1. Effective on-site evaluation of the entire range of medical services is accomplished while using the physician's time in an efficient manner;
2. The addition of operating units will expand the system to serve a growing patient population;
3. The attending physician, by receiving informal notification from the reviewer of an impending disapproval, has the opportunity for meaningful rebuttal, which also tends to lessen the possibility of embarrassment;
4. Delays are reduced to a minimum;
5. Checks and cross-checks of physician's diagnoses and proposed treatments are maintained.[125]

Laboratory Control

The laboratory department operation is controlled by dividing the effort into four distinct phases:

Phase 1 - begins daily at 8 A.M. when abridged master patient cards are keypunched from the midnight admission and discharge lists. The cards are read into the computer to update the in-house patient master file. This process is completed by 9 A.M. at about 9:30 A.M., all the blood specimens arrive in the laboratory accompanied by requisition slips with patient data imprinted. The specimens are separated and assigned consecutive laboratory numbers. The slips and blood tubes then follow separate routes. The specimens are centrifuged and stored in a central patient rack. The slips are keypunched together with the requested test codes per patient.

---

[123] Ibid.

[124] Ibid., p. 78.

[125] Ibid.

The cards are then fed into the computer to create a technologist's schedule. Each card is first checked against the master file, which is organized by chart number using a terminal digit method. Both the chart number and admission number have to match before the name is read and inserted into the work schedule as it is being created. Mismatches are printed out as errors.[126]

Phase 2 - The technologists set up their auto analyzers, checking out all components: reagents and controls are constituted and standards prepared for the daily run. As soon as a steady baseline is reached, the lab requests on-line monitoring of all lab channels. The computer operator initiates the monitoring. Extensive input editing procedures ensures that the proper channels are started.

Following the steady baseline is a series of standards which the computer scans every two seconds, establishes peak values, and computes a statistical "best-fit" line through all the points. In this process, incorrect peaks are spotted and messages printed out in the lab. The program is capable of eliminating a wrong standard value and recalculating the standard line.[127]

Following the standards is a series of human serum controls, the concentrations of which are calculated from the previously found standard line fit. If the values are within acceptable tolerances, the process proceeds with the actual patient samples. Otherwise the scanning is stopped until the problem is identified and corrected.

All patient samples are scheduled in groups of eight, followed by a known control value and a water sample. If during the daily run the control value deviates by plus or minus five per cent, a message to the technologist is printed out in the lab. The water sample in each group of ten is used for baseline monitoring and drift correction to the patient samples.

The quality control programs can also detect contaminated samples, excessive process drift, rate of flow variations, continuous flow interruptions, loss of sensitivity and certain dialyzer problems. All quality control problems are detected and reported on a real time basis. The calculated patient results are transferred to the patient history file, whenever there is available computer time.[128]

Phase 3 - At about noon, the computer prints a temporary list of results for glucose, urea and the four electrolytes. These test results are used for reporting to the nursing floors. In addition, as soon as a channel completes the daily run, the technologist receives a complete listing of

---

[126] D. Kanon, "Computer Analyzes Lab Tests, Does Own Quality Control," Modern Hospital, November 1969, p. 105.

[127] Ibid., p. 106.

[128] Ibid.

patient results in the order in which they wereprocessed. This list is checked for possible errors and the edited results are returned to the computer room for correction.[129]

Close to 4 P.M. the computer prints the daily run of cumulative reports. This is phase 4. These reports undergo a final random output edit before release to the floor.[130]

The hospital laboratory measures actual specimens to control specimens. The quality assurance program causes everyone involved to do additional work. For example, at least three specimens which have a known sugar value are simultaneously tested with every analysis of patient's blood sugar levels.[131] These known specimens are the standards or control specimens. They are processed with the specimens obtained from the patients, and their values must agree with their predetermined values.[132] If the results obtained on these "known" specimens are off significantly, testing the entire set of patients' specimens and controls is repeated until the control material agrees with its own true values.[133]

The objective of these checks is threefold. First, the procedure or method itself is being tested, in order to make certain that the most reliable testing methods have been chosen.[134] Next, the calibration of the precision instruments is constantly being checked, since such instruments occasionally require adjustment.[135] Third, the human element is tested, in order to determine that all personnel are performing properly.[136]

From the description of the laboratory control procedure, it is clear that the management and function of the hospital laboratory can be aided by the use of computerized data processing.[137] Ever increasing routine clinical and clerical laboratory tasks can be relegated to the machine. The computer handles easily, many individual information-handling tasks time after time, without error.[138]

Medication Distribution

The principle concern in medication distribution is controls. The physician writes his medication orders in a composite, nursing division order book containing the physician's order sheets for all patients receiving a particular service or under the care of a nursing team. The pharmacist

---

[129]Ibid., p. 107.

[130]Ibid.

[131]Ibid.

[132]J. E. Moon, op. cit., p. 120.

[133]Ibid.

[134]Ibid., p. 122.

[135]Ibid.

[136]Ibid.

[137]Marty Juel, op. cit., p. 16.

[138]Ibid.   493

transcribes all orders for or involving medications from physicians' original orders onto a patient medical profile which serves as the master information source. In this way, pharmacy assumes complete responsibility for filling the order, and nursing personnel no longer need to transcribe the order onto a nursing Kardex and to patient's chart.

After the pharmacist has copied the physician's orders, the nurse checks the physician's original order against the entry made by the pharmacist and initials. Two professional people have thus checked the physicians' orders.[139]

Cart Has 12-Hour Supply. Each unit has two sets of carts, one in use at all times in the nursing divisions, the other in the central unit dose dispensary being prepared for the next dosage administration time. These carts are exchanged every four hours and are in readiness one-half hour before the major dosage times from 8 A.M. to 8 P.M. (at which time a 12-hour medication supply is placed in the cart). The pharmacy technician maintains a profile from which he prepares the medication cart for scheduled doses with the prepackaged unit dose medications.

The technician in the central unit dose dispensary places the individually packaged, labeled and ready-to-administer medication in each patient's drawer. The technician does not prepare the medication but handles individual units much as a wholesale "order picker."[140]

The pharmacist checks the cart after it is received on the nursing unit. After checking the contents of the cart against the medication profile, the cart is released to the nurse, who administers the medication. A third check is made just before the empty cart is returned to the central unit dose area. To guard against errors of omission, the pharmacist checks whether any medications have been left in the drawer.[141]

Recurring (PRN) medications are handled slightly differently. The pharmacist transcribes the physician's order onto the medication profile and onto a PRN card. Solid oral dosage forms are attached directly to the card and placed in the appropriate patient drawer along with liquid and injectable pins. When a patient requests or needs an ordered PRN medication, the nurse selects the card, with the medication attached, and administers the dose. Since the date and time of administration are recorded on the back of the PRN card after each dose is given, the nurse can immediately determine how long it has been since the previous dose was administered.[142]

After giving the medication, the nurse makes the appropriate entries on the medication profile and then puts the PRN card in a box in the medicine

---

[139]Winston Durant, op. cit., pp. 106-107.

[140]Ibid.

[141]Ibid.

[142]Ibid.

cupboard for replacement by the technician. This person attaches a new dose of the medication to the card, and it is ready for the next administration.

With the exception of additional records, narcotics are handled in the same way as PRN medications. Under this system, however, the department of pharmacy is responsible for proof of use sheets and for perpetual inventory.

A limited number of intravenous fluids are maintained in the nursing division and may be administered by the nurse according to a procedure similar to that used for PRN medications. Fluids that require additives are prepared by a pharmacist. If they are needed immediately, the pharmacist can prepare them in the nursing division. In most cases, however, they are prepared in the additive area of the central pharmacy, where a laminar flow hood and sufficient information on drug compatibilities help to maintain conditions optimum for their preparation.[143]

A stock status report, issued weekly, consists of a complete alphabetical listing, by vendor, of all the drugs in the pharmacy, including both chemicals and wholesale drugs. Included in the listing are: average cost per base unit, number of units on hand, extended cost value of these units, reorder point, indication of whether the reorder point was not previously, and month-to-date and year-to-date usage figures.[144]

All drug ordering is done from this report, with the exception of the wholesale items, which are ordered with a conventional order book.[145]

An ancilliary report lists those items that have fallen below the reorder point for the first time. It specifies the item, reorder point, vendor and item code.

A prescription analysis report lists the totals of new and refilled prescriptions and the dollar amount per employee, intern, resident, nurse, compensation and discharge prescription. This report is used by the business office for cost accounting purposes, and give accurate information for any of the listed categories.

A weekly report, by vendor, listing the drugs received, total units, total cost, a new computed unit cost for each drug, unit cost variance, and new quantity on hand, is produced by the computer. It provides most of the data on inventory ledger cards.

Other statistical reports used for control purposes include drugs transferred to other departments within the H.M.O. and the drugs used by both out and inpatients. All of these reports result in increased control of drugs, including automated ordering and control of narcotics. The need for frequent physical inventory counts to verify manual records is diminished greatly.[146]

---

[143]Ibid.

[144]Ibid.

[145]Ibid.
[146]Ibid.

Figure VIII - 3 shows the mechanics of a medication distribution system employing a high level of quality control.

CORRECTIVE MEASURES FOR DEVIATIONS

Reliability of the System

Many of the issues dealt with in the previous section raise important technologic and legal problems. It is evident, for example, that if the information system were charged with an increasing number of responsibilities in the delivery of health care, a point would be reached, eventually, at which a major system failure would have disastrous consequences.[147]

Dependence on the computer for storage and retrieval of medical records, for provision of medication, for assistance in diagnostic and therapeutic decisions, for processing of laboratory data, and for a host of other more mundane housekeeping functions would carry with it the potential for serious disruption of clinical care if a breakdown of more than brief duration should occur.[148]

The vulnerability of a computer-based information network is apparent. Not only would continued operation depend upon the uninterrupted availability of electrical power, but also on the smooth functioning of a multitude of vital machine, program, and communications components. The incorporation of features designed to minimize the likelihood of operational failure would thus loom as a prominent issue in the design of the system.[149]

Some considerable degree of protection would be provided by an "active" and a "stand-by" computer complex, but even this approach could not ensure against partial or even total failure of the system.[150] Dependence on the system would therefore require accepting as a potential social cost the problems of sporadic deteriorations in function.

In anticipation of partial failures, assignments of priorities would be necessary to assure most effective utilization of remaining computer capacity - automated anesthesia and patient monitoring taking precedence, for example, over automated history taking or record retrieval. In anticipation of total or near total failure (loss of all but emergency power, for example), contingency plans would be required for return to manual operation. Because of the relatively small staff of the H.M.O., emergency measures involving

---

[147]William Schwartz, "Medicine and the Computer," New England Journal of Medicine, Vol. 283, No. 23, p. 1262.

[148]Ibid.

[149]Ibid.

[150]Ibid.

FIGURE VIII - 3

FLOW DIAGRAM OF MEDICATION DISTRIBUTION SYSTEM[a]

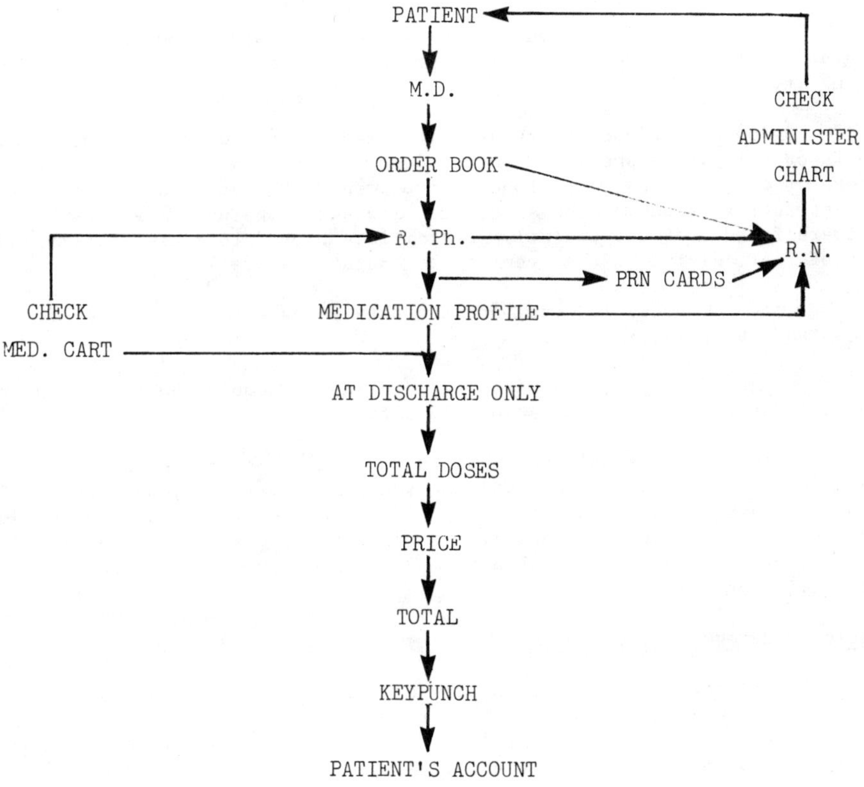

(a) Winston Durant, "A New Medication Distribution System", Hospital Progress (May, 1969), 105.

manual operations could only be employed for about a week before the entire medical administration would be hopelessly bogged down, and quality controls for patient care would have disappeared. However, in a system such as the one described, the possibility of the entire apparatus becoming inoperative for an entire week is extremely remote.[151]

Nevertheless, it is foreseeable that each of the complex decisions involved in the design and planning effort would involve compromise and risk.[152]

Reliability of System Hardware

Hardware for the system consists of standard components made by reputable manufacturers. Special components should be built to high standards of quality.

Communications errors are minimized by character and block parity checks on all data transmitted to the computer, and by character parity checks on all messages to peripheral equipment. Detection of a parity error will cause repetition of the associated message. The universal check-restart software feature of the executive system is employed to minimize time and cost of reprocessing in the event of an operational failure.[153]

The computer rejects incoming data messages with improper format or contradictory entries.

The AMHT system requires technicians to double check each entry of abnormal data, and reject unreasonable data.

The system should be designed to acquire patient data on machine-readable backup forms, so that malfunction of hardware will not prevent continued patient testing. No hardware malfunction results in a need to repeat more than the tests in progress at the time of failure. In the event of failure, repetition for more than 80 medical history questions for each patient is not required.[154]

Privacy and Legal Issues

Privacy. The threat to privacy posed by computer-based medical records represents one facet of the more general threat to personal privacy raised by the prospect of a centralized all-encompassing data bank. Protection of the medical record presents a special problem. However, the

---

[151] Ibid.

[152] Ibid.

[153] Marketing Paper on "Specification for the MS5110 AMHT System,"(New York: Sperry-Rand Corp.) March 1971, p. 3.

[154] Ibid.

effort to safeguard privacy would have to be balanced in system design against the need to make information available to the physician quickly and easily.[155]

The most practical solution involves the classification of information according to its degree of sensitivity, access to highly confidential data achievable only through relatively complex procedures. For access to psychiatric findings, for example, the simultaneous use of separate passwords by patient and physician might be required - much as two keys are used to open a safe-deposit box. It must be recognized, however, that no matter how many safeguards might be established to restrict the use of computerized data, all computer banks are potentially penetrable.[156]

Legality. There is a problem of developing a new legal code that must assign liability for difficulties arising from system errors or failure.[157] If technical problems within the network should lead to the delivery of inaccurate information to the physician (for example, the wrong record or incorrect laboratory data), who would be held responsible for resulting missteps in management - the manufacturer, the programmer, the medical personnel, or all three? If a program that has been used in guiding therapy proves to have a previously unrecognized flaw and the patient suffers in consequence, who is legally at fault: the physician who prepared the program, the panel that approved it, the physician who employed it, or all of them jointly? What is the liability of health-care specialists and nurses led into error by their use of the information system?[158]

It is not the subject of this paper to delve into the legal ramifications posed by an automated information system. The important point to be considered is that new legal problems may arise from a breakdown of the quality control mechanisms discussed in this paper.

The Problem-Oriented Medical Record

The data made available by the AMHT to assist the physician in making diagnoses is the first step in providing total medical care for the patient. Facilitating quality control is the physician's use of a problem-oriented medical record. This requires the group's doctor, examining the patient following completion of the AMHT tests, to identify and list all of the patient's problems. These include psychiatric and social problems, as well as physical. The problems are placed at the front of the chart, much like a table of contents. All subsequent data, including the physician's plans, orders, progress notes, and even the hospital discharge summary, are cross-referenced to the numbered problems. The list is then modified as

---

[155] L. Fosburgh, "23 to Study Computer Threat," New York Times, March 12, 1970.

[156] Ibid.

[157] Fano, R. M., Quoted by Fosburgh.

[158] William Schwartz, op. cit., p. 1263.

problems are classified, altered or diagnosed; those resolved or dropped are marked accordingly and their corresponding numbers left unused thereafter.[159]

Computer Input. Such structured records lend themselves to computer storage and CRT display. By keying in the patient's number on the CRT terminal, the physician can direct the patient's problem record to appear on the screen. The doctor "leafs through" the record, turning the "pages" by touching a button on the keyboard and keying in proposed drug therapy, for example. The computer automatically presents a suggestion of displays entitled, "check problem for," "side effects to watch for," and "metabolism and excretion" on any one of perhaps 150 different pharmaceuticals stored in the computer memory.[160]

"Information recorded in this fashion can be readily retrieved and reviewed," says Dr. Lawrence L. Weed, Professor of Medicine at the University of Vermont Medical Center in Burlington. "It should help the doctor become more efficient in managing his patient's multiple problems because he is constantly reminded of all the difficulties which may or may not interact."[161]

Developing the Medical Record. The term problem, in the total system, is all-inclusive. The patient has a problem - "doctor, I have pain." The physician has a problem - he is working toward a diagnosis. A problem could also be an abnormal or inconsistent laboratory finding.

The complete list, however, constitutes only one of the four major steps in developing the problem-oriented medical record, as set forth by Dr. Weed. These steps are:

1. Establishment of a data base;
2. Formulation of all problems;
3. Plans for each problem;
4. Follow-up on each problem-progress notes.[162]

The first step is accomplished completely by the test results of the AMHT. The second step is partially accomplished by the AMHT tests as a result of the normal and abnormal ranges in the system that are compared to actual values. The balance of the problems are determined by physical examination of the patient by the group's physician following completion of all tests. Additional problems uncovered by the doctor are added to the list. Impressions and guesses are not included.

Only after examining the entire list can the physician intelligently proceed to step three and devise the initial plan of action. Each problem has its own plan. Additional tests can be ordered to "rule out" conflicting

---

[159]"The Problem-Oriented Medical Record," Medical World News, May 7, 1971, pp. 31-33.

[160]Ibid.

[161]Ibid., pp. 33-34.

[162]Ibid., p. 35.

diagnostic possibilities or aid in deciding how best to manage an illness. Specific therapies are instituted for clear-cut problems.

The section containing progress notes represents the most crucial part of the quality control system. The doctor describes the results of his actions in a structured form: subjective, objective, assessment and plan.[163]

The Structured Form. First, the physician notes the subjective results of his work from the patient's own comments, and then records any objective aspects noticed. Under assessment, he analyzes these effects and finally sets down his new plans for therapy.

By applying this structured form to all progress notes, the clinician records his thoughts and approach so that other members of the Health Care Team can understand the strategy.[164]

The usual diagnostic categories and standard protocols of therapy contain artificial and false discontinuities, as every patient represents a unique combination of problems. Within the structured record, the physician can explain why he may have deviated from the usual management criteria for a single problem due to conflicts with other interacting problems.[165]

All entries to the structured form are input to the AMHT computer through the CRT display, and becomes an integral part of the patient's medical record. The total record then becomes the basis for comprehensive patient care, a continuing, auditable account of the clinician's management. It also becomes a basic instrument for continuing the education of the physician in logical, objective assessment and management of his patient's problems.[166]

Dr. Forst E. Brown, a plastic surgeon at the Hitchcock Clinic in Hanover, N.H., says that group practice has found value in the problem-oriented record. He believes that he can now review a patient's problems and determine a course of action faster when called in for consultation.[167]

The Interactive System

Sources of Information. The subscriber provides the medical group with basic data (name, address, phone number, etc.) upon entry to the plan. Additional data, including demographic and historical information, are provided by the patient at the initial testing phase of AMHT.[168]

The computer generates reports detailing the results of the medical protocol, flagging abnormalities and summarizing pertinent facts. A hard copy is sent to the patient's physician, while a duplicate microfilm set is sent to the central files of the medical group, for review by the

---

[163]Ibid., pp. 36-40.

[164]Ibid.

[165]Ibid.

[166]Ibid.

[167]Ibid.

[168]"Laboratory Information System," p. 12.

group's administration. The data is stored by the computer on disk files, for the purpose of updates by the physician, using remote terminal input.[169]

When the physician examines the patient, he places the examination results, diagnoses and treatment into the computer from his office, by accessing the CRT display. The data on disk file is immediately updated. New reports are produced reflecting the revised data. This process continues indefinitely: the AMHT workups create analytical data;the physician provides subjective analyses and treatment; the AMHT measures the effectiveness of the treatment by repetition of testing; the physician applies stronger corrective measures when treatment is not effective. At all times, the data, both analytical and subjective, are made available by the computer in hard copy, microfilm, and disk storage form. These are available to the physician, administration,health educator and peer review group.

The computer produces control reports, such as medical summaries, numbers of patients tested, patients with reports and tests due, and patient test status. These are necessary to keep track of the mass population and assist the AMHT and physicians in offering total care to each subscriber.[170]

Exhibit VIII - 3 shows the flow of quality control information thoughout the H.M.O. It should be noted that the primary objective of the quality control data flow is to continually update the medical records as fast as possible using data processing techniques. In this manner, quality controls can be applied by the physicians in the regional medical centers, the testing center, or the hospital. The review committees, meanwhile, are reviewing the practices of the physicians by also using the medical records as a basis for their reviews. In this manner, a closed-loop information flow is established throughout the entire organization.[171]

FINANCIAL CONSIDERATIONS

Data Processing

Capital Requirements. To supply the necessary data system equipment (refer to Table VIII - 1) will require a capital outlay of about $525,000.[172] If the assumption is made that a separate data processing center and testing facility will be established, an additional $415,000[173] will be required for the building and furnishings. This is a total of about $940,000 to be expended for capital equipment, if purchased new. This outlay will build a computer center capable of handling 5000 patients a

[169]Ibid.

[170]"Specification for the MS5110 AMHT System," pp. 2-2 through 2-13,

[171]Sperry-Rand, "Multiphasic Testing Center," Unpublished Report, 1971, p. 27.

[172]Ibid.

[173]Ibid.

EXHIBIT VIII - 3(a)

FLOW DIAGRAM OF INFORMATION FOR QUALITY CONTROL

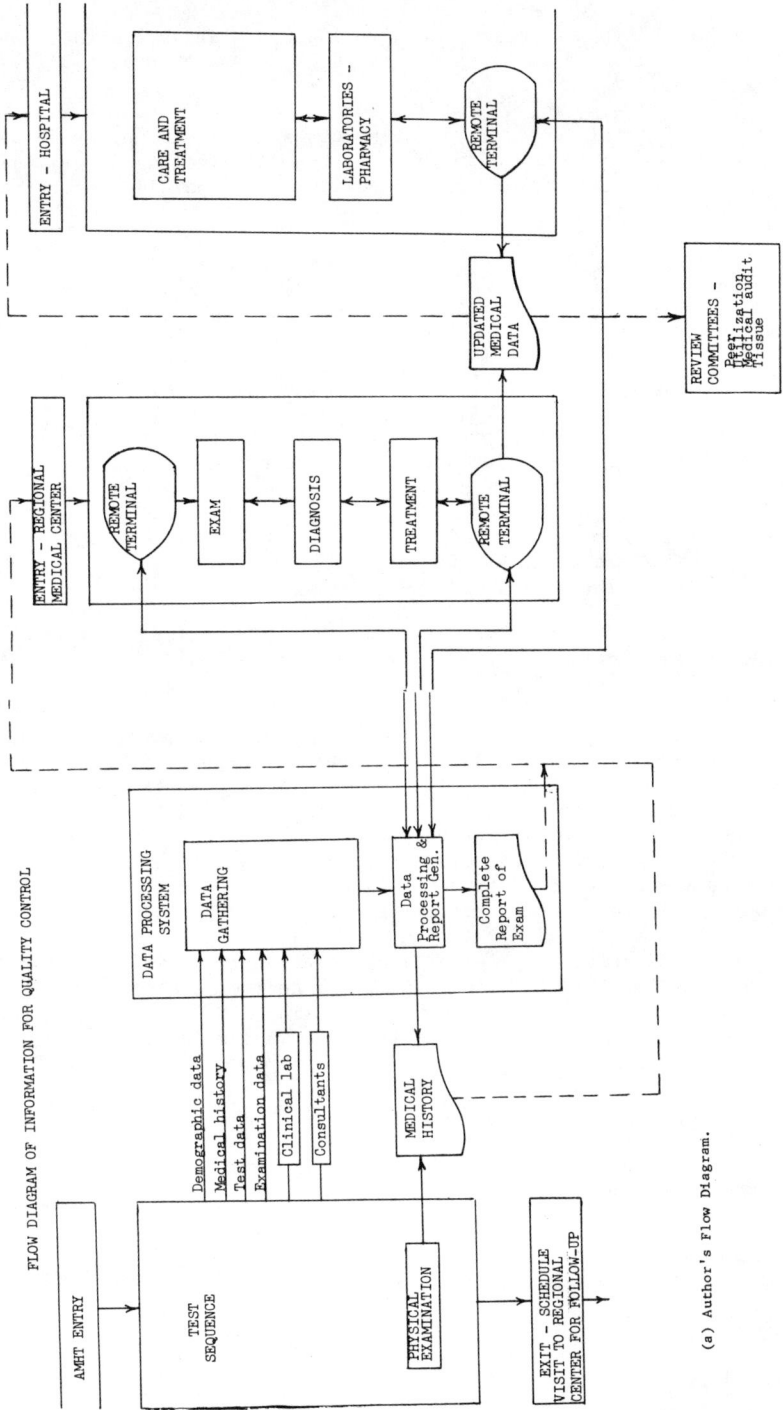

(a) Author's Flow Diagram.

month for multiphasic testing and full storage and retrieval capacity for 50,000 participants of the H.M.O. plus good control over quality of health care.

Initial Expense. Start-up costs for the computer system are estimated to be $80,000.[174] These costs would include program design and testing, consultant fees, system modifications, parallel operation and systems and procedures.

Ongoing Costs. Salaries to operate the testing center and data processing facility will average about $30,000 per month, including 25 per cent for fringe benefits.[175] Disposable supplies and other overhead will amount to $40,000 per month.[176]

Cost per Patient. From the above data, and assuming that the H.M.O. deals with 5,000 patients per month, the per-patient cost to cover the expenses of the data processing center, including amortization of the capital equipment over five years at six per cent is $16.87, broken down as follows:

1. Capital   - $ 3.62;
2. Start-up   - $ .15;
3. Labor, etc.- $13.10.[177]

For 2000 patients per month, the per-patient cost rises to $28.48, based on the fact that the total fixed expense would be spread among a fewer number of patients.[178]

Subjective Analysis. For an H.M.O. just forming, the initial outlay of capital for a full data processing capability and multiphasic testing may be prohibitive. It is more likely that the organization will not have these capabilities to begin with, but will build slowly to this goal as the number of subscribers increases to the point that the burden of record-keeping, individual examinations and manual work-ups, together with the need for measurable standards of quality to effectively handle a large number of people, becomes prohibitive.

The critical point will be reached at a level of about 2,000 patients per month. At this volume, the cost of the patient for the data processing equipment is reasonably low. The H.M.O., at that point, could well consider the purchase of their own computer and testing facilities.

---

[174] Ibid., p. 28.

[175] Ibid., p. 27.

[176] Ibid.

[177] Ibid., p. 26.

[178] Ibid., p. 29.

Managerial Aspects

The plan to implement a program of quality control for the H.M.O., which includes peer review, medical audit, utilization review committees, product analysis committees, certification by specialty boards, etc., is of such a nature that cost analysis is difficult. Little data regarding the analysis of cost versus quality controls offered has been made available.

Because the managerial aspects of quality control involve personnel rather than equipment (data processing cost is covered in the prior section of this paper), cost will depend upon the number of personnel in the organization required to effect good quality control. Obviously, if the personnel necessary to develop standards in the various departments of the H.M.O. are not made available, there will be no basis of actual performance measurement against the criteria. Hence, quality control will suffer. An individual to oversee the creation of standards will cost approximately $25,000 a year.[179] If the various department heads create their own standards, the incremental cost is zero, as their salaries are already being absorbed through the application of their everyday work.

The use of committees to evaluate and criticize the various functions of the medical practice is standard operating procedure throughout the profession. The number of committees and the vigor with which their business is prosecuted bears a direct relation to the number of people available for committee work and the time available to devote to these efforts.

From a cost viewpoint, the H.M.O. would not hire personnel to sit on committees. The medical personnel required to do committee work will come from the existing medical staff, together with volunteers from the community. Consequently, the amount of committee work will be restricted initially, due to the limited staff. To avoid overburdening the staff with committee work, assignments should be set up on a rotating basis. Physicians can be compensated for their extra effort by a special allowance of $20 or $25 for each hour of service on one of the committees.

As the organization grows, quality control requirements will become critical to the continuing operation of the H.M.O. Hence, it may become necessary to hire outside assistance for the important review work of the organization. Here, in this regard, standard practice of remuneration, but a figure of $10 to $25 per hour would probably not be unreasonable for each hired committee member.[180]

CONCLUSIONS

Factors for Success

To enable the quality control system described in this chapter to be successful, there are important factors to be observed by the group in

---

[179]Author's estimate.

[180]Author's estimate.

providing for such a system. Among these factors are:

1. Planning;
2. Economy of scale;
3. Integration into a delivery system;
4. Acceptability to physicians;
5. Acceptability to subscribers and the community.

Planning. The purpose of controls must be clear. The population to be reached must be defined, the aides and technicians must be trained and the instrumentation to be used must be reliable. Space must be properly designed, optimum patient flow established, and the entire process designed to function semi-automatically.

Economy of Scale. It is essential that the scale of utilization be great enough to make the program economical. Unless sufficient volume is achieved, the program will be unjustifiably costly and wasteful of both trained personnel and expensive instrumentation.

Integration into a Delivery System. The relationship between the AMHT program and the rest of the H.M.O. must be operational. The ready transfer of data and information within the system must be facilitated and feedback of information to the patient must be rapid and responsive.

Acceptability to Physicians. The program must be acceptable to the physicians who participate in the program if the controls are to be enforceable.

Acceptability to Patients and Community. The entire program should be acceptable to the persons it is intended to serve. This acceptance depends upon an adequate explanation of the purpose to be served, the manner in which the program is carried out, the liaison between the program's sponsors and the community, and the resultant quality of the services rendered.

Difficulties

Applying quality control procedures to medical practice is a difficult task, because: the standards of measurement constantly change; the initial measurements can number in the thousands; corrective actions are subjective in many cases; and the results are perceivable only after a lapse of time.

Nonetheless, despite problems, a closed-loop quality control system for a mass group practice is achievable and practical, although the disciplines involved are not easy to master.

Future Strategy

The Computer Used to Appraise the Physician. As the computer comes to play a major part in diagnoses and treatment, the system itself can readily be used to evaluate physician performance. Special programs could collect information on the frequency with which consultations are requested, and the numbers and types of questions asked, and could generate at regular intervals a profile defining the character and intensity of the interaction between physician and machine. These data could serve the constructive purpose of guiding review panels to the areas in which the programming repertoire needed strengthening.[181]

Future H.M.O. Whether dealing with quality or with cost, the quality assurance system (or lack of one) has a large impact on both areas. The H.M.O. of the future has been described in other papers and the focal point through which health services of the community are to be integrated. When this has been accomplished, H.M.O. will be in a position to influence the quality of care through the entire spectrum of health services.[182]

Certainly the need for strong management in health care delivery systems was never more apparent or the consequences of weakness potentially more disastrous. A revolution in the delivery of health services to the population is in the making.[183] Some reorganization of medical practice seems inevitable. It is incumbent on physicians and hospitals to make common cause for the betterment of the health care system.[184]

------

[181] Ibid., p. 1260.

[182] Smits, loc.cit.

[183] Ibid.

[184] Ibid.

BIBLIOGRAPHY

American College of Surgeons, Manual of Hospital Standardization, (1966), p. 8.

Anderson, J. "Health Education Aspects of a Multiphasic Screening Program," California Health, Vol. 8, (December 31, 1950), pp. 91-93.

_____. "Implementation of a System - Automated Multiphasic Health Testing," Hospitals, J.A.H.A., Vol. 45, (March 1, 1971), pp. 49-56.

_____. "The Multitest Laboratory in Health Care of the Future," Hospitals, J.A.H.A., Vol. 41 (May 1967), pp. 119-124.

_____. "Periodic Health Examinations Using an Automated Multitest Laboratory," J.A.M.A., Vol. 195, March 7, 1966, pp. 830-833.

_____. "Provisional Guidelines for Automated Multiphasic Health Testing and Services," Operational Manual, Washington, D.C.: U.S. Government Printing Office, 1960.

Commission on Professional and Hospital Activities. Length of Stay in PAS Hospitals, United States, Pre- and Post-Medicare, Ann Arbor, Michigan, 1969, Extract.

Daiger, Stephen. "Peer Review - Cost Control or Quality Control? California Medicine, (December 1970), pp. 75-79.

Durant, Winston J. "A New Medication Distribution System," Hospital Progress, (May 1969), pp. 104-114.

Editorial on "Peer Review," Medical World News, (August 20, 1971), pp. 45-52.

Editorial on "The Problem-Oriented Medical Record," Medical World News, (May 7, 1971), pp. 31-40.

Eisele, C. W. "Methods of Evaluating Medical Care in Hospitals," Rocky Mountain Medical Journal, Vol. 53 (December 1956), pp. 1117-1121.

Fosburgh, L. "23 to Study Computer Threat," New York Times, (March 12, 1970).

Herring, Carron. "Ohio Hospitals' Quality Control and Staff Utilization Program," Hospital Progress, (July 1970), pp. 38-44.

Holden, William. "Specialty Board Certification as a Measure of Professional Competence," J.A.M.A., Vol. 213, (August 10, 1970), pp. 1016-1018.

Juel, Marty. "Maintaining High Lab Standards Through a Quality Assurance Program," Hospital Progress, (July 1970), pp. 14-16.

Kanon, D. "Computer Analyzes Lab Tests, Does Own Quality Control," Modern Hospital, (November 1969), pp. 105-107.

Katz, S. "Chronic Disease Classification in Evaluation of Medical Care Programs," Medical Care, Vol. 7, (1969), pp. 139-140.

Lembcke, Paul S. "Evolution of the Medical Audit," J.A.M.A., Vol. 199, No. 8, (February 20, 1967), pp. 114-117.

_____. "Measuring the Quality of Medical Care Through Vital Statistics Based on Hospital Service Areas: 1. Comparative Study of Appendectomy Rates," American Journal of Public Health, Vol. 42, (March 1952), pp. 276-286.

_____. "A Scientific Method for Medical Auditing," Modern Hospitals, Vol. 33, (June 16, 1959 and July 1, 1959), pp. 65-71.

Makover, H. B. "The Quality of Medical Care, Methodology of Survey of the Medical Groups Associated with the Health Insurance Plan of New York," American Journal of Public Health, Vol. 41, (July 1951), pp. 824-832.

Marketing Report on Laboratory Information System, Report by Systems Management Division, New York: Sperry-Rand Corp., March 1971.

Moon, J. E. "Computerized Pharmacy System Solves Hospital's Drug Inventory Problem," Modern Hospitals, (November 1969), pp. 118-122.

Myers, R. S. et al. "Medical Audit," Modern Hospitals, Vol. 85 (September 1955), pp. 77-83.

O'Connell, J. A. "Product Analysis Committee, Yes, Standards Committee, No," Hospital Progress, (February 1969), pp. 68-72.

Rosenfeld, L. S. "Quality of Medical Care in Hospitals," American Journal of Public Health, Vol. 47, (July 1957), pp. 856-865.

Schapiro, B.D. "Multiphasic Testing in the Hospital Environment," AMHT Workshop Joint Meeting of College of American Pathologists and the American Society of Clinical Pathologists, September 17-18, 1970, pp. 17-20.

Schwartz, William. "Medicine and the Computer," New England Journal of Medicine, Vol. 283, (December 3, 1970), p. 1262.

Shapiro, S. "Efficacy of the Concept," Hospitals, J.A.H.A., Vol. 45, (March 1, 1971), pp. 45-48.

Slee, V. N. et al. "Can the Practice of Internal Medicine be Evaluated," Ann. Intern. Med., Vol. 44, (January 1956), pp. 144-161.

Smits, J. E. "Strong Management and Quality Control," Hospital Progress, (February 1969), p. 56.

Soghikian, K. and Collen, F. B. "Acceptance of Multiphasic Screening Examinations by Patients," Bull. of N.Y. Acad. of Medicine, 2d Ser., Vol. 45, (December 1969), p. 1366.

Southmayd, H.J. et al. Small Community Hospitals, New York: Commonwealth
    Fund, Div. of Publications, 1944.

Sperry-Rand, "Multiphasic Testing Center," Unpublished Marketing Report,
    1971, pp. 26-29.

U.S. Congress, Senate, Subcommittee on Health of the Elderly, Detection and
    Prevention of Chronic Diseases Utilizing Multiphasic Health
    Screening Techniques, Hearing, 89th Congress, 1st sess.
    Washington, D.C.: U.S. Government Printing Office, 1966.

U.S. National Center for Health Services Research and Development,
    Provisional Guidelines for Automated Multiphasic Testing and
    Services, Report of the AMHT Advisory Committee, Washington,
    D.C.: U.S. Government Printing Office, 1970.

ABOUT THE AUTHOR

Allan Easton is Professor of Management at the School of Business of Hofstra University in Hempstead, New York. He has also taught management, marketing, and business decision making at Columbia University's Graduate School of Business. He also has ten years of experience as an executive in industry.

Dr. Easton has published widely in the areas of marketing, management, decision analyses, and public affairs. He is the author of Complex Managerial Decisions Involving Multiple Objectives (Wiley 1973) and editor of several Hofstra Business Yearbooks including Community Support for the Performing Arts, Managing Organizational Change, Current Problems in Mergers and Acquisitions. In addition he has published articles in The Journal of Marketing, Journal of Marketing Research, Journal of Human Relations, Journal of Systems Management, Proceedings of the American Institute of Decision Sciences, and others.

Dr. Easton holds a B.S. in Industrial Management from Hofstra College and a Ph. D. from Columbia University.

RELATED TITLES

Published by Praeger Special Studies

CHANGING THE MEDICAL CARE SYSTEM: A Controlled Experiment in
Comprehensive Care
                              Leon S. Robertson, John Kosa,
                              Margaret C. Heagherty, Robert J.
                              Haggerty and Joel J. Alpert
                              Foreword by Charles A. Janeway

HEALTH CARE TEAMS: An Annotated Bibliography
                              Monique K. Tichy

THE PHYSICIAN'S ASSISTANT: A National and Local Analysis
                              Ann Suter Ford

HOSPITAL EFFICIENCY AND PUBLIC POLICY
                              Harry I. Greenfield

THE POLITICS OF HEALTH CARE: Nine Case Studies of Innovative Planning
in New York City
                              edited by Herbert Harvey Hyman

POVERTY, POLITICS AND HEALTH CARE: An Appalachian Experience
                              Richard Couto

MENTAL HEALTH AND RETARDATION LOBBIES
                              Daniel A. Felicetti